Cardiac Rehabilitation:
Basic Theory and Application

This book is dedicated
to the memory of
August and Ethel Quinet
and
Lona M. Brannon

Cardiac Rehabilitation: Basic Theory and Application

Frances J. Brannon, Ph.D.
Professor and Coordinator
Exercise Physiology Laboratory
Slippery Rock University
Slippery Rock, Pennsylvania

Mary J. Geyer, M.S.
Owner-Director
Bio-Energetiks Rehabilitation Clinics
Prospect, Pennsylvania

Margaret W. Foley, M.S.N.
Assistant Administrator
Nursing Services
Florida Keys Memorial Hospital
Key West, Florida

Steven L. Wolf, Ph.D., F.A.P.T.A.
Editor-in-Chief
Associate Professor
Department of Rehabilitation Medicine
Emory University School of Medicine
Atlanta, Georgia

 F. A. DAVIS COMPANY • Philadelphia

Contemporary Perspectives in Rehabilitation
Volume 1, Thermal Agents in Rehabilitation
Volume 2, Cardiac Rehabilitation: Basic Theory and Application

Printed in the United States of America

LIBRARY OF CONGRESS
Library of Congress Cataloging-in-Publication Data

Brannon, Frances J., 1935–
    Cardiac rehabilitation: basic theory and application / Frances J. Brannon, Mary J. Geyer, Margaret W. Foley.
        p.   cm. — (Contemporary perspectives in rehabilitation; v. 2)
    Includes bibliographies and index.
    ISBN 0-8036-1121-8
    1. Exercise therapy.   2. Heart—Diseases—Patients—Rehabilitation.   I. Geyer, Mary J., 1950–
. II. Foley, Margaret W., 1954–   III. Title.   IV. Series.
    [DNLM: 1. Exercise Therapy.   2. Heart Diseases—rehabilitation.
W1 C0769NS v. 2 / WG 200 B821c]
RC684.E9B73 1988
616.1'2062—dc19
DNLM/DLC
for Library of Congress   87-30095
                                                                                                                                    CIP

Foreword

There have been several recent advances in the progression toward clinical excellence in physical therapy. In 1983, the Board for Certification of Advanced Clinical Competencies in Physical Therapy, created by the American Physical Therapy Association, approved the competencies developed by the Specialty Council of the Cardiopulmonary Section of the APTA. By 1985, this Council saw their first advanced certificants approved by the Board. This significant milestone parallels the achievements in the testing of advanced knowledge levels for cardiology already promulgated by the American College of Sports Medicine. These advances acknowledge that non-physicians have gained a prominent place in the provision of services to patients with respiratory or cardiac disorders. However, individuals wishing to provide service to clients with cardiopulmonary pathology need an informational base that comprehensively reviews relevant anatomy and physiology, and also meaningfully assesses laboratory values from functional tests so that correct clinical decisions regarding intervention can be made.

Cardiac Rehabilitation: Basic Theory and Application fulfills this strenuous demand. This second volume in the *Contemporary Perspectives in Rehabilitation (CPR)* series is intended to guide the novice allied health student through a basic understanding of cardiac rehabilitation, followed by a comprehensive review of cardiac anatomy, physiology, and pathology designed to supplement materials learned in more basic courses. The authors then challenge the reader to problem solve issues related to abnormal cardiograms and laboratory findings, and provide extensive crossreferencing to earlier material to facilitate the decision-making process. This content will not only hold interest for the student but also tax the inquisitive mind of the cardiac rehabilitation clinician. This unique format facilitates the process by which clinicians assimilate data and call upon basic knowledge in order to make educated decisions for provision of optimum care. Through this process, clinicians will enhance their capabilities for dealing more effectively with cardiac patients in both inpatient and outpatient settings.

Cardiac Rehabilitation: Basic Theory and Application integrates basic theory from various disciplines relevant to cardiac rehabilitation programing and obviates the need to refer to a number of disparate sources. Based upon the objectives in the classroom, laboratory, or clinic, it provides a knowledge base that is relevant to undergraduate students in physical therapy, health sciences, physical education, nursing, sports medicine, and athletic training; to graduate students studying physical therapy cardiopulmonary specialization, exercise physiology, or nursing; and to any clinician responsible for monitoring, generating, or evaluating the status of rehabilitation programs among patients with cardiac or pulmonary disorders.

Steven L. Wolf, Ph.D., F.A.P.T.A.
Series Editor

Preface

Recent innovations in health care delivery systems and a more informed public have contributed to an unprecedented interest in health, wellness, fitness, and nutrition; in the prevention of degenerative diseases, such as cardiac disease; and in the rehabilitation of individuals with such diseases. This timely text fills a void for many allied health professionals involved in providing scientifically-based exercise programs for healthy populations as well as those with cardiac disease. The specialized field of cardiac rehabilitation attracts many health professionals, including physical therapists, exercise physiologists, respiratory therapists, nurses, psychologists, nutritionists, and certainly physicians. Although each specialist brings unique skills to the field, the knowledge that an individual clinician possesses regarding cardiac rehabilitation programming is often incomplete. Therefore, we have written this book to enhance the allied health professionals' understanding of the basic scientific theory and principles associated with outpatient (Phases II, III) cardiac rehabilitation. Specific innovations in instrumentation, surgical procedures, pharmacology, and behavioral medicine techniques are presented. Every effort has been made to include the most current references and research available regarding the information presented.

Our goal is to offer a comprehensive description (which integrates information from a variety of disciplines) of the current state of knowledge and clinical practices in the field of cardiopulmonary rehabilitation for both the student and the experienced clinician. The text begins with an overview of cardiac rehabilitation; Chapters 2 and 3 present Cardiac and Circulatory Anatomy and Physiology; Chapter 4 discusses Pathophysiology of Coronary Heart Disease (CHD); Chapter 5 explores Surgical and Pharmacological Management of the CHD Patient; Chapter 6, on ECG Interpretation, includes sample rhythm strips illustrating arrhythymias that the clinician must be able to readily identify as either benign or life-threatening. A self-test is included, which is valuable as a review of the material and considerably enhances the identification process. We then discuss Physiologic Assessment in Chapter 7, The Exercise Prescription in Chapter 8, and The Exercise Training Session in Chapter 9. The last chapter is devoted to Risk Factor Modification. The Appendix contains a variety of sample forms for patient, physician, and cardiopulmonary rehabilitation staff, along with health risk appraisals, stress inventories, and dietary information.

Another major goal of our book is to facilitate the acquisition and development of decision-making skills. The depth and breadth of the content provide the means for acquiring these skills. We also have provided nine case studies to which we refer in the later chapters in order to integrate the information from chapter to chapter and to foster the development of problem-solving skills. In this way, the learner may follow the course of treatment described for a specific individual beginning with physiologic assessment and criteria for test termination, followed by the writing of the exercise prescription, and ending with the progression through the training program. This method of presentation is unique to this book and has not been so utilized in any text in this field.

Throughout the text, illustrations are provided to clarify complex technical data such as formulae, physiologic processes, and algorithms. Photographs of specific procedures have been included as needed and anatomical illustrations have been chosen for their simplicity and their pedagogic value.

It should be emphasized that the concepts presented are to be utilized as "guidelines" to assist the clinician in the evaluation and treatment process since no one method applies to all situations. We hope that the practical nature of the text will aid the decision-making process of the clinician who is responsible for conducting the outpatient cardiac rehabilitation program and is, therefore, responsible for making the ultimate decisions regarding patient care.

ACKNOWLEDGMENTS

The task of completing a major text of this nature was made easier by the support and encouragement of our families and friends. We would especially like to thank the following:

Dr. Kathleen Byrne
Elise and Clovis Faltot
Joan Faltot
Lt. Terry Foley
Claudia Hickly
Marjorie Stephens
Peggy and Jim Wiley

A special thanks also goes to all the patients, Program Directors, and Medical Directors (Dr. Herbert Gray, Dr. Wilfredo Rubio, Dr. Surendra Sethi, Dr. Michael Wusylko) of the Bio-Energetiks Rehabilitation Clinics.

We wish to offer our gratitude to the following reviewers who read various drafts of the manuscript: Carolyn Burnett, Jane Golden, Thomas W. Hare, Thomas Hon, Nancy Humberstone, Althea Jones, Steven L. Wolf, Lana K. Woods, and finally, our thanks go to the staff at F. A. Davis who contributed to make the book a reality: Susan Ferragino, Mary Helen Bond, Herbert Powell, Jr., Philip Ashley, and Jean-François Vilain.

FJB
MJG
MWF

Contents

CHAPTER 1

Cardiac Rehabilitation: Overview

HISTORICAL PERSPECTIVE

Thirty years ago persons with cardiovascular disease were given little hope of leading normal lives.[1] Cardiac patients were treated as invalids, and the prospects of returning to full-time work were dismal. Perhaps the Framingham Study[2] provided the impetus to change the direction for treatment and hence prognosis for the cardiac patient. With the examination of 5200 men and women at regular intervals, a pattern of the etiology of cardiovascular disease began to appear. Of course, very little can be done to change family history, but other risk factors indicated life-style might exacerbate the incidence of coronary heart disease (CHD). Elevated blood pressure, blood fats, and blood sugar, cigarette smoking, and lack of exercise seem to be interrelated and to lead to the increased risk of developing CHD.[2] Could CHD be prevented or the age of CHD onset delayed if those risk factors that seem to be responsible could be modified? The answer to this question remains to be found, but current research[3] indicates that regular exercise of the appropriate type and intensity and modification of other risk factors contribute to longevity in a normal population,[4-10] as well as to the secondary prevention of cardiac events in CHD populations.[11-14]

Exercise has become an integral part of medicine by assisting in the diagnosis of cardiopulmonary disease and by serving as an adjunct to traditional medical practice in the treatment of persons with CHD.[15-18]

Despite the recent declines in CHD mortality, cardiovascular disease remains the single most prevalent cause of death in the United States today.[19] Although research and advances in surgical and medical treatment have most likely contributed to the declining death rates from CHD (approximately 24 percent between 1968 and 1977[19]), modifications of factors related to coronary risk are also important. However, behavioral ap-

1

proaches to induce individuals to modify negative health habits have only recently been given appropriate attention.[20]

Current trends in cardiac rehabilitation indicate that programs are changing to include a multispecialty approach with the emphasis on exercise therapy followed by intervention that addresses various risk factors. Risk factor modification is becoming increasingly scientific and requires the specialized skills of many health professionals working as a team to provide effective rehabilitative services. This multispecialty approach is not new to inpatient rehabilitation programs, and both free-standing and hospital-based outpatient cardiac rehabilitation programs are also increasing their specialized services to include the expertise of the physical therapist, the respiratory therapist, the exercise physiologist, the psychologist, the registered dietitian or nutritionist, the nurse cardiac specialist, and various exercise specialists and health educators. Regardless of the specialization of the health professionals who, under the supervision of the physician medical director(s), provide the rehabilitative services in a specific setting, current trends in cardiac rehabilitation emphasize more professional approaches to stress management, nutritional counseling, and smoking cessation. Unfortunately, insurance reimbursement for largely "educational" approaches to risk factor modification is virtually nonexistent. In many cases, the cost of utilizing the skills of all the aforementioned professionals thus becomes prohibitive. Overlap in the educational backgrounds of these professionals and education of existing staff may, however, provide quality programming in many areas of specialization; for example, a nurse cardiac specialist can be trained in the theory and practice of cardiac exercise physiology. It is for this purpose that this text was written—to provide the basic theory of outpatient cardiac rehabilitation and the practical application of this theory so that allied health professionals at various educational levels might gain sufficient information to function optimally as cardiac rehabilitation specialists.

INPATIENT CARDIAC REHABILITATION

The inpatient exercise program (Phase I) is begun in the hospital, usually in the coronary care unit (CCU). Persons with uncomplicated myocardial infarctions (MI), coronary artery bypass grafts (CABG), pulmonary disease, or peripheral vascular disease may begin their programs early during their hospital stays. Needless to say, the inpatient exercise program must begin at a low intensity (1 to 2 METs) and gradually progress to a level of 2 to 3 METs (2 to 3 times resting O_2 consumption). Usually a person has been transferred out of the CCU when ambulation activities are begun. Table 1–1 illustrates an example of activities and progressions that have been used in an inpatient rehabilitation program to help patients achieve functional capacity that permits self-care.

OUTPATIENT CARDIAC EXERCISE TRAINING PROGRAMS
Supervised Programs

Outpatient (Phase II) exercise training ideally should be provided in a facility which offers continuous ECG monitoring, emergency equipment, and medically supervised exercise.[10] Outpatient treatment is usually initiated within a few weeks following hospital discharge.

However, to qualify for insurance reimbursement, rehabilitation should begin sometime within the first year following a diagnosis of coronary artery disease, coronary artery bypass surgery, a myocardial infarction, coronary angioplasty, or other cardiac events that warrant rehabilitative services. Unsupervised programs are not recommended for the majority of cardiac patients, as the safety of unsupervised exercise programs is yet to be determined.[21] Patients with the following characteristics should be trained in a medically supervised setting:

1. Low maximal functional capacity
2. Severely depressed left ventricular function
3. Complex ventricular arrhythmias
4. Exercise-induced hypotension
5. Exertional angina
6. Inability to self-monitor exercise heart rate

Patients with these characteristics are at increased risk for adverse cardiac events during exercise.[22]

Most increases in cardiorespiratory functional capacity occur in outpatient exercise programs. Because Phase I (inpatient) patients are discharged from the hospital as soon as they are stable, there is insufficient time for significant physiologic adaptation to occur.

Patients are generally referred to supervised outpatient cardiac rehabilitation programs by their cardiologists or primary physicians. The medical director of the outpatient program must supervise all laboratory assessment and exercise therapy sessions. The medical director is responsible for the medical management of the patient's rehabilitation program. Physicians conduct and interpret routine ECG monitoring, interpret laboratory assessment results, and are responsible for administering emergency medical care with the assistance of trained, qualified staff.

Generally, the program director (exercise physiologist, physical therapist, nurse cardiac specialist) is responsible for administering stress tests and other laboratory evaluations (under the direct supervision of a physician), writing exercise prescriptions, revising exercise prescriptions (after physician review), and most administrative and managerial functions. The program director must have a thorough understanding of human anatomy and the physiology of exercise, as well as a knowledge of basic ECG interpretation, pathophysiology, and pharmacology, so that exercise prescriptions and patient progression may proceed as safely as possible.

A consulting nutritionist may counsel patients about proper diet, and a consulting psychologist may work with patients on management of stress and other risk factor modifications, such as cessation of smoking. These tasks may also be assigned to health educators or specialists in the field who have been trained to provide such services.

In most cases, the outpatient program is begun soon after the patient is discharged from a hospital. Continuous monitoring of the patient during the early stages of the rehabilitation program is standard procedure. During the course of the exercise therapy program, stable patients are gradually weaned from continuous monitoring in order to effect self-regulation of the recognition of their exercise limitations in preparation for Phase III or home exercise programs. Stable patients learn to count their own pulse rates in order to learn how to modify their exercise intensities to reach target heart rates (see Chapters 7 and 8) and to reinforce knowledge of the contraindications to exercise.

TABLE 1–1. Inpatient Rehabilitation: Seven-Step Myocardial Infarction Program (Grady Memorial Hospital and the Emory University School of Medicine)

Step	Date	MD Initials	Nurse/PT Notes	Supervised Exercise	CCU/Ward Activity	Educational-Recreational Activity
CCU						
1				Active and passive ROM all extremities, in bed Teach patient ankle plantar and dorsiflexion — repeat hourly when awake	Partial self-care Feed self Dangle legs on side of bed Use bedside commode Sit in chair 15 min 1–2 times/day	Orientation to CCU Personal emergencies, social service aid as needed
2				Active ROM all extremities, sitting on side of bed	Sit in chair 15–30 min 2–3 times/day Complete self-care in bed	Orientation to rehabilitation team, program Smoking cessation Educational literature if requested Planning transfer from CCU
Ward						
3				Warm-up exercises, 2 METs: Stretching Calisthenics Walking 50 ft and back at slow pace	Sit in chair ad lib To ward class in wheelchair Walk in room	Normal cardiac anatomy and function Development of atherosclerosis What happens with myocardial infarction 1–2 METs craft activity

	Exercise	Ward activity	Educational, recreational activity
4	ROM and calisthenics, 2.5 METs Walk length of hall (75 ft) and back, average pace Teach pulse counting	OOB as tolerated Walk to bathroom Walk to ward class, with supervision	Coronary risk factors and their control
5	ROM and calisthenics, 3 METs Check pulse counting Practice walking few stairsteps Walk 300 ft bid	Walk to waiting room or telephone Walk in ward corridor prn	Diet Energy conservation Work simplification techniques (as needed) 2–3 METs craft activity
6	Continue above activities Walk down flight of steps (return by elevator) Walk 500 ft bid Instruct on home exercise	Tepid shower or tub bath, with supervision To OT, cardiac clinic teaching room, with supervision	Heart attack management: Medications Exercise Surgery Response to symptoms Family, community adjustments on return home Craft activity prn
7	Continue above activities Walk up flight of steps Walk 500 ft bid Continue home exercise instruction; present information regarding outpatient exercise program	Continue all previous ward activities	Discharge planning: Medications, diet, activity Return appointments Scheduled tests Return to work Community resources Educational literature Medication cards Craft activity prn

From Wenger, NK and Fletcher, GF: Rehabilitation of the Patient with Symptomatic Atherosclerotic Coronary Heart Disease. In Hurst, JW, et al (eds): The Heart, ed 6. © 1986, McGraw-Hill Book Company. Used by permission.

Generally, exercise therapy is conducted three times per week over a minimum period of 3 months. At the end of 12 weeks, a re-evaluation, including a stress test, is administered. This re-evaluation provides valuable information about improvement in cardiorespiratory function, allows for exercise prescription revisions, and serves as an important motivator for the patient.

Decisions as to when the patient may progress to a medically unsupervised (less intensely monitored Phase III or community program) or home program are based on: (1) the patient's functional classification at re-evaluation (an aerobic capacity of at least 5 METs as determined by the stress test[10]), (2) the patient's ability to self-monitor his or her exercise program, (3) the stability (or absence of contraindications to exercise) of the patient, and (4) the psychological and emotional status of the patient. The decision to recommend a patient for home or Phase III exercise is usually made by the rehabilitation team as a whole after carefully considering the patient's safety, functional and medical status, and the likelihood of patient compliance. Many patients develop a dependency on the rehabilitation staff and must be slowly phased from the supervised program by decreasing the frequency of supervised visits over a period of time and encouraging unsupervised exercise at home. In this way, the more dependent patients can build confidence in their own abilities to make decisions regarding their exercise programs as the staff provides feedback regarding their conduct during unsupervised exercise (see next section on home exercise). This process helps to eliminate the feeling of abandonment that many patients report following the sudden cessation of a formal supervised program.

Even though a patient may no longer be actively involved in the supervised exercise therapy program, periodic re-evaluations should be scheduled to ensure that the exercise program and cardiorespiratory function are being maintained. Re-evaluations also help in the early detection of conditions for which further medical evaluations are indicated.

HOME EXERCISE PROGRAMS

Usually the exercise program at home is begun in conjunction with an outpatient program. When the staff deems it feasible (based on exercise and lab data), the patient can be assigned simple exercise activities to be done at home. The patient returns to the outpatient site with a record of heart rates and problems that may have occurred during the homework assignment. The staff analyzes these data, adjusts the homework prescription as necessary, and suggests methods for more accurate self-monitoring of the home program. If no contraindications occur, the staff advises the patient to continue with the home program. Progression of patient to home programs is an ultimate goal of the outpatient program. Once patients reach the level of functional capacity where maintenance becomes the primary goal, they should be encouraged to continue exercising at home with periodic re-evaluations, so that maintenance of cardiorespiratory functional capacity may be achieved.

PHASE III (COMMUNITY) PROGRAMS

Persons with CHD who are exercising without medical supervision should probably do so only after "graduating" from a medically supervised program. With the current increase in knowledge and continued research into the science of exercise, it seems irresponsible for patients to be advised "to do what you feel like doing" without exercise evaluations and concrete guidelines as to their exercise target heart rates. Once patients have completed programs in which they learn what is necessary to maintain their cardiorespiratory function, they should be able to engage in unsupervised programs fairly safely. At the Phase III level, maintenance of cardiorespiratory function is the primary goal; therefore, many such programs are ineligible for third-party reimbursement.

A criticism of unsupervised programs is that they often lack personnel with the ability to give sound advice about exercise prescriptions and progressions. In order to improve compliance, these centers often employ recreational games as a part of the rehabilitation process, a procedure that is discouraged by those who seek closer controls over exercise heart rates and emphasize avoidance of emotional responses to exercise and similar competitive situations that may affect the safety of CHD patients. Physicians should decide whether the unsupervised program in their area meets the standards necessary for patient safety. These decisions should be made on an individual basis in accordance with the guidelines previously discussed.

A MULTISPECIALTY APPROACH TO CARDIAC REHABILITATION

The primary goals of cardiac rehabilitation programs should be to increase the functional capacity of CHD patients and to assist them in attaining normal function, insofar as possible, in their daily lives. To be more effective in achieving these goals, rehabilitation centers must utilize personnel from several allied health disciplines. The knowledge that exists today as to the risk factors leading to CHD dictates that few persons, if any, have all the knowledge required to meet the medical, physical, social, and psychological needs of the patient. The physician, nurse, exercise physiologist, physical therapist, nutritionist, psychologist, and others must all work together with the health of the patient foremost in their thoughts if cardiac rehabilitation programming and risk factor modification is to be effective.

SUMMARY

This chapter has presented a basic overview of cardiac rehabilitation programs. Inpatient rehabilitation programs (Phase I) are begun during a patient's hospitalization and are of insufficient length and intensity to allow dramatic physiologic change. Most of the increase in cardiorespiratory functional capacity occurs during the outpatient (Phase II) rehabilitation program. Phase II programs are physician-supervised and may employ persons from several allied health disciplines. The outpatient program is usually conducted 3 times a week for a period of 12 weeks. Patients are gradually phased from the outpatient program and encouraged to begin home exercise or unsupervised (Phase III) programs that include periodic re-evaluations by the outpatient rehabilitation staff.

REFERENCES

1. Wenger, NK: Exercise and the Heart. FA Davis, Philadelphia, 1978.
2. Dawber, TR: The Framingham Study: The Epidemiology of Atherosclerotic Disease. Harvard University Press, Cambridge, 1980.
3. MacKeen, PC, et al: A Thirteen Year Follow-Up of a Coronary Heart Disease Risk Factor Screening and

Exercise Program for 40–59 Year-Old Men: Exercise Habit Maintenance and Physiologic Status. J Cardio-pulmonary Rehabilitation 5:510–525, 1985.

4. Paffenbarger, RS, Jr., et al: A Natural History of Athleticism and Cardiovascular Health. JAMA 252:491–5, 1984.
5. Eichner, ER: Exercise and Heart Disease: Epidemiology of the "Exercise Hypothesis." Am J Med 75:1008–23, 1983.
6. Kannel, WB and Sorlic, P: Some Health Benefits of Physical Activity: The Framingham Study. Arch Intern Med 139:857–61, 1979.
7. Costas, R, et al: Relation of Lipids, Weight, and Physical Activity to Incidence of Coronary Heart Disease: The Puerto Rican Heart Study. Am J Cardiol 42:653–8, 1978.
8. Smith, EL, Reddan, W, and Smith, PE: Physical Activity and Calcium Modalities for Bone Mineral Increase in Aged Women. Med Sci Sports Exerc 13:60–4, 1981.
9. Wallace, JP: Physical Conditioning. In Regelson, W and Sinex, FM (eds): Intervention in the Aging Process, Part A. Alan R. Liss, New York, 1983, pp 307–323.
10. American College of Sports Medicine: Guidelines for Exercise Testing and Prescription. Lea & Febiger, Philadelphia, 1986, p 58.
11. Sparrow, D, et al: The Influence of Cigarette Smoking on Prognosis After a First Myocardial Infarction. J Chronic Dis 31:425–532, 1977.
12. Mulcahy, R, et al: Factors Affecting the Five-Year Survival Rate of Men Following Acute Coronary Heart Disease. Am Heart J 93:556–559, 1977.
13. Coronary Drug Project Research Group: Influence of Adherence to Treatment and Response of Cholesterol on Mortality in the Coronary Drug Project. N Eng J Med 303:1038–1041, 1980.
14. Dyer, AR and Stamler, PJ: Alcoholic Consumption and 17 Year Mortality in the Chicago Western Electric Study. Prev Med 9:78–90, 1980.
15. Fletcher, GF and Cantwell, JD: Exercise and Coronary Heart Disease. Charles C Thomas, Springfield, 1979.
16. Blocker, WP and Cardus, D: Rehabilitation in Ischemic Heart Disease. Spectrum Publications, New York, 1983.
17. Wilson, PK, Fardy, PS and Froelicher, VF: Cardiac Rehabilitation, Adult Fitness and Exercise Testing. Lea & Febiger, Philadelphia, 1981.
18. Froelicher, VF: Exercise Testing and Training. LeJacq Publishing, New York, 1983.
19. Garrison, RJ, et al: Epidemiology of CHD: New Trends. Department of Epidemiology, National Heart, Lung and Blood Institute, NIH, Bethesda, MD.
20. Blumenthal, JA, et al: Continuing Medical Educator: Cardiac Rehab: A New Frontier for Behavioral Medicine. J Cardiac Rehab 3:637–56, 1983.
21. Wenger, NK and Fletcher, GF: Rehabilitation of the Patient with Symptomatic Atherosclerotic Coronary Heart Disease. In J Hurst, et al (eds): The Heart, ed 6. McGraw-Hill, New York, 1986.
22. Williams, RS, et al: Guidelines for Unsupervised Exercise in Patients with Ischemic Heart Disease. J Cardiac Rehab 1:213, 1981.

CHAPTER 2

The Heart and Circulation

THE HEART

The heart is a hollow organ weighing approximately 250 to 300 grams. It is not positioned in the center of the chest cavity; most of it lies to the left of center. The base of the heart is broad and is located superiorly, and the apex is at the inferior end and points anteriorly and approximately 45° to the left. The heart is enclosed in a fibrous protective sac called the pericardium. The major portion of the heart itself is composed of muscle referred to as the myocardium. The inner surface of the myocardium is lined with a smooth epithelial tissue called the endocardium, which allows the blood to pass through the chambers of the heart without damage to the blood cells.[1]

The outer, external surface of the myocardium is covered with a fibrous membrane, the epicardium, which merges at the base of the heart with the pericardium. The muscular tissue of the myocardium is arranged in layers that run in indefinite, circular, and oblique directions.[1]

The four chambers of the heart are the right and left atria and the right and left ventricles. The apex of the heart is formed by the tip of the left ventricle.[2]

The surfaces of the heart are the sternocostal, the diaphragmatic, and the posterior. The sternocostal surface (anterior) is formed primarily by the right atrium and the right ventricle. The diaphragmatic (inferior) surface of the heart is formed by the right and left ventricles. The posterior (base) surface of the heart is formed primarily by the left atrium, although the right atrium forms a small part of the posterior surface.[2]

The four borders of the heart are the right, left, superior, and inferior. The right border is formed by the right atrium; the left border is formed mainly by the left ventricle, but a small part is formed by the left atrium. The superior border is formed by both atria and is located in the area where the great vessels unite with the heart. The inferior border is formed primarily by the right ventricle and to a lesser extent by the left ventricle (Figure 2–1).

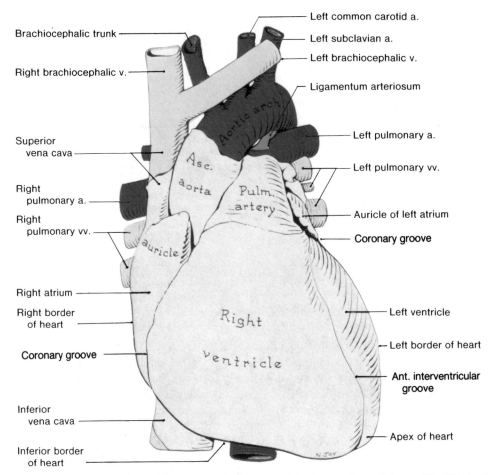

FIGURE 2–1. Illustration of the sternocostal aspect of the heart. (From Moore, KL: Clinically Oriented Anatomy, ed 2. Williams & Wilkins, Baltimore, 1985, with permission.)

Heart Chambers

The heart has four chambers that are arranged in pairs. The two atria are thin-walled cavities designed to receive blood into the heart. The right atrium receives blood from the systemic circulation through two openings, the superior and inferior venae cavae. During systole of the atria, blood from the right atrium is sent through the right atrioventricular orifice to the right ventricle. This orifice contains the tricuspid valve, which opens to allow the blood to pass into the ventricle during atrial systole.[3]

During ventricular systole, the tricuspid valve closes so that blood will not be pumped back into the atrium (Figure 2–2).

The left atrium is also thin-walled. It has four openings at its superior and posterior wall (Figure 2–3). These openings accommodate the four pulmonary veins that carry oxygenated blood from the lungs to the left atrium. Blood passes from the left atrium through the left atrioventricular orifice, which is controlled by the bicuspid or mitral valve.

During ventricular contraction, the mitral valve is tightly closed to prevent blood surging back to the atrium.[4]

The walls of the ventricles are much thicker and stronger than those of the atria and are well suited to pump the blood greater distances. The right ventricle forms most of the front of the heart and pumps the blood through the pulmonary orifice into the pulmonary artery (Figure 2–4). The blood flow to the pulmonary artery is controlled by the semilunar or pulmonary valve, which prevents the flow of blood back to the right ventricle during systole. The right ventricle contracts to send the blood via the pulmonary artery through the pulmonary circulation to be oxygenated; hence, the right ventricle is referred to as the pulmonary pump.[4,5]

The walls of the left ventricle are thicker and stronger than the walls of the right ventricle. The left ventricle forms most of the left margin and the apex of the heart and is responsible for pumping blood throughout the entire systemic circulation; it is the systemic pump. Blood enters the systemic circulation from the left ventricle through the aortic orifice, guarded by the aortic valve, and into the aorta. The aorta is the largest artery in the body.[4,5]

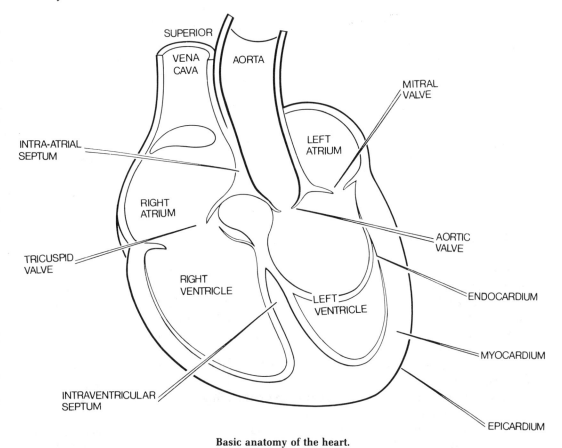

Basic anatomy of the heart.

FIGURE 2–2. Illustration of the heart and chambers. (From Phillips, RE and Feeney, MK: The Cardiac Rhythms, ed 2. WB Saunders, Philadelphia, 1980, p 11, with permission.)

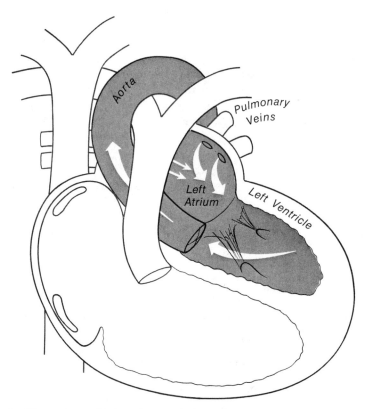

FIGURE 2-3. Illustration of left atrium and the pulmonary veins. (From Phillips, RE and Feeney, MK: The Cardiac Rhythms, ed 2. WB Saunders, Philadelphia, 1980, p 9, with permission.)

THE CORONARY ARTERIES

The two major arteries that supply the heart with blood arise directly from the aorta at a point near the aortic valve (Figure 2-5). Although there is considerable variation, the right coronary artery branches to send blood to the right atrium, the right ventricle and, in most persons, to the inferior wall of the left ventricle, the atrioventricular (AV) node, and the bundle of His. The sinoatrial (SA) node receives its blood supply from the right coronary artery in about 60 percent of human beings.[6]

The left coronary artery branches into two main divisions within approximately two centimeters from its point of origin. The left anterior descending (LAD) artery supplies the left ventricle, the interventricular septum, the right ventricle and, in most persons, the inferior areas of the apex and both ventricles.[4,6]

The second main division of the left coronary artery, the left circumflex, supplies blood to the inferior walls of the left ventricle and to the left atrium. In about 40 percent of humans, the left circumflex supplies the SA node with blood.[4,6]

Circulation to the Heart

Blood circulating to the heart muscle itself via the coronary arteries must do so while the muscle fibers are relaxed, during diastole of the heart. This is an important fact to remember when considering whether the heart muscle has adequate blood flow during exercise and in order to prevent the occurrence of an ischemic state. Although blood is forced into the coronary arteries from the heart during systole, that blood cannot enter the cardiac muscle fibers to supply oxygen to the tissue until the heart is in diastole and the fibers are relaxed.[1] Perhaps this is the greatest single reason for keeping the exercising heart rate low in a coronary patient.

METABOLISM OF CARDIAC TISSUE

Cardiac tissue contains large amounts of myoglobin, the enzymes of the Krebs cycle and the electron transport system, and is thus well suited for aerobic metabolism. In order for

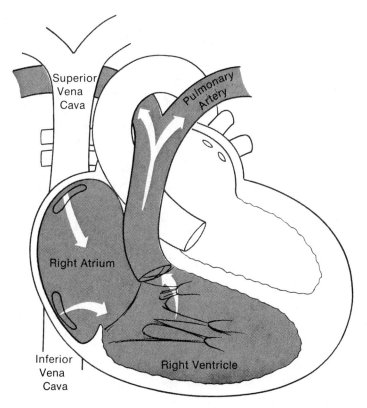

FIGURE 2–4. Illustration of blood flow from right ventricle to the lungs. (From Phillips, RE and Feeney, MK: The Cardiac Rhythms, ed 2. WB Saunders, Philadelphia, 1980, p 9, with permission.)

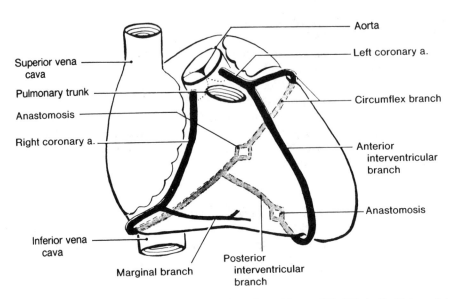

FIGURE 2–5. Illustration of the coronary arteries. (From Moore, KL: Clinically Oriented Anatomy, ed 2. Williams & Wilkins, Baltimore, 1985, with permission.)

the heart to function properly, it must receive a constant supply of oxygen to support its almost exclusively aerobic metabolism. The principal source of energy production for cardiac muscle is the oxidation of free fatty acids. Although acetoacetic acid and lactic acid can be metabolized to produce energy, the energy of preference of the heart is through fatty acid metabolism.[6,7] Examples of the anaerobic and aerobic pathways for adenosine 5'-triphosphate (ATP) production can be seen in Table 2–1.

The most common fatty acids have chains of 16 and 18 carbons. Through B-oxidation (oxidizing 2 carbons at a time), a 16-carbon-chain fatty acid could produce approximately

TABLE 2–1. Anaerobic and Aerobic Metabolic Pathways for Production of ATP

Anaerobic Metabolism

1. Coronary circulation delivers glucose to cardiac tissue
2. Glucose via Glycolysis (in cytoplasm) $\longrightarrow$ Pyruvate + 2 ATP
OR
3. Lactate delivered by coronary circulation to cardiac tissue
4. Lactate (in cytoplasm) $\longrightarrow$ Pyruvate + 2 ATP

Aerobic Metabolism

1. Coronary circulation delivers free fatty acids to cardiac tissue
2. Free fatty acids undergo B-oxidation $\longrightarrow$ ~ 4 ATP + Acetyl Co A (Mitochondria)
3. Acetyl Co A enters Krebs cycle + O_2 $\longrightarrow$ ~ 12 ATP (approximately 6 total ATP with *each* 2-carbon oxidation) + H_2O + CO_2
OR
4. Pyruvate (from cytoplasm) $\longrightarrow$ Acetyl Co A (Mitochondria)
5. Acetyl Co A $\longrightarrow$ Krebs cycle + O_2 $\longrightarrow$ 36 ATP + H_2O + CO_2

128 ATP when completely metabolized (16 ATP $\times$ 16 carbon/B-oxidation) = 16 ATP $\times$ 8 = 128 ATP.[6]

The importance of a continuous O_2 delivery to the cardiac muscle can be seen in the relative contributions of anaerobic and aerobic metabolism to the production of ATP. During rest, cardiac tissue extracts approximately 70 percent of the O_2 that is delivered to it via the coronary arteries. This leaves a very limited reserve for increasing oxygen extraction during increased myocardial work. The increased demand for more oxygen during work is met by increasing the blood flow to the cardiac tissue. Consequently the rate and force of cardiac contraction and therefore cardiac output increases in response to increased activity. Increased coronary blood flow is also achieved through a reduction in the resistance (dilation) of the coronary vessels.[6]

CONDUCTION

Although there are structural and functional similarities between cardiac and skeletal muscle, there are major differences between these two types of muscle.[8] In addition to ordinary muscle tissue, cardiac muscle has two other major types of tissue: nodal tissue and Purkinje tissue. The nodal tissue is located at the junction of the superior vena cava and the right atrium (sinoatrial node) and at the junction of the right atrium and the right ventricle (atrioventricular node). The Purkinje fibers are the specialized conducting tissues of both ventricles.

Sinoatrial Node

The sinoatrial (SA) node (Figure 2–6) is composed of small, slender, spindle-shaped cells that contain very few myofibrils but large amounts of thick connective tissue. The SA node is called the pacemaker of the heart and has sympathetic and parasympathetic innervation, although at rest the SA node is under continuous parasympathetic control via the vagus nerve. Small strands of fibers extend out from the main region of the SA node and are continuous with the ordinary muscle fibers of the atrium. Through this arrangement, once the SA node initiates an impulse (sinus rhythm), that impulse can spread from muscle fiber to muscle fiber throughout both atria (functional syncytium).[1,9]

Atrioventricular Node

The atrioventricular (AV) node is a band of fibers located at the lower end of the interatial septum of the right atrium (Figure 2–7). The AV nodal tissue merges with the atrioventricular bundle of His near the origin of the ventricles. The AV node normally functions to receive the impulse that originates from the SA node and conducts it to the bundle of His. In cases of impaired SA node function, the AV node can become the pacemaker of the heart and send out its own impulses to keep the heart beating (nodal rhythms). The AV node is also supplied with nerves from the sympathetic and parasympathetic systems.[1,9]

**Atrial
Depolarization**

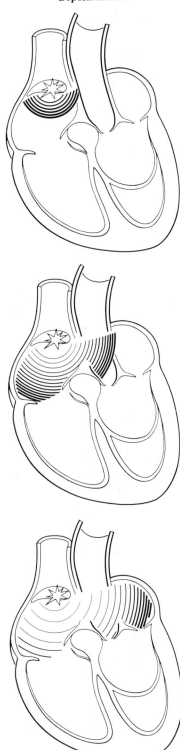

FIGURE 2–6. Illustration of atrial impulse conduction. (From Phillips, RE and Feeney, MK: The Cardiac Rhythms, ed 2. WB Saunders, Philadelphia, 1980, p 21, with permission.)

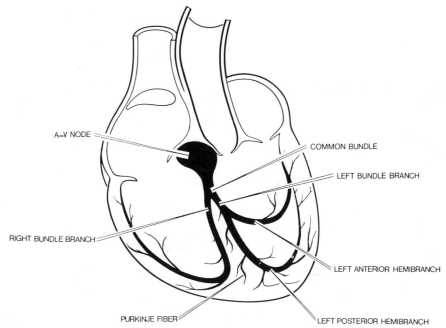

FIGURE 2–7. Illustration of ventricular conduction. (From Phillips, RE and Feeney, MK: The Cardiac Rhythms, ed 2. WB Saunders, Philadelphia, 1980, p 23, with permission.)

Purkinje Tissue

The AV bundle of His has two branches, the right and the left, located along either side of the intraventricular septum (Figure 2–7). These branches terminate in the Purkinje fibers, which are the specialized conducting tissues of both ventricles. The fibers that comprise the Purkinje system have sarcoplasm that contains large amounts of glycogen but few myofibrils. The fibers of the Purkinje system terminate in twigs that penetrate the ventricles and are intimately associated with the contractile fibers of the ventricle muscles.[1,9]

Origin and Conduction of Heart Beat

The origin of the electrical impulse that precedes the contraction of the heart is in the SA node (myogenic). This impulse spreads quickly through both atria, which then contract simultaneously. This wave of electrical activity next stimulates the AV node, which transmits the impulse down the bundle of His to the Purkinje fibers. Because the Purkinje fibers merge with the walls of the ventricles, the impulse spreads through the Purkinje system to the cells of the ventricles, and the ventricles contract together (Figure 2–8). This rhythmical sequence of events occurs, on the average, 72 times per minute.[1]

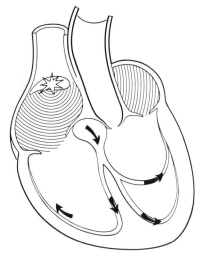

Pathways of conduction.

FIGURE 2–8. Schematic illustration of conduction system of cardiac muscle. (From Phillips, RE and Feeney, MK: The Cardiac Rhythms, ed 2. WB Saunders, Philadelphia, 1980, p 23, with permission.)

Myocardial Fibers

The microscopic appearance of cardiac muscle fibers is similar to that of skeletal muscle fibers. Both types of muscle appear to be striated, as their myofibrils have well identified A, I, and Z bands.[8] Compared to skeletal muscle, cardiac tissue has numerous mitochondria and its T-tubules are larger, but the sarcoplasmic reticulum (SR) is not well developed.[8] A major functional difference between skeletal and cardiac muscle is that cardiac muscle exhibits a rhythmicity (myogenicity) of contraction whereas skeletal muscle contracts in response to direct neural stimulation. This inherent rhythmicity of cardiac tissue originates in the SA node.

GENERAL MYOLOGY

Muscle Tissue

The protoplasm of muscle cells has the ability to contract, and because most muscle cells are elongated, individual cells are called fibers. There are three types of muscle tissue in the body: smooth, skeletal, and cardiac. (Skeletal or striated muscle is sometimes divided into two categories: skeletal and cardiac.[5])

Smooth muscle is closely associated with connective tissue structures and is found in the walls of the digestive tract, urinary tract, and blood vessels. Contraction of smooth muscle in these areas causes the structures to change in size and volume. Smooth muscle is also called involuntary or visceral, and the terms are used interchangeably. Each individual muscle fiber (cell) of smooth muscle tissue has a single oval nucleus. Unlike cardiac and skeletal muscle, smooth muscle can regenerate quite well following injury.[3]

The basic cellular structure of skeletal muscle may be described as a multinucleated cylinder that varies in length and may be longer than 30 centimeters. Skeletal muscle cells appear striped and have light (isotropic) and dark (anisotropic) bands throughout. Synonymous terms for skeletal muscle are somatic, voluntary, and striated muscle. These muscles are responsible for moving the various parts of the skeleton.[3]

The individual cells of cardiac muscle are irregular in shape, contain a single oval nucleus, and seem to have incomplete cell membranes. Like skeletal muscle, cardiac muscle is striated. Unlike skeletal muscle, individual cardiac cells are joined through intercalated disks. Because cardiac cells have branches that appear to connect with adjacent fibers, the cells contract as a unit to act as a syncytium (a functional rather than an anatomical syncytium). The heart has two such functional syncytia, the atria and the ventricles.[1,3,8]

Although the muscles of the body are composed of three different types of contractile tissues, they are similar in that they all are affected by the same kinds of stimuli, they will atrophy in response to inadequate activity, and they will hypertrophy as a result of increased work. Current theory regarding muscle contraction indicates that skeletal and cardiac muscle contraction are similar physiological processes.

PROTEINS OF THE MUSCLES

Chemical study of muscle tissue indicates that a large portion of the solid material in muscle is protein. For instance, skeletal muscle is 75 percent water and 25 percent solid material. Of that solid material, 20 percent is protein and the remaining 5 percent is other material.[1]

Classification of Proteins. Considerable variation exists in classifying proteins, but a convenient method is according to their function. The majority of proteins found in muscle tissue are either enzymes (approximately 40 percent) or structural (almost 60 percent).[10,11] The remaining muscle proteins are the stroma proteins, which function to hold various structures intact.[11-13]

Enzymes. The protein enzymes are located primarily in the sarcoplasm and in the membranes of intracellular organoids. They control the metabolic processes of muscle metabolism. Thus glycolysis (occurring in the sarcoplasm) and the Krebs cycle (occurring in the mitochondria) are controlled by protein enzymes.

Structural Proteins. The structural proteins constitute almost 60 percent of total muscle proteins and are abundant in the myofibrils.[13] The major proteins of the contractile process are myosin, actin, tropomysin and troponin.[14] Other minor proteins of uncertain function which may influence contraction are: A-actinin, B-actinin, C-protein, M-protein, and desmin.[15] Desmin is particularly abundant in cardiac muscle. Myoglobin (muscle hemoglobin) is a protein found in the sarcoplasm.[14,16]

THE MUSCLE FIBER

The membrane of a muscle cell is the sarcolemma. Each muscle cell has at least one nucleus. It is surrounded by the cytoplasm, which, in muscle cells, is called the sarcoplasm. The myofibrils are those structures in the sarcoplasm of muscle cells that give stability, and they are directly responsible for muscle contraction (Figure 2–9). The function of the mitochondria found in muscle cells is the same as that for other cells of the body, that of

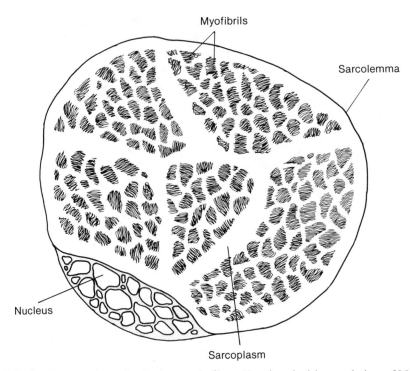

FIGURE 2-9. Cross section of a single muscle fiber. (Reprinted with permission of Macmillan Publishing Company from Grollman, S: The Human Body. Copyright © 1978 by Sigmund Grollman.)

energy production. There are abundantly more mitochondria in cardiac fibers than there are in skeletal muscle fibers. Skeletal muscle fibers respond to aerobic training by increasing the number and size of mitochondria in their cells, a response which apparently does not occur in cardiac tissue.[17]

Two important tubular systems found in muscle fibers are the transverse tubules (T-tubules) and the sarcoplasmic reticulum (Figure 2-10). The T-tubules occur at regular intervals along the fibers and function to conduct waves of depolarization from the sarcolemma to deeper regions of the fiber. The numerous sac-like structures that comprise the sarcoplasmic reticulum (SR) are located next to the T-tubules.[18] The SR seems to be a storage place for the calcium (Ca^{++}) that is necessary for muscle contraction to occur. The T-tubules in cardiac tissue are significantly larger than the T-tubules in skeletal muscle. Conversely, the SRs of cardiac muscle are not as abundant as in skeletal muscle. The amount of Ca^{++} released into the fiber during the contractile process seems to relate to the force of contraction that is generated by that fiber.[19]

The Myofibril. Muscle fibers contain numerous myofibrils, those filaments directly responsible for the contractile process. The smallest functional unit of the myofibril is the sarcomere, which is characterized by alternating light (I-band) and dark (A-band) bands. The A-band contains mainly the protein myosin, a thick, dark filament. The I-band is composed primarily of the protein actin, a much thinner filament than myosin (Figure

2–10). During muscle contraction, cross bridges located on myosin connect to the actin filaments. The thin actin filaments slide inward toward the center of the sarcomere and the sarcomere shortens.[12,17,18,20,21]

Myosin. Chemical studies of myosin indicate several forms and several large components. The fundamental unit of myosin is a protein with an average molecular weight of 470,000.[22] The ATPase (ability to split ATP) activity of the myofibril is confined to myosin; this ATPase ability is activated by Ca^{++} and inhibited by Mg^{++}.[23,24]

Actin. Actin has been found to exist as G-actin (globular) and as F-actin (fibrous). It has a molecular weight of approximately 42,000. The conversion of F-actin to G-actin and vice versa involve a process of polymerization, which is necessary for muscle contraction. ATP has been found to bind to actin, and this binding is stronger to F-actin than to G-actin.[13,21,22]

The Regulatory Proteins. The two major proteins in the myofibril that exert a regulatory effect on contraction are tropomyosin and troponin.[12] In the resting state,

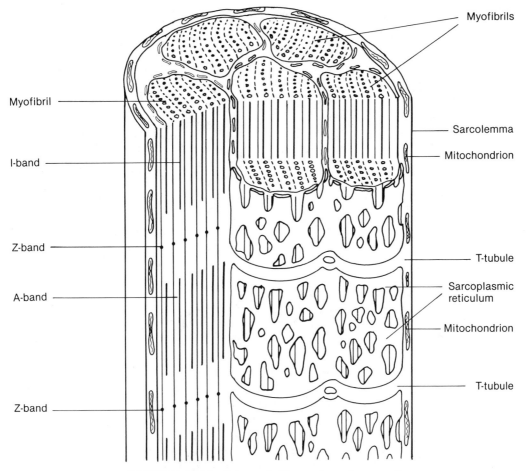

FIGURE 2–10. Schematic illustration of myocardium.

tropomyosin seems to prevent actin and myosin from interacting. Once calcium enters the cell, it binds with troponin to remove the inhibiting effect of tropomyosin. At this point, actin and myosin can interact and muscle contraction occurs (Figure 2–11).

Ca^{++} plays a role in the contraction of skeletal and cardiac muscle. In the resting state, the regulatory protein tropomyosin prevents actin and myosin from interacting. When muscle cells are stimulated, Ca^{++} is released from the SR and binds to the regulatory protein troponin, which removes the inhibiting effect of tropomyosin. Actin and myosin are now free to interact to cause contraction.[8]

Contraction Theory

Once a nerve impulse enters the muscle fiber, Ca^{++} is released by the SR. Some of the Ca^{++} combines with myosin to form an "activated myosin," which now has the property of the enzyme ATPase. This activated ATPase is able to react with ATP to remove its energy. This energy, in turn, is utilized to "pull" the actin filaments in among the myosin filaments; this is the sliding filament theory of contraction.[8]

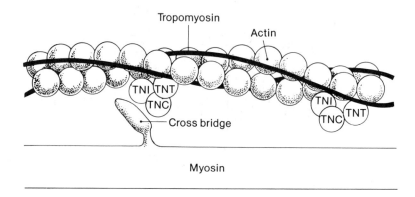

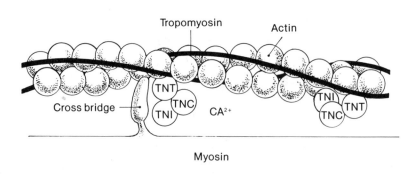

FIGURE 2–11. Schematic illustration of the regulatory proteins, TNI (troponin), TNT (tropomyosin, troponin), TNC (calcium-binding troponin). (Reprinted with permission of Macmillan Publishing Company from Grollman, S: The Human Body. Copyright © 1978 by Sigmund Grollman.)

TABLE 2–2. Energy Formation in Muscle Cells

1. ATP–F-actomyosin $\xrightarrow[\text{Ca}^{++}]{\text{nerve impulse}}$ G-actomyosin + ATP
2. ATP $\rightleftharpoons$ ADP + Pi (H_3PO_4) + E (energy used for contraction)
3. Phosphocreatine $\rightleftharpoons$ creatine + Pi (H_3PO_4) + E (energy used for resynthesis of ATP)
4. Glycogen (Glycolysis) $\rightleftharpoons$ Lactic acid + E (energy used for resynthesis of phosphocreatine)
5. ⅕ Lactic acid + O_2 (Krebs cycle) $\longrightarrow$ CO_2 + H_2O + E (energy to drive reaction 6)
6. ⅘ Lactic acid + E $\longrightarrow$ Glycogen

In the resting muscle cell, the myofibril is composed of F-actomyosin with ATP strongly attached to it to form an ATP–F-actomyosin complex. As a result of the ionic events that occur in response to nerve impulses, the ATP–F-actomyosin linkage is broken and G-actomyosin is formed. Table 2–2 summarizes the energy-forming events.

NEURAL CONTROL OF HEART RATE AND BLOOD VESSELS

The heart is regulated by the autonomic nervous system, which has two major divisions, the parasympathetic and the sympathetic (Figure 2–12).

Parasympathetic Center. The parasympathetic system innervates the heart via the vagus nerve (X cranial). The center for this system, located in the medulla, is considered a cardioinhibitory center. Stimulation of the parasympathetic nerves (Figure 2–13) causes a release of acetylcholine (cholinergic), which in turn both slows the heart from its normal intrinsic rate and decreases the force of its contraction. Vagal stimulation also causes the coronary arteries to dilate, which enhances coronary blood flow. At rest, the normal heart is under continual vagal control.[1,9]

Sympathetic Center. The sympathetic center (adrenergic) is located in the medulla oblongata. Stimulation of this center causes an increase in the rate and the force of contraction of the cardiac muscle. The chemical mediator for sympathetic stimulation is primarily norepinephrine, although epinephrine is also released (Figure 2–13). The sympathetic system has two types of receptors that respond to stimulation, the alpha and beta (β_1 and β_2) receptors. The majority of alpha receptors, when stimulated, cause coronary arteriolar vasoconstriction. In contrast, the beta receptors when stimulated cause coronary arteriolar vasodilation. A balance between the alpha and beta receptors is necessary for the heart to function properly.[1,9]

Additional Control of the Heart Beat. Although the neural regulation of the heart seems to be its main mode of control, other factors influence heart action. The pressoreceptors (baroreceptors) located in the aorta and carotid sinus are sensitive to changes in blood pressure. When blood pressure is increased, the pressoreceptors send this information to the medulla oblongata and stimulate the parasympathetic system to decrease the rate and force of the cardiac contraction.

The chemoreceptors located in the carotid body are sensitive to changes in blood chemicals such as O_2, CO_2 and lactic acid. For instance, either an increase in CO_2 (and decreased amounts of O_2) or lactic acid concentration (causing decreased pH) will cause the heart rate to increase. Increased levels of O_2 will cause the heart action to decrease.[25]

Body temperature plays an important role in controlling the rate of heart action.

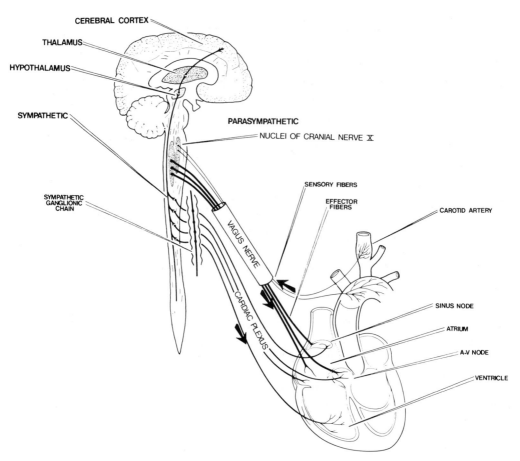

FIGURE 2 – 12. Illustration of the autonomic nervous system innervating cardiac muscle. (From Phillips, RE and Feeney, MK: The Cardiac Rhythms, ed 2. WB Saunders, Philadelphia, 1980, p 63, with permission.)

Increased body temperature causes the heart rate to increase, whereas a decrease in body temperature causes the heart rate to decrease.[8]

The concentration of ions in the blood is important in proper heart action. Increased concentration of potassium (hyperkalemia) decreases the rate and force of contraction. Hypokalemia causes arrhythmias.[8]

Excessive calcium concentration (hypercalcemia) increases the action of the heart and produces prolonged contractions.[26] Hypocalcemia depresses heart action. All these factors govern heart action, and proper balance among them is necessary for normal cardiac function.[8]

PERIPHERAL CIRCULATION

Blood circulates when the pressure in one area or structure of the body is higher than in another. Blood flows from an area of higher pressure to one of lower pressure. Blood pressure can be defined as the pressure exerted by the blood against the walls of the vessels.[27] During systole (contraction) of the ventricles, the pressure exerted against the walls of the vessels is greater than during diastole (relaxation) of the ventricles. Measurements of systolic and diastolic arterial blood pressure are usually determined indirectly by the auscultatory method with the bell of the stethoscope applied to the brachial artery. Average systolic arterial blood pressures usually range from 90 mmHg to 120 mmHg (millimeters of mercury), and the average diastolic arterial pressure range is from 60 mmHg to 90 mmHg. Resting arterial systolic blood pressures consistently above 140 mmHg and resting diastolic arterial blood pressures in excess of 100 mmHg are considered to be abnormal.[27] Although blood pressures vary with such factors as age, emotional

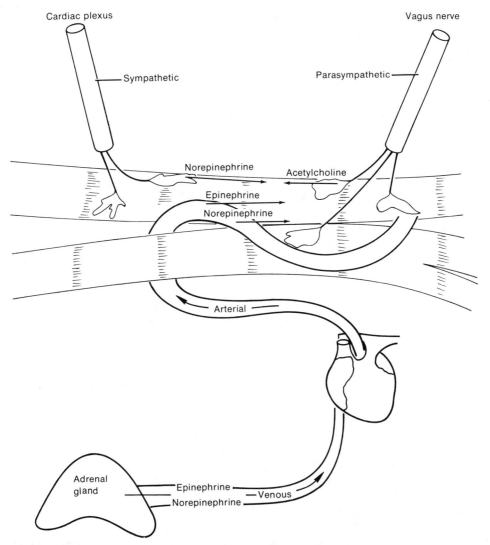

FIGURE 2-13. Illustration of sympathetic and parasympathetic influence on heart rate. (From Phillips, RE and Feeney, MK: The Cardiac Rhythms, ed 2. WB Saunders, Philadelphia, 1980, p 66, with permission.)

states, and exercise, a primary determinant of blood pressure is the volume of blood in the arteries. Thus, an increase in the blood volume in the arteries tends to cause an increase in arterial pressures and, conversely, a decrease in volume tends to cause a decrease in arterial pressure. Two important factors affecting blood volume, and thus blood pressure, are cardiac output and peripheral resistance.[4,28]

CARDIAC OUTPUT

An increase in cardiac output (amount of blood ejected from the heart per minute) tends to increase arterial blood volume and, therefore, increase blood pressure. The volume of blood pumped per minute depends upon the number of contractions (heart beats) per minute and the amount of blood pumped with each contraction. The amount of blood pumped per beat (stroke volume) depends on the force of ventricular contraction. The greater the force of contraction, the greater the stroke volume and the systolic pressure tend to be.[4,28]

Increases in heart rate result in increases in cardiac output. This causes arterial blood volume and therefore arterial blood pressure to increase. Conversely, when the heart beats more slowly and/or with less force, there are decreases in cardiac output, arterial volume, and arterial blood pressure.[4,28]

Regulation of Cardiac Output

Stroke volume is directly related to contractility and, consequently, to the strength of the heart beat. The main regulator for stroke volume is the ratio of sympathetic to parasympathetic impulses innervating the heart. An increase in sympathetic impulses causes a more forceful contraction of the heart. This increases its stroke volume. Blood concentrations of epinephrine also affect stroke volume in that increases in blood epinephrine increase stroke volume.[4,28]

The pressoreceptors (baroreceptors) in the aortic arch and in the carotid sinus are the main mechanisms responsible for controlling heart rate. If the blood pressure within these areas increases, impulses are sent to the cardioinhibitory center in the medulla oblongata, which causes the heart rate to slow. A decrease in the blood pressure in the aortic arch or carotid sinus causes a reflex acceleration of the heart.[4,28]

Pressoreceptors in the right atrium of the heart also affect heart rate. When right atrial blood pressure increases, there is a reflex acceleration of the heart beat; decreases in right atrial pressure cause reflex slowing.[4,28]

Other factors affecting heart rate, and therefore cardiac output, include emotions, exercise, blood temperature, and hormones. Anxiety, fear, and anger tend to increase heart rate and cardiac output, whereas grief tends to decrease heart rate and cardiac output. Increases in heart rate are observed during exercise, with increases in the temperature of the blood, and with increased levels of epinephrine.[4,28]

Peripheral Resistance

A change in peripheral resistance (resistance to blood flow) tends to cause the volume of blood within the arteries to change and thus changes blood pressure. An increase in peripheral resistance tends to increase arterial blood volume and, therefore, to increase arterial blood pressure. A decrease in peripheral resistance tends to cause decreased blood volume and, therefore, decreased arterial blood pressure. Peripheral resistance is influenced by the viscosity of the blood and the diameter of the arterioles and capillaries. When the amount of blood that flows from the arteries into the arterioles decreases, more blood is left in the arteries. This increases blood volume and tends to cause an increase in arterial blood pressure.[4,28]

REGULATION OF PERIPHERAL RESISTANCE

The amount of resistance encountered by the peripheral circulation depends primarily on the viscosity of the blood and the diameter of the arterioles. The viscosity (thickness) of the blood determines to a large extent the ease with which the blood flows. The hematocrit, or the ratio of the formed elements (red blood cells, white blood cells, and platelets) to the plasma content of whole blood, exerts a great influence on viscosity as does the number of plasma proteins circulating in the blood. If the formed elements (mainly red blood cells) increase, then viscosity increases and so does peripheral resistance. Normally, blood viscosity changes very little. In cases such as hemorrhage, viscosity decreases (as does total blood volume), lowering peripheral resistance and arterial blood pressure. In cases where the hematocrit rises above 50 percent (as in polycythemia), the corresponding increase in blood viscosity causes decreased blood flow and also increases the work of the heart.[28]

Arteriole diameter (vasoconstriction and vasodilation) is influenced by many factors, among which are arterial blood pressure, oxygen and carbon dioxide content of the blood, pH of the blood, and substances such as hormones (epinephrine, norepinephrine), histamines, and lactic acid. Decreases in arteriole diameters (vasoconstriction) increase the peripheral resistance and therefore increase blood pressure. Increases in arterial blood pressure stimulate the aortic and carotid baroreceptors, causing parasympathetic impulses to be sent to the cardioinhibitory system in the medulla oblongata, which inhibits the vasoconstriction center. As a result, impulses are sent to the heart and blood vessels, causing the heart rate to decrease and the arterioles to dilate, thereby reducing arterial blood pressure. Decreases in arterial blood pressure have the opposite effect.[4,28]

SUMMARY

This chapter has dealt with the basic structure and function of the heart, the proteins and protein enzymes responsible for cardiac contraction, and similarities between skeletal muscle and cardiac tissue.

A discussion of muscle fiber structure included the comments that more mitochondria are found in cardiac fibers than in skeletal fibers and that aerobic training does not appear to increase the number and size of mitochondria in cardiac muscle cells. The T-tubules in cardiac tissue are larger than those in skeletal muscle but the sarcoplasmic reticulum is not as abundant in cardiac tissue.

The ultra structure of the myofibril and the A- and I-bands and their relationships to actin and myosin were presented. Muscle contraction theory, including the role of tropomyosin and troponin as regulatory proteins, was discussed.

In presenting the function of the heart, particular attention was given to the fact that the heart has three kinds of tissue: nodal tissue, Purkinje tissue, and ordinary muscle tissue. The origin and conduction of the heart beat are functions of the coordination of these three tissues.

A discussion of the anatomy of the heart included the four chambers (two atria and two ventricles), the three surfaces (sternocostal, diaphragmatic, and posterior), and the four borders (right, left, superior, and inferior). Circulation to the heart is provided by two major arteries — the right and left coronary arteries.

Metabolism of the heart was described as primarily aerobic, with the preferred substrate being fatty acids. The importance of a continuous O_2 delivery to cardiac muscle was emphasized.

Factors controlling the rate and force of cardiac contraction were shown to be primarily neural (cholinergic or adrenergic). Other factors influencing heart action are the pressoreceptors, chemoreceptors, body temperature, and the concentration of ions (potassium and calcium) in the blood.

A primary determinant of peripheral blood pressure is the volume of blood in the arteries. Increases in arterial blood volume tend to increase blood pressure. Factors affecting blood volume and thus blood pressure are cardiac output and peripheral resistance. Increases in heart rate and stroke volume increase cardiac output, which tends to increase arterial blood pressure. Increases in peripheral resistance tend to increase arterial blood volume and therefore to increase arterial blood pressure. Peripheral resistance is influenced by the viscosity of the blood and the diameter of the arterioles and capillaries. The blood viscosity is determined largely by the hematocrit, and the arteriole diameter is influenced by blood pressure, blood concentration of oxygen, carbon dioxide, pH, hormones, lactic acid, and histamine.

REFERENCES

1. Grollman, S: The Human Body, ed 4. Macmillan, New York, 1978, pp 85–262.
2. Moore, L: Clinically Oriented Anatomy, ed 2. Williams & Wilkins, Baltimore, 1985.
3. Sinclair, D: An Introduction to Functional Anatomy, ed 5. JB Lippincott, Philadelphia, 1975, pp 50–53.
4. Anthony, CP and Thibodeau, GA: Textbook of Anatomy and Physiology, ed 11. CV Mosby, St. Louis, 1983, pp 14–422.
5. Vick, RL: Contemporary Medical Physiology. Addison-Wesley, Menlo Park, CA, 1984, pp 160–195.
6. Amsterdam, EA and Mason, DT: Coronary Artery Disease: Pathology and Clinical Correlations. In Amsterdam, EA, et al (eds): Exercise in Cardiovascular Health and Disease. Yorke, New York, 1977, pp 13–18.
7. Devlin, TM (ed): Textbook of Biochemistry with Clinical Correlations. John Wiley & Sons, New York, 1982, p 1017.
8. Guyton, AC: Textbook of Medical Physiology, ed 7. WB Saunders, Philadelphia, 1986, pp 121–162.
9. Phillips, RE and Feeney, MK: The Cardiac Rhythms, ed 2. Philadelphia: W. B. Saunders Co., 1980, pp 21–68.
10. Dowhen, RM: In Mountcastle, VB (ed): Medical Physiology, ed 14. CV Mosby, St. Louis, 1980, p 83.
11. Orten, JM and Neuhaus, OW: Human Biochemistry, ed 10. CV Mosby, St. Louis, 1982, pp 27–59.
12. Bell, GH, Emslie-Smith, D and Paterson, CR: Textbook of Physiology and Biochemistry, ed 9. Longman Group, London, 1976, pp 10–329.
13. Keele, CA, et al: Samson Wrights' Applied Physiology, ed 13. Oxford University Press, New York, 1982, p 249.
14. Schottelius, BA and Schottelius, DD: Textbook of Physiology. CV Mosby, St. Louis, 1978, pp 87–1097.
15. Gordon, AM: Muscle. In Ruch, T and Patton, HD (eds): Physiology and Biophysics. WB Saunders, Philadelphia, 1982, p 182.

16. Mannberg, HG and Goody, RS: Proteins of Contractile Systems. Annual Review of Biochemistry 45:427, 1976.
17. Amsterdam, EA, Wilmore, JH and DeMaria, AN: Exercise in Cardiovascular Health and Disease. Yorke, New York, 1977, pp 70–94.
18. Edington, DW and Edgerton, VR: The Biology of Physical Activity. Houghton Mifflin, Boston, 1976, pp 23–26.
19. Jensen, D: The Principles of Physiology, ed 2. Appleton-Century-Crofts, New York, 1980, p 75.
20. Buchthal, F, Svensmark, O and Falck, PR: Mechanical and Chemical Events in Muscle Contraction. Physiological Reviews 36:503–538, 1956.
21. Harrington, WF: Contractile Proteins of Muscle. In Neurath, H, et al (eds): The Proteins, ed 3, vol 4. Academic Press, New York, 1979, pp 246–393.
22. White, A, et al: Principles of Biochemistry, ed 6. McGraw-Hill, New York, 1978, pp 1085–1103.
23. Taylor, EW: Mechanism of Actomyosin ATPase and the Problem of Muscle Contraction. Current Topics in Bioenergetics 5:201, 1973.
24. Taylor, EW: Chemistry of Muscle Contraction. Annual Review of Biochemistry 41:577, 1972.
25. Smith, JJ and Kampine, JP: Circulatory Physiology, ed 2. Williams & Wilkins, Baltimore, 1984, p 360.
26. Bigger, JT: A Primer on Calcium Ion Antagonists. Knoll Pharmaceutical, 1980.
27. Thomas, CL (ed): Taber's Cyclopedic Medical Dictionary, ed 15. FA Davis, Philadelphia, 1985.
28. West, JB (ed): Best and Taylor's Physiological Basis of Medical Practice, ed 11. Williams & Wilkins, Baltimore, 1985.
29. Tortora, GJ: Principles of Human Anatomy, ed 4. Harper & Row, New York, 1986.

CHAPTER 3

Physiologic Adaptations to Aerobic Exercise

Rehabilitation management of CAD is designed to reduce the physical and psychological impact of a disabling disease, as well as to increase the individual's functional capacity. However, to meet increased demands for energy placed upon the body during exercise, several physiologic adjustments must be made. Muscular contractions of the isometric type usually evoke the Valsalva maneuver, increase muscle pressure on the arteries, increase blood pressure, and do not benefit the cardiovascular system. For these reasons, activities involving sustained contractions and dynamic overhead arm work are not generally recommended as a major part of cardiac rehabilitation programs or for older adults.[1-5] This discussion of physiologic adaptations to exercise (acute and chronic) will thus be limited to changes that occur during dynamic, rhythmical, and continuous activities of an aerobic nature.[6-11]

ACUTE RESPONSES TO AEROBIC EXERCISE

The acute responses to exercise include those physiologic adjustments that normally occur in response to a single bout of exercise. The major adjustments that must be made include cardiac adaptations, coronary and systemic circulatory adjustments, blood pressure and blood volume changes, and metabolic adaptations.

Cardiac Adaptations

The rate of contraction of the heart begins to increase before exercise begins (anticipatory rise). As exercise commences and continues, the increase in heart rate is proportional to the intensity of the activity.[3,10,12] If the intensity of the activity is too great, the maximum heart rate will be achieved, exhaustion will ensue, and the exercise will be anaerobic. Aerobically, there is a linear relationship between heart rate and oxygen consumption (see section on metabolic adaptations).

The cardiac muscle responds to exercise not only by increasing its rate of contraction, but also by increasing its force of contraction. The increased force of contraction results in an increase in the stroke volume or the amount of blood ejected by the heart per beat. The normal ejection fraction is .6 to .75; this increases during exercise.[2,13]

As a result of the increased heart rate and stroke volume that accompanies exercise, the cardiac output increases. Cardiac output is equal to the volume of blood pumped by the heart per minute and is a product of the stroke volume and the heart rate. As presented in Chapter 2, the rate and force of cardiac contraction is regulated by the autonomic system, chemoreceptors, pressoreceptors, and body temperature.[10,14]

Two important observations concerning heart rate and cardiac output should be noted. The first is that the maximal heart rate an individual can attain decreases with increasing age, that is, an inverse relationship. The second is that both heart rate and stroke volume increase when an individual is exercising at 40 to 60 percent of his or her maximum capacity. However, at higher levels increased cardiac output is accomplished by an increase in heart rate only; stroke volume does not increase.[1,15] Keeping in mind that coronary circulation (circulation to the heart muscle itself) occurs primarily during diastole, it is important to remember that for people with limited ability to increase heart rate (coronary and/or older patients) exercise must be done at comparatively low heart rates.[2,15,16]

Coronary Circulation Adjustments

In response to exercise, the heart muscle must increase its work and therefore needs more oxygen so that its metabolism can produce the energy for it to continue to contract. At rest, the cardiac muscle extracts approximately 70 percent of the oxygen that is delivered to it via the coronary circulation. This leaves little reserve for increasing oxygen delivery to the cardiac muscle by this mechanism. The increased coronary demands of exercise are met by increasing the rate at which blood flows through the coronary arteries so that more oxygen will be delivered per unit of time. Increasing coronary flow is accomplished primarily by increased cardiac output, dilation of the coronary arteries, and increased aortic blood pressure, all of which force more blood into the coronary arteries. Any obstruction to coronary blood flow decreases the amount of oxygen delivered to the cardiac tissues and could precipitate an ischemic condition. The literature suggests that high exercising heart rates in coronary and older patients make it difficult for the myocardium to continue receiving adequate amounts of oxygen, therefore, the value of graded exercise testing with ECG-monitoring, a scientifically developed exercise prescription based upon the exercise test and careful monitoring during exercise sessions are factors that can help to avoid creating situations where there may be inadequate blood flow to the myocardium.[3,10,12]

Systemic Circulation Adjustments

During aerobic exercise, the muscles that are actively working need an increased oxygen supply to produce the energy needed for continuing muscular contraction. This increased need for oxygen is supplied to the working muscles not only by an increase in the cardiac output, but also by an increase in blood flow to the active muscles. Because a limited amount of blood must supply all the tissues of the body, the amount of blood flowing to any specific tissue depends upon the oxygen need of that tissue. Thus, during exercise, blood is directed away (shunted) from tissues that are less active (such as digestive organs) and shunted to muscles that are actively working and have increased metabolic activity. This shunting is accomplished by a series of chemical (increased CO_2 and lower pH) and reflex adjustments (sympathetic nervous system firing) that cause the dilation of arterioles in the working muscles and a constriction of vessels in inactive regions of the body.[2]

Because blood is shunted to areas of increased activity during exercise, there is also an increased blood flow to the lungs with increased activity. To meet the metabolic demands of the body, the rate and depth of ventilation and the diffusion of oxygen from the alveoli into the pulmonary capillaries increase with increasing activity.[6]

The increased blood flow to active muscles during exercise thus improves oxygen delivery to the active tissues. Additionally, there are increases in the oxygen consumption (metabolism) of the muscle cells and better oxygen extraction by those cells.[10]

To dissipate the heat that is produced during exercise, blood flow to the skin also increases. The hypothalamus is responsive to changes in the temperature of the blood. When blood temperature increases, the hypothalamus signals the blood vessels supplying the skin to dilate. More blood can then flow to the surface of the skin so that evaporation of sweat can occur. Evaporation of perspiration cools the skin, which, in turn, cools the blood. Exercising in an environment of high humidity impairs the cooling process owing to decreased ability to evaporate sweat. Cardiac patients should be warned of the dangers of exercising in an environment of high humidity, particularly when high humidity is combined with a high environmental temperature.

Blood Pressure Adjustments

In the active muscles during aerobic exercise, the blood vessels dilate. This dilation decreases the resistance to blood flow and tends to cause a decrease in blood pressure. However, the trend toward lower blood pressure during exercise is negated by an increase in cardiac output. The net effect is that the systolic blood pressure increases in normotensive individuals. The increase in systolic blood pressure is normally proportional to the intensity and oxygen demand of the activity. In normotensive individuals, there is little or no increase in diastolic blood pressure with increased aerobic work.[2]

Dramatic declines in systolic blood pressure can be seen when an individual has been exercising intensively and suddenly stops. The resultant pooling of blood in the lower extremities decreases venous return and cardiac output. It may cause fainting associated with poor perfusion to the brain. To avoid this result, especially with cardiac patients, all aerobic exercise sessions should include a "cool down" phase.[2,15]

Exercises involving the arms evoke a greater rise in blood pressure than exercises with the legs. Apparently this difference is at least partially due to the smaller muscles being utilized for the activity. Although there is dilation of the blood vessels in the arms, there is constriction of the vessels in the inactive, larger leg muscles, and blood pressure increases during arm exercises. For persons with cardiovascular disease and older individuals, aerobic activities involving the arms should be cautiously administered. Prolonged intense arm exercises are to be utilized with care, and patients should be cautioned about performing daily activities involving continued arm work such as shoveling, digging, raking, lifting, and carrying. However, since many leisure and vocational activities require arm activity, arm training may be included as part of a rehabilitation program. Rehabilitation programs should emphasize aerobic activities utilizing the larger leg muscles—walking, jogging, cycling.[1,2,5,10,12,17]

Blood and Fluid Adaptations

The body cools itself by evaporation of perspiration. Continued aerobic exercise can cause significant loss of body fluid. Consequently, the plasma volume (approximately 90 percent water) may decrease while the protein and cellular components remain relatively unchanged. This state is referred to as hemoconcentration because the solid particles of the blood constitute a relatively higher percentage of whole blood. Hemoconcentration results in "thicker" blood. It can increase the resistance to blood flow and increase blood pressure. Exercises performed in an environment of high temperature and high humidity can promote further dehydration and fluid loss and are to be avoided.[2]

Metabolic Adaptations

To meet the increased metabolic demands of exercise, the amount of oxygen delivered to the tissues increases as a result of increased cardiac output and increased blood flow to the working muscles.[12] (This assumes that the hemoglobin concentration of the blood is normal and provides adequate oxygen transport.) Upon delivery to the individual cells, oxygen must be utilized by those cells to provide energy for continued muscle contraction. Oxygen utilization (oxygen uptake) is determined not only by delivery, but also by the number of mitochondria in the cells, the amount of myoglobin, the enzymes of metabolism, the substrates available for metabolism, and probably many other factors. The maximal amount of oxygen (VO_2 max) that can be consumed by an individual is commonly considered to be the best and most accurate indication of cardiorespiratory fitness.[1,3,10,12] VO_2 max is usually expressed as milliliters of oxygen utilized per kilogram of body weight per minute. Direct measurements of VO_2 max can be made if the arterial-venous oxygen difference is found by sampling inspired and expired air. Because of the expense of the necessary measuring equipment, it is considered acceptable to predict VO_2 max. Predictions are based on heart rate responses to a standard exercise workload as both VO_2 max and heart rate increase in a linear manner in response to increases in exercise intensities.[2,10,18]

It has been suggested that the limiting factor in exercise performance is the ability of the tissues to utilize oxygen.[2,12,18] Compared with the resting state, the arterial-venous oxygen difference during exercise increases by as much as threefold.[1] This ability to utilize more oxygen during exercise by the active muscles keeps the heart from having to work too hard to supply the necessary circulation for continued muscular contractions. Increased oxygen extraction by the tissues during exercise is enhanced by chemical, temperature, and hormonal changes in the blood.[8]

CHRONIC RESPONSES TO AEROBIC EXERCISE

In recent years, considerable interest has developed concerning the long-term physiologic benefits an individual derives from engaging in a program of dynamic, rhythmic, and continuous activities over a period of time. Although there is considerable controversy on the subject, many researchers feel that coronary heart disease can be prevented and/or reversed with cessation of smoking, regular aerobic exercise (training), and elimination or reduction of the amount of fat, salt, caffeine, and the like from the diet.[12,14,19-22] There seem to be different opinions, because of lack of information, as to the constituents of a good training program. For clarity, the information presented in this text will be for the purpose of training the cardiovascular-impaired individual and will not deal with the training of athletes.

Cardiac Adaptations to Aerobic Training

The individual fibers of cardiac muscle may adapt to aerobic training by becoming larger (hypertrophy) and stronger.[23] Unlike skeletal muscle, cardiac tissue does not seem to respond to training by increasing the number of mitochondria or by increasing the oxidative capacity of the respiratory enzymes.[12]

The hypertrophy of cardiac muscle as a result of aerobic training is accompanied by a larger stroke volume. Thus, at any given workload, the heart does not have to beat as often to supply an adequate volume of blood, and the cardiac output at submaximal work levels may not change compared with pretraining conditions. At maximal workloads, the cardiac output increase is due to the increased stroke volume, whereas the maximal heart rate does not appear to change. Endurance training also causes an increase in recovery heart rates from all levels of work.[10,12]

As yet, there is no clear explanation for the bradycardia that results from aerobic training. Bradycardia is observed at rest and at all levels of work. Bradycardia may be partially due to the increased strength of the myocardial fibers, so that more blood is pumped per beat and the heart does not have to beat as often to supply the same amount of blood. Recent studies indicate an increased vagal tone in response to aerobic training.[1,2,10] This results in a shift away from the sympathetic nervous system's influence (the catecholamines) on the heart in favor of the parasympathetic system, which enhances the influence of the vagus nerve and results in bradycardia. In cardiac patients, the bradycardia that results from training is a major factor in raising the angina threshold — the level of work at which angina occurs.[1,2,10,15,21]

Coronary Circulation Responses

Because aerobic training does not seem to increase the oxygen extraction ability of the myocardium, the increased need of the myocardium for oxygen during exercise must be supplied by increases in coronary blood flow. Increases in coronary blood flow result from increases in heart rate, stroke volume, and vasodilation. However, relatively speaking, the bradycardia and increased stroke volume that accompany training result in a longer period of diastole between beats so that there is enhanced perfusion in the coronary arteries as a result of training. These physiological adaptations to aerobic training are major factors in the improvement of ischemic ECG changes in patients with coronary artery disease (CAD).[10]

Considerable controversy exists as to whether there is an increase in the diameter of the coronary arteries and/or increased collateral circulation as a result of aerobic training.[12,24] Such increases have been demonstrated to occur in animal experimentation and in some studies with humans, but as yet not consistently in humans.[10,20,25] Current methodologies to determine increased collateral circulation in humans may not be sensitive enough to detect improvements.[9,26,28,29]

Changes in Systemic Circulation

The capacity for blood flow to skeletal muscles is increased in response to aerobic training by an increase in the number of capillaries that supply the muscle fibers. There is also an increase in the number and size of the mitochondria and the enzyme systems in skeletal muscle that supply energy for contraction.[12] These changes in skeletal muscles account for a greater arterial-venous oxygen difference in response to training. However, during submaximal work, blood flow to the active muscles does not seem to be as important as metabolism in the observed arterial-venous oxygen difference. During maximal work, blood flow and metabolism are considerably increased in response to aerobic training. These physiologic adaptations to training allow for better delivery and utilization of oxygen at the tissue site so that, relatively speaking, the heart does not have to work so hard to deliver an adequate blood supply to the active muscles.[10]

Blood Pressure Changes

Although considerable controversy exists about the long-term effects of aerobic exercise on blood pressure, recent studies have reported a decrease in both systolic and diastolic resting and working blood pressures following periods of consistent training.[30-34] These changes have also been reported in individuals who are hypertensive and medicated.[31,32] In some cases the blood pressure decreases were so dramatic that the individuals were able to discontinue their medications. The physiologic mechanisms whereby these changes occur are yet to be determined. It may be that aerobic training directly causes improvements in the smooth muscles of the circulatory system, or the reported decreases in blood pressure may be a result of reduction of the risk factors that often accompany training, such as reduced body fat, cessation of smoking and the like.[18,32,34,35]

Blood and Fluid Responses

Endurance training causes an increase in the total blood volume of the body. This increase is due largely to an increase in the amount of the plasma portion of whole blood. As a result, aerobic training allows a person to adjust better to environments of high temperatures and high humidities by improving the sweating mechanism.[2,36]

Aerobic training increases the number of red blood cells slightly. Consequently, the amount of hemoglobin increases, although the hematocrit remains relatively unchanged. Whether training causes decreased aggregation of the platelets and thus lessens the chance of forming an intravascular thrombosis remains to be demonstrated, but increasing evidence indicates that exercise enhances fibrinolytic activity.[27,37-39]

Metabolic Adaptations

The increase in VO_2 max that results from aerobic training is due to increases in cardiac output and in the arterial-venous oxygen difference.[10] Measurements of VO_2 max are utilized extensively in the diagnosis of cardiovascular diseases and in the prescription of appropriate exercise programs for persons with cardiovascular disease. Tests for VO_2 max are discussed in chapter 7.

Training increases the number of mitochondria in the working muscles and enhances the utilization of oxygen. During submaximal exercise, the lactic acid concentration of the blood does not increase as it does in maximal work because of an adequate oxygen supply and utilization by the mitochondria (steady state). Exercise prescriptions for the cardiac patient should elicit work of a submaximal nature so that metabolic energy comes from aerobic metabolism (Krebs cycle) rather than from anaerobic sources (glycolysis).[10]

Body Composition Changes

It is well established that regular aerobic exercise can be an important factor in helping individuals lose and/or control body fat. Weight loss through exercise is accompanied by a decrease in the percentage of body fat and an increase in lean body mass. For best results, cardiac patients needing to lose body fat should combine an aerobic exercise program with restricted caloric intake.[14,33,40,41]

Changes in Blood Lipids

The lack of agreement in the literature about the effects of aerobic training on total blood cholesterol, triglycerides, and high density lipoprotein cholesterol (HDL) most likely is due to lack of control over the experimental variables.[12,22,42-44] Several sources have reported that regular exercise is effective in lowering total blood cholesterol and triglyceride levels and in increasing the HDL levels.[31,32,43,45] These results may be due to dietary modifications that reduce saturated fat intake rather than to exercise effects. Whether dietary modifications can alter cholesterol and other blood lipid levels is itself controversial, although several sources indicate a positive response.[3,43] Current thinking favors a combination of proper nutrition (with reduced fat intake) and proper exercise to reduce blood lipid concentration and to prevent or reverse the atherosclerotic process that leads to heart disease. Although more research is needed in this area, significant positive correlations have been reported that link HDL levels with number of aerobic miles run per week.[27,31,32,42,46-49]

Training and Stress

Evidence exists that correlates personality traits with incidents of ischemic heart disease. Individuals with Type A personalities have been found to have higher levels of blood catecholamines, higher heart rate, and higher blood pressure responses than those with Type B personalities when both types are subjected to the same stress situation. Individuals with Type A personalities have been reported to experience twice the ischemic heart disease than Type B individuals.[3,50-53] Recent research indicates that Type A personalities harboring anger and hostility may be the significant factors in predisposing an individual to CHD.[51]

Emotional states such as anxiety and depression have also been found to adversely affect the cardiovascular system.[54,55] It is theorized that these emotional stresses can cause platelet aggregation, evoke an ischemic state, or even precipitate an acute attack. Persons subjected to prolonged adverse emotional states may have a higher chance for developing ischemic heart disease than do nonstressed individuals.[4,52,53,56-58]

Although more research is needed in this area, aerobic exercise is valuable to some people in helping to relieve some personality and emotional tensions, perhaps as a result of a decreased catecholamine secretion.[20,25,40,59-61] Speculations about the "runners' high" include increased levels of endorphins in the blood in response to training. If for no other reason, the fact that aerobic activity undertaken on a regular basis gives individuals a sense of well-being may be sufficient justification in itself to recommend training for persons in stressful situations or those with personalities of the A type.[55,59-61]

Training and Ischemic Heart Disease

Ischemia occurs when the myocardial demand for oxygen exceeds the supply and the muscle cells must rely on anaerobic metabolism (glycolysis) for its energy. Ischemia usually is thought to result from atherosclerosis of the coronary arteries, although recent evidence suggests that coronary artery spasm may be responsible for ischemia in some individuals.[62]

Angina occurs when an individual reaches his or her ischemic threshold—a phenomenon dependent on systolic blood pressure and heart rate.[12] Anything that causes an increase in either systolic blood pressure or heart rate can precipitate an attack of angina. Physical activity increases both these parameters and can also cause an anginal attack. Regular aerobic activity, however, has been found to cause physiologic changes that lower the heart rate and blood pressure for any given submaximal workload and thus raise the ischemic threshold.[2,15,21,31]

Other beneficial effects of regular exercise include a decreased catecholamine production, increased coronary perfusion, increased functional work capacity, decreased peripheral resistance, possible increased collateral circulation, increased fibrinolysis, and decreased ST-T wave changes. Some cases have been reported in which there is an apparent reversal of the symptoms of ischemic heart disease in individuals who exercise on a regular basis and restrict their dietary fat consumption. More research is needed in this area, as it is a relatively new concept to consider aerobic training seriously as a viable adjunct to traditional medical therapy in the treatment of ischemic heart disease.[3,10,12,17,31,32,38,55,63,64]

SUMMARY

This chapter has presented the major physiologic adaptations made by the body in response to acute and chronic bouts of aerobic exercise. During an acute bout of activity, the heart rate rises in proportion to the intensity of the workload. Cardiac output, dilation of coronary arteries, and blood pressure all increase to allow for increased coronary blood flow. Because coronary circulation occurs during diastole of the cardiac cycle, coronary and/or older patients should be exercised at relatively low heart rates to allow for adequate coronary perfusion.

Blood flow during exercise is directed (shunted) away from less active tissues to the more active muscle tissues in which there is also dilation of the blood vessels. Increased rate and depth of ventilation and increased cellular metabolism also occur. The hypothalamus responds to increased heat production by stimulating the sweat glands to increase their output so that evaporation of sweat can promote the cooling process.

Exercise involving the arms and isometric activities should be used with caution in cardiac patients owing to the dramatic increases in systolic blood pressure that may result. Rehabilitation programs should emphasize aerobic activities that utilize the larger leg muscles (walking, jogging, and cycling).

In response to chronic bouts of aerobic exercise, cardiac muscle fibers hypertrophy and become stronger. This results in a greater stroke volume and an increase in recovery heart rate. The bradycardia that also results from training seems to be a major factor in raising the angina threshold. It remains to be clearly demonstrated whether or not increased collateral circulation occurs.

Skeletal muscle capillarization and the number and size of skeletal muscle mitochondria all increase in response to aerobic training. As a result, there is better O_2 delivery and utilization with less lactic acid concentration in the working muscles, and the workload on the heart is reduced. Beneficial effects of aerobic training on both systolic and diastolic blood pressures and better adjustments to high temperatures have been reported.

Aerobic exercise has been found to be very effective in helping individuals control body weight and in increasing the HDL cholesterol levels of the blood. It has also been proven beneficial to persons who are subjected to stress and similar tensions. Chronic aerobic activity has been found to raise the ischemic threshold, decrease catecholamine production, increase coronary perfusion, increase work capacity, decrease peripheral resistance and decrease ST-T wave ECG changes. It has also been reported that regular aerobic activity can prevent or reverse the symptoms of CHD when combined with dietary and other risk factor modifications and life-style changes.

REFERENCES

1. Astrand, P and Rodahl, K: Textbook of Work Physiology, ed 3. McGraw-Hill, New York, 1986, pp 178–473.
2. deVries, HA: Physiology of Exercise, ed 4. WC Brown, Dubuque, IA, 1986, pp 113–514.
3. Smith, JJ and Kampine, JP: Circulatory Physiology, ed 2. Williams & Wilkins, Baltimore, 1984, pp 219–278.
4. Strasser, AL: Heart Ailments and Workplace Stress Mistakenly Called Occupational Diseases. Occupational Health and Safety 54 (9):59, 1985.
5. Zamfirescu, NR, et al: Modifications Cardiovasculaires Determinees Par L' Effort Isometrique (Handgrip) Chez Les Malades Avec Hypertension Arterielle. Physiologie 22 (3):197–202, 1985.
6. Berman, LB and Sutton, JR: Exercise for the Pulmonary Patient. J Cardiopulmonary Rehabilitation 6:52–61, 1986.
7. Dehn, MM: Rehabilitation of the Cardiac Patient: The Effects of Exercise. American Journal of Nursing 80:435, 1980.
8. Dehn, MM and Mitchell, JH: Exercise. In The American Heart Association Heartbook. EP Dutton, New York, 1980.
9. Ferguson, RJ, et al: Coronary Blood Flow During Isometric and Dynamic Exercise in Angina Pectoris Patients. J Cardiac Rehabilitation 1:21, 1981.
10. Hammond, HK: Exercise for Coronary Heart Disease Patients: Is It Worth the Effort? J Cardiopulmonary Rehabilitation 5:531–539, 1985.
11. Taylor, JL, et al: The Effect of Isometric Exercise on the Graded Exercise Test in Patients with Stable Angina Pectoris. J Cardiac Rehabilitation 1:450, 1981.
12. Fletcher, GF and Cantwell, JD: Exercise and Coronary Heart Disease, ed 2. Charles C Thomas, 1979, pp 11–60.
13. Schlant, RC and Sonnenblick, EH: Normal Physiology of the Cardiovascular System. In Hurst, JW (ed): The Heart, ed 6. McGraw-Hill, New York, 1986.
14. McGandy, RB and Remmell, PS: The Dietary Management of Coronary Heart Disease. In Brest, AN (ed): Coronary Heart Disease. FA Davis, Philadelphia, 1969.
15. Franklin, BA, et al: Exercise Prescription for the Myocardial Infarction Patient. J Cardiopulmonary Rehabilitation 6:62–79, 1986.
16. Getchell, LH: Exercise Prescription for the Healthy Adult. J Cardiopulmonary Rehabilitation 6:46–51, 1986.
17. Hammond, HK: Regression of Atherosclerosis: A Review. J Cardiac Rehabilitation 3:347, 1983.
18. Auchincloss, JH, et al: Cardiac Output Reserve at Exercise. J Cardiopulmonary Rehabilitation 5:468–473, 1985.
19. Doyle, JT: The Prevention of Coronary Heart Disease. In Brest, AN (ed): Coronary Heart Disease. FA Davis, Philadelphia, 1969.
20. Ferguson, RJ, et al: Effects of Physical Training on Treadmill Exercise Capacity, Collateral Circulation and Progression of Coronary Disease. American J Cardiology 34:764, 1974.
21. Kattus, AA and McAlpin, RN: Role of Exercise in Discovery, Evaluation and Management of Ischemic Heart Disease. In Brest, AN (ed): Coronary Heart Disease. FA Davis, Philadelphia, 1969.
22. Miettinen, TA, et al: Multifactorial Primary Prevention of Cardiovascular Disease in Middle-Aged Men. JAMA 254:2097–102, 1985.
23. Hagan, RD, et al: The Problems of Per-Surface Area and Per-Weight Standardization Indices in the Determination of Cardiac Hypertrophy in Endurance-Trained Athletes. J Cardiopulmonary Rehabilitation 5:554–560, 1985.
24. Nitzberg, WD, et al: Collateral Flow in Patients with Acute Myocardial Infarction. American J Cardiology 56 (12):729–736, 1985.
25. Conner, JF, et al: Effects of Exercise on Coronary Collateralization: Angiographic Studies of Six Patients in a Supervised Exercise Program. Medicine and Science in Sports 8:145, 1976.
26. Andersen, KL, et al: Habitual Physical Activity and Health. World Health Organization, Copenhagen, 1978, p 186.
27. Froelicher, VF: Exercise Testing and Training. Le Jacq, New York, 1983, p 180.
28. Schaper, W and Pasyk, S: Influence of Collateral Flow on the Ischemic Tolerance of the Heart Following Acute and Subacute Coronary Occlusion. Circulation 53 (Suppl 1):57, 1976.
29. Scheel, KW: The Stimulus for Coronary Collateral Growth: Ischemia or Mechanical Factors? J Cardiac Rehabilitation 1:149, 1981.
30. Aaron, DJ: The Effects of a 12-Week Exercise Program on the Functional Capacities, Cardiovascular

Responses and Body Weights of Individuals Medicated With Beta-Blockers. Unpublished Thesis, Slippery Rock University, Slippery Rock, PA, 1985.

31. Barnard, JR, et al: Effects of an Intensive, Short-Term Exercise and Nutrition Program on Patients with Coronary Heart Disease. J Cardiac Rehabilitation 1:99, 1981.
32. Hall, JA and Barnard, RJ: The Effects of an Intensive 26-Day Program of Diet and Exercise on Patients with Peripheral Vascular Disease. J Cardiac Rehabilitation 2:569, 1982.
33. Hoglund, JL: The Effects of a 12-Week Cardiovascular Exercise Program on the Resting Blood Pressure, Body Weight and Resting Heart Rate Levels of Hypertensive Individuals. Unpublished Thesis, Slippery Rock University, Slippery Rock, PA, 1984.
34. McHenry, D: The Effects of a Twelve-Week Cardiac Rehabilitation Program on Body Composition, Heart Rate and Blood Pressure. Unpublished Thesis, Slippery Rock University, Slippery Rock, PA, 1981.
35. Brannon, FJ and Geyer, MJ: Fitness After Fifty-Five. Unpublished Study, Bio Energetiks Rehabilitation, Prospect, PA, 1980.
36. Lamb, DR: Physiology of Exercise, ed 2. Macmillan, New York, 1984, p 160.
37. Froelicher, VF and Brown, P: Exercise and Coronary Heart Disease. J Cardiac Rehabilitation 1:277, 1981.
38. Taylor, HL: Results of Physical Conditioning in Healthy Middle-Aged Subjects. In Cohen, LS, et al (eds): Physical Conditioning and Cardiovascular Rehabilitation. John Wiley & Sons, New York, 1981.
39. Williams, RS, Scott, E and Andersen, J: Reduced Epinephrine Induced Platelet Aggregation Following Cardiac Rehabilitation. J Cardiac Rehabilitation 1:127, 1981.
40. Bubb, WJ, et al, Predicting Oxygen Uptake During Level Walking at Speeds of 80–130 m/min. J Cardiopulmonary Rehabilitation 5:462–65, 1985.
41. Lampman, RM, et al: Exercise as a Partial Therapy for the Extremely Obese. Medicine and Science in Sports Exercise 18:19–24, Feb. 1986.
42. Arnold, JD, et al: Lipid Profile, Physical Fitness, and Job Activity of Canadian Postal Workers. J Cardiopulmonary Rehabilitation 5:373–7, 1985.
43. Boyd, GS and Craig, IF: Biochemistry of Degenerative Vascular Disease. In Williams, DL and Marks, V (eds): Biochemistry in Clinical Practice. Elsevier, New York, 1985.
44. McManus, BM: Defining Coronary Risks in a Reference Range for Total Cholesterol and Lipoprotein Values: A Problem Yet to be Solved. American J Cardiology, Dec. 31, 1985.
45. MacKeen, PC, et al: A 13-Year Follow-Up of a Coronary Heart Disease Risk Factor Screening and Exercise Program for 40- to 59-Year-Old Men: Exercise Habit Maintenance and Physiologic Status. J Cardiopulmonary Rehabilitation 5:510–523, 1985.
46. Allison, TG, et al: Failure of Exercise to Increase High Density Lipoprotein Cholesterol. J Cardiac Rehabilitation 1:257, 1981.
47. Hagan, RD and Gettman, LR: Maximal Aerobic Power, Body Fat, and Serum Lipoproteins in Male Distance Runners. J Cardiac Rehabilitation 3:331, 1983.
48. Haskell, WL: Influence of Habitual Physical Activity on Blood Lipids and Lipoproteins. In Cohen, LS, et al (eds): Physical Conditioning and Cardiovascular Rehabilitation. John Wiley & Sons, New York, 1981.
49. Rotkis, TC, et al: Relationship Between High Density Lipoprotein Cholesterol and Weekly Running Mileage. J Cardiac Rehabilitation 2:109, 1982.
50. Byrne, DG, et al: Consistency and Variation Among Instruments Purporting to Measure the Type A Behavior Pattern. Psychosomatic Medicine 47:242–261, 1985.
51. Dembroski, TM, et al: Components of Type A, Hostility and Anger. In: Relationship to Angiographic Findings. Psychosomatic Medicine 47:219–33, 1985.
52. Velasco, JA, et al: Rehabilitation After Myocardial Infarction: Prognostic Features and Psychosocial Considerations. J Cardiopulmonary Rehabilitation 5:427–8, 1985.
53. Williams, RB and Gentry, WD: Psychological Problems in the Cardiopathic State. In Long, C (ed): Prevention and Rehabilitation in Ischemic Heart Disease. Williams & Wilkins, Baltimore, 1980.
54. Adler, HM and Hammett, VBO: The Psychosomatics of Coronary Heart Disease. In Brest, AN (ed): Coronary Heart Disease. FA Davis, Philadelphia, 1969.
55. Shephard, RJ, et al: Mood State During Postcoronary Cardiac Rehabilitation. J Cardiopulmonary Rehabilitation 5:480–4, 1985.
56. Blocher, WP: Coronary Risk Factors. In Blocher, WP and Cardus, D (eds): Rehabilitation in Ischemic Heart Disease. SP Medical and Scientific, New York, 1983.
57. Leon, GR: Behavior Modification in Reducing Risk Factors for Ischemic Heart Disease. In Long, C (ed): Prevention and Rehabilitation in Ischemic Heart Disease. Williams & Wilkins, Baltimore, 1980.
58. Willerson, JT, Hillis, LD and Buja, LM: Ischemic Heart Disease. Raven Press, New York, 1982.
59. Dracup, K: A Controlled Trial of Couples Group Counseling in Cardiac Rehabilitation. J Cardiopulmonary Rehabilitation 5:436–42, 1985.
60. Goldwater, BC and Collis, ML: Psychologic Effects of Cardiovascular Conditioning. Psychosomatic Medicine 47:174–81, 1985.

61. Roth, DL and Holmes, DS: Influence of Physical Fitness in Determining the Impact of Stressful Life Events on Physical and Psychological Health. Psychosomatic Medicine 47:164–73, 1985.
62. Tortora, GJ: Principles of Human Anatomy, ed 4. Harper & Row, New York, 1986, p 317.
63. Dressendoifer, RH, Amsterdam, EA and Mason, DT: Therapeutic Effects of Exercise Training in Angina Patients. In Cohen, LS, et al (eds): Physical Conditioning and Cardiovascular Rehabilitation. John Wiley & Sons, New York, 1981.
64. Levenkron, JC, et al: Chronic Chest Pain with Normal Coronary Arteries: A Behavioral Approach to Rehabilitation. J Cardiopulmonary Rehabilitation 5:475–9, 1985.
65. Neill, WA: Coronary and Systemic Circulatory Adaptations to Exercise Training and Their Effects on Angina Pectoris. In Amsterdam, EA, et al (eds): Exercise in Cardiovascular Health and Disease. Yorke, New York, 1977.
66. Rulli, V: Normal Cardiovascular/Pulmonary Responses to Exercise. In Amsterdam, EA and James, WE (eds): Coronary Heart Disease, Exercise Testing and Cardiac Rehabilitation. Symposia Specialists, Miami, 1977.

CHAPTER 4

Pathophysiology of Coronary Artery Disease

The American Heart Association estimated that in 1984, 550,000 individuals died in the United States from myocardial infarctions and approximately 4.6 million others (or 20 of every 1000 individuals) experienced some morbidity associated with coronary artery disease (CAD). Although the overall incidence of mortality as a result of coronary artery disease has declined since 1968, it remains the number one cause of sudden death in adults.[1,2]

Coronary artery disease is an atherosclerotic process that manifests itself in one or more of four clinical syndromes — angina pectoris, myocardial infarction, heart failure, or sudden death. Beginning as early as the second decade of life, atherosclerosis may affect any arterial system in the body, with the most common sites being the aorta, coronary arteries, and cerebral, femoral, and other large- to middle-sized arteries.[3,4] This disease is characterized by a thickening in the intimal layer of the blood vessel wall owing to the localized accumulation of lipids.

The actual pathogenesis of atherosclerosis remains unknown at this time. Establishing cause and effect has been difficult because the disease begins and progresses insidiously, existing from months to years prior to the onset of symptoms.[4] Past and current research have closely tied the development of atherosclerotic plaque to a group of coronary risk factors. Risk factors (as discussed in chapter 10) are certain characteristics that through systematic observation and clinical study have been shown to have a significant relationship between their presence and the subsequent development of CAD.[6] The major risk factors are high blood pressure, hyperlipidemia, and cigarette smoking. Risk factors are also classified as either modifiable (smoking, blood lipid levels, obesity, inactivity, stress) or nonmodifiable (age, sex, family history of CAD, previous medical history). The presence of more than one risk factor has a synergistic effect on the other risk factors in predicting an individual's risk of CAD.[6]

This chapter reviews the pathophysiology of CAD, beginning with the normal arterial wall structure, and describes the changes that occur with atherosclerosis. The hypothesized pathogenesis of atherosclerosis is briefly reviewed, with the majority of the chapter devoted to the clinical manifestations of coronary artery disease.

THE ARTERIAL WALL

The normal arterial wall is a smooth muscular wall made up of three distinct layers of tissue: the intima, media, and adventitia. The wall and the individual layers vary in thickness depending on the caliber of the vessel (the larger the inner diameter, the thicker the arterial wall). The layers become progressively less distinct as the vessels reach the level of the arteriole (Figure 4–1).[8,9]

The intima is a single layer of endothelial cells lining the vascular lumen. It is impermeable to proteins circulating in the blood and is separated from the second layer, the media, by a continuous boundary of elastic fiber known as the internal elastic lamina. The media constitutes the bulk of the arterial wall and is composed almost entirely of smooth muscle cells, interspersed with collagen, elastin fibers, and proteoglycans. The media makes the dilation and contraction of the vessel wall possible. The outer layer, the adventitia, is separated from the media by a noncontinuous elastin fiber boundary called the external elastic lamina. The adventitia consists primarily of fibrous tissue that gives the arterial wall strength and at the same time provides for some distensibility to prevent rupture in the presence of hypertension.[7]

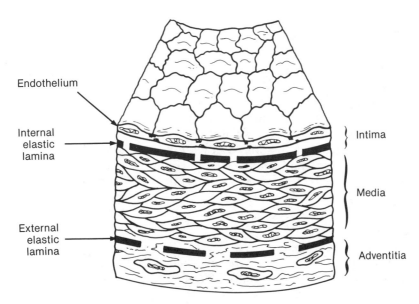

FIGURE 4–1. Structure of normal muscular artery. (From Ross, R and Glomset, JA. N Engl J Med 295:370, 1976, with permission.)

ATHEROSCLEROTIC LESIONS

Atherosclerosis is a progressive disease with the lesions (or plaque) going through what is hypothesized to be a series of changes that alter both arterial structure and functional capacity.[12,13] The intimal layer of the vessel wall is primarily affected by the atherosclerotic degeneration. The media undergoes some secondary changes as the atheromatous plaque extends into it, weakens the wall, and possibly causes localized dilatation or aneurysm formation.[3] These lesions are classified into three morphologic types: fatty streak, fibrous plaque, and complicated plaque or lesion.

Fatty Streak

The atherosclerotic process begins as a recognizable fatty streak in the intima of the blood vessel. The lesion does not impinge on the lumen of the artery. There are no symptoms at this time. Fatty streaks have been found throughout the arterial tree in individuals from infancy through late adulthood. They most commonly involve the aorta, coronary and cerebral arteries, and the arteries of the lower extremities.[3] Microscopically, these intimal lesions consist of smooth muscle cells with varying proportions of lipid material and fat droplets. These are commonly referred to as "foam cells" because of their tendency to "balloon out."

The lipids are composed mainly of cholesterol, cholesterol ester, phospholipid, and neutral fat. Because of the predominantly fatty content, they are often soft and yellow in appearance.[14] It remains controversial as to whether this lesion progresses to a raised fibrous lesion or is reversible.[8]

Raised Fibrous Plaque

The raised fibrous plaque is the characteristic lesion of atherosclerosis. This lesion is a yellowish-gray elevated lump that thickens and begins to impinge on the lumen of the vessel. As the plaque develops muscle cells from the intima and media proliferate, and lipids are deposited from the plasma into the lesions. A matrix of collagen, elastin, and connective tissue cells surrounds the plaque and gives it a fibrous cap.[3,9] The central core of the plaque remains mainly a lipid material with various plasma components including white blood cells, albumin, fibrin, fibrinogen, and cellular debris. Although most pathologists believe this plaque is irreversible, some feel that its progression may be slowed.[3,12]

Complicated Plaques

The complicated plaque is a fibrous plaque that has undergone one or more of the following pathological changes: calcification, necrosis, internal hemorrhage, rupture of the plaque, or thrombus formation over the plaque. The lumen of the vessel is impinged upon by these plaques, and the individual may often demonstrate symptoms of decreased or inadequate blood flow in the organ fed by the affected arteries. These structural changes in the intima may progress to affect the medial layer of the wall. Degeneration of a medial muscular layer further affects the arteries' ability to distend and meet the oxygen demand of the cells.[10] The weakened arterial wall may permit localized arterial dilation or ballooning out, that is, an aneurysm, which may rupture and cause hemorrhage. Other complications arise if the plaque has broken through the intima and comes in contact with the flowing blood. The rough surface of the complicated plaque provides a site for platelet aggregation, fibrin deposition, and clot formation. The clot further impinges the vessel's lumen and may either completely occlude the artery or embolize to occlude a more distal, smaller vessel and cause ischemia. If ischemia is prolonged, infarction may occur.[15]

All three types of lesions may be present at the same time, at various sites in the arterial tree. Unaffected segments may be interspersed with diseased segments.[16] Postmortem studies indicate that when the coronary arteries are affected, the majority of lesions occur at proximal points in the three major coronary arteries at the points of bifurcation of the arteries.[18] Symptoms in coronary patients usually correlate with lesions that result in more than 70 percent occlusion of the coronary arterial lumen.[11]

PATHOGENESIS OF ATHEROSCLEROSIS

Although the pathogenesis of atherosclerosis is unknown, there are six accepted hypotheses: response to injury, monoclonal, clonal-senescence, lipid-insudation, thrombogenic, and hemodynamic. Some factors of these hypotheses are interchangeable and have been combined with one another through years of speculation and research. Two hypotheses currently predominate — the response to injury and monoclonal hypotheses. These hypotheses are briefly discussed here; the reader is referred to other sources for further explanation of these and the remaining four hypotheses.[4,5,12,13,17]

Response to Injury Hypothesis

This theory suggests that plaque formation begins in response to some type of trauma to the endothelial lining of the vessel wall. The damage may result from any one of a number of mechanical, chemical, hormonal, or immunologic stressors. The turbulence of arterial blood flow in an individual with hypertension, the hydrocarbons from cigarette smoke, and circulating plasma cholesterol have all been hypothesized as causative agents.[14,17] The damaged endothelium then becomes permeable to substances in the blood and provides a site for platelet aggregation. As the platelets aggregate, they release substances that may interact with plasma constituents and cause a proliferation of smooth muscle cells into the intima, forming new connective tissue. Also, in response to the injury, the endothelial cells proliferate to repair the damage. Ross and Glosmet[12,13] proposed that, in limited injury, the regeneration of the endothelial layer may limit the smooth muscle proliferation. However, in repeated injury, this relationship may be thrown out of balance, and continual proliferation of smooth muscle and connective tissue cells and additional lipid deposition into the intima may result. The final result is the "growth" of fibrous plaques within the intimal layer of the arterial wall.[4,12]

Monoclonal Hypothesis

The second hypothesis suggests that each lesion is a result of the proliferation of one smooth muscle cell that has acquired a selective advantage. Benditt[14] suggests that this is a result of some mutagenic agent such as cigarette smoke or a virus. Microscopically, however, neither fibrous plaques nor fatty streaks are of one type of cell origin, which raises serious questions as to the validity of this theory.[4,14]

ATHEROSCLEROSIS AND CORONARY ARTERY DISEASE

Atherosclerosis is a disease that affects people in the middle-to-older age brackets. Although it has been stated that the initial lesions can be isolated in infants, the onset of symptoms is usually in the fourth to fifth decade of life for men and approximately 10 years later in women.[15] Although atherosclerotic changes and plaque formation can occur in any artery, this text is specifically concerned about its effect on the coronary arteries and the clinical manifestations of atherosclerosis in coronary artery disease (CAD).

As CAD progresses, the atherosclerotic lesions develop in the intima of the coronary arteries. As these lesions grow, they thicken and harden the walls of the artery, reduce arterial wall elasticity, and impinge upon the lumen of the vessel. These structural changes in the wall result in a decrease in coronary artery blood flow and a decrease in oxygen distribution to the myocardium.

With the coronary circulation compromised and the arteries inelastic, the normal adaptive mechanism (local dilation of the coronary arteries) to increase blood flow through the coronary arteries in response to increasing oxygen requirements is diminished. As the lesions progressively occlude the vessels' lumen and without adequate collateral circulation to provide blood flow to the area by another vessel, the demands of the heart cannot be met. This causes an ischemic episode (an inadequate supply of oxygenated blood to the muscle) to occur.

Initially individuals with CAD may be asymptomatic but, as the atherosclerotic lesions progress, the individual becomes symptomatic. Although symptomatology and the progress of the atherosclerotic disease process vary tremendously from one individual to the next, the functional inability of the artery to supply oxygenated blood remains the same. The resulting imbalance in myocardial oxygen demand versus supply is known as *ischemia*.

Ischemia and Infarction

Ischemia occurs when blood flow to the cell is insufficient to meet cellular needs. Ischemia may be the result of some obstruction to blood flow, an increased metabolic demand that the heart is unable to meet, inadequate hemoglobin content in the blood, or pulmonary disease. The duration and severity of ischemic imbalance determine the pathological injury to the involved tissue. Transient ischemia is completely reversible. The ischemic tissues do not sustain any permanent damage.[8] When ischemia is prolonged, the tissues undergo a series of changes, including a shift from aerobic to anaerobic metabolism. It may ultimately result in irreversible injury or infarction.[9]

Manifestations of ischemia and infarction include pain, elevated serum enzymes (enzymes that are released by the damaged cells into the circulation), and symptoms related to the function of the affected organ or tissues (decreased renal function with renal ischemia; intermittent claudication or muscle cramps with peripheral ischemia). Chronic ischemia may produce a dull pain, whereas acute occlusion causes an intense pain often followed by numbness or absence of sensation. The mechanism of ischemic pain is not fully understood. It may be a result of one of two phenomena. The peripheral nerve endings may be stretched and stimulated by swelling of the cell caused by the ischemia, or the nerve endings may be stimulated by the localized release of kinins and other chemical mediators that result in the pain sensation.[9]

The transition from ischemia to infarction is not inevitable. Several factors determine whether or not infarction will result. Those factors include the rate of onset of the ischemia, the ability of the ischemic tissue to compensate for decreased blood flow, the oxygen requirements of the particular tissue, and the availability of oxygen in the blood.[22] Ischemia that has developed gradually is usually better tolerated because collateral circulation (communicating channels that serve as an alternate pathway to blood flow) may develop and supply the otherwise ischemic areas. Tissues also compensate for decreased oxygen supply by increasing their oxygen extraction from whatever blood flow is available. The heart is unable to compensate in this manner because at rest the heart muscle extracts 65 to 70 percent of the available oxygen, leaving little for reserve in response to decreased blood flow or increased oxygen demand.[9] The overall oxygen requirement of the affected tissue also determines its vulnerability to infarction. Some tissues, like the brain, are very sensitive to decreased oxygen supply. Skeletal muscle, however, has a longer survival time in the presence of decreased oxygen. Finally, the quality of the individual's blood influences the ischemia-to-infarction progression. Anemia, decreased oxygen-carrying capacity, and decreased oxygen diffusion into the blood all reduce potential oxygen availability to the tissue and increase vulnerability to infarction.[22]

Infarction, or cellular death, is identified as a central core of necrotic cells that are electrically and functionally silent. Surrounding this core are cells with gradations of function dependent on the severity of the ischemia to the surrounding area.[20]

Treatment is aimed at reversing the ischemia and preventing further infarction by promoting oxygen supply to the affected area. This is achieved by removing any physical impedance to blood flow and removing any stimulus that may increase metabolic demands to the tissue. Oxygen and pharmacologic agents may be used, as appropriate, to relieve ischemia. If the individual is anemic, transfusion of red blood cells may be necessary to provide sufficient hemoglobin to transport oxygen adequately.

Despite all interventions, cell necrosis may still result. When cells die, they release enzymes that promote cellular destruction and the inflammatory response. Cellular debris is removed via phagocytosis, and the tissues undergo a series of changes ending in the formation of fibrous scar tissue.

Myocardial Ischemia and Infarction

Ischemia occurs when the oxygen demand of a tissue exceeds the oxygen supply. Myocardial ischemia results when an inadequate amount of oxygen is supplied to the heart.

The myocardial oxygen demand (MVO_2) is determined by the heart rate, the myocardial contractility, and the ventricular wall tension.[4,21] The heart rate is the frequency at which the heart pumps. The faster the heart rate, the greater the demand for oxygen. The myocardial contractility is the actual mechanical work of the heart. The workload is determined by the oxygen demands of the tissues. The heavier the workload, the harder the pump has to work and the greater its own demand for oxygen. Ventricular wall tension is directly influenced by preload (the ventricular volume or filling pressure) and afterload (the resistance, primarily the systemic blood pressure, against which the ventricle must pump to expel the blood). As the workload increases, the ventricular wall tension also increases, resulting in an increased myocardial oxygen demand.

The supply of oxygen to the myocardium depends on many factors, including the integrity of the pulmonary system, the hemoglobin content of the blood, the health of the coronary arteries, the heart rate, the blood pressure, and the resistance of the coronary arteries.[4,5,21,25]

An intact pulmonary system ensures that oxygen will diffuse from the lungs into the blood, where it is bound to the hemoglobin and carried to the tissues. If the hemoglobin level is low (anemia), the oxygen-carrying capacity is reduced.

The health of the coronary arteries refers to their ability to dilate in response to demand. In exercise they may need to carry 4 to 5 times their normal capacity. Coronary atherosclerosis not only impairs vessels' ability to dilate, but also affects redistribution of blood and oxygen within the heart.

Since myocardium is perfused during diastole, the heart rate is a factor in myocardial oxygen supply and demand. The faster the heart rate, the shorter the period of time for perfusion during diastole (see Chapter 2) and the greater the myocardial demand.

Hypotension (low blood pressure) inhibits adequate coronary artery perfusion. Hypertension (high blood pressure) affects the ventricular wall tension by increasing the afterload against which the heart must pump (increasing oxygen demand).

Resistance within the coronary circulation depends on the ventricular wall pressure. During systole, the ventricular wall pressure collapses the coronary arterial walls and occludes the blood flow to the myocardium (see Chapter 2). The greatest external wall pressure is on the subendocardial vessels, making the subendocardium particularly vulnerable to ischemia.[5,20,21]

The six factors previously discussed emphasize the interrelatedness of myocardial oxygen demand and supply. The heart's initial response to increased demand (increased heart rate) increases the oxygen supply as well as further increasing the oxygen demand. If the demand continues to exceed the supply, a vicious cycle is established.

When the oxygen demand is increased sixfold to eightfold, the healthy heart responds by increasing the coronary artery flow 4 to 5 times its normal level and by increasing its oxygen extraction to make up for the relative deficiency.[5] In a heart with CAD, the diseased vessels are not able to dilate to provide an increased blood flow and, therefore, the muscle supplied by the stenotic artery becomes ischemic.

CORONARY ARTERY DISEASE: CLINICAL MANIFESTATIONS

Coronary artery disease is manifested in any of four clinical syndromes: angina, myocardial infarction, sudden cardiac death, and congestive heart failure.[7] These manifestations are the results to varying degrees of the ischemia-infarction process on the myocardial muscle, which is extremely sensitive to decreased oxygen supply, particularly in the presence of coronary atherosclerosis.

Angina Pectoris

Angina pectoris (literally "strangling of the chest") is a reversible ischemic process caused by a temporary inability of the coronary arteries to supply sufficient oxygenated blood to the heart muscle. There are three basic categories of angina: stable angina, unstable angina, and variant or Prinzmetal's angina. All are a result of ischemia to the myocardium and occur secondarily to the arterial changes brought on by CAD.[6,28,29] All three are characterized by the sudden onset of anterior chest pain that is relatively diffuse. It is usually described as a "squeezing" or pressure sensation. It can also manifest itself as burning in the throat or jaw, discomfort between the shoulder blades, shortness of breath, or many other equivalent symptoms. The three types of angina differ in their duration, intensity, pattern of occurrence, and precipitating factors.

STABLE ANGINA

Stable angina is known as effort angina in that it is most often precipitated by exercise or stress. Individuals who experience stable angina quickly become aware of the specific activities that bring on the pain. Some of the most common precipitating events include exercise (particularly after a large meal), emotional stress, cigarette smoking, and exposure to cold temperatures.[23,28] The angina "attack" is characterized by substernal chest pain or pressure that may or may not radiate. The duration of pain is 5 to 10 minutes. Cessation of the activity is often sufficient to relieve the pain; otherwise, rest and sublingual nitrates completely relieve the angina.[7] In stable angina, the episodes of pain are very similar in cause, character, and method of relief.[23,27] Angina brought on by emotional stress may be more difficult to relieve because the stressor itself is more difficult to eliminate.[28]

UNSTABLE ANGINA

Unstable angina is also effort-related. However, the episodes of pain occur with increased frequency, intensity, and duration. Angina pectoris occurring for the first time, present less than 60 days, or occurring at rest may also be defined as unstable angina. It is also known as crescendo or preinfarction angina. Crescendo angina may indicate progressive CAD and an increased risk of impending myocardial infarction.[21,23]

The symptoms are less responsive to rest and nitrates. Individuals may require hospitalization for rest and treatment with intravenous nitrates to prevent the myocardial ischemia from progressing to myocardial infarction. Unstable angina is a transient phase because either it progresses to a myocardial infarction or the condition stabilizes because the individual develops collateral circulation,[5,18] or receives appropriate medical intervention.[28]

PRINZMETAL/VARIANT ANGINA

Prinzmetal/variant angina, commonly known as rest angina, is caused by coronary artery spasm.[27,28,30] The pain often occurs while the individual is at rest and most frequently in the early morning or upon arising. The anginal episodes are cyclic and often occur at the same time each day. Variant angina is unaffected by exertion, but it may be relieved by rest and nitrates. The pain is usually more intense and of longer duration than in stable angina. It more frequently leads to a myocardial infarction.[15,21,27,33] Individuals with variant angina present often with both pain and related complaints of syncope and palpitations. Cardiac arrhythmias occur more frequently during episodes of variant angina than during effort angina.[21]

Although variant angina may be seen in individuals without CAD, it is often seen in the presence of significant CAD.[7,27] With the advent of coronary arteriography, actual coronary artery spasm has been visualized and documented. During the cardiac catheterization, coronary artery spasm has been provoked by use of ergonovine, an ergot alkaloid that exerts a strong vasoconstricting effect on the coronary vascular system. The spasm of variant angina has been successfully relieved by use of nifedipine, a calcium channel blocker.

DIAGNOSIS AND TREATMENT

The frequency and characteristics of angina attacks vary. The attacks may depend upon the degree of coronary insufficiency, the collateral circulation, the response to treatment, and physical and emotional characteristics of the individual.[18,23] Angina provoked by emotional stress may last longer than episodes brought on by physical activity.

The diagnosis of angina is usually by history alone, as anginal episodes do not usually occur during the physical exam.[7,28] If the individual is examined during an episode of pain, tachycardia and hypertension will be found. During auscultation of the heart, an S_3 or S_4 gallop or a mitral murmur may be heard. These sounds may be secondary to ischemia of the papillary muscle.[21,28] ECG findings during episodes of pain reveal ST-segment elevation in variant angina and ST depression in unstable angina.[21] Exercise tolerance tests and cardiac radionuclide imaging may reveal areas of decreased perfusion. Cardiac catheterization provides a means of definitive diagnosis. Its use is usually limited to evaluation of atypical chest pain or for localizing and quantifying a lesion and evaluating left ventricular function in order to determine suitability for coronary artery bypass graft surgery. Cardiac catheterization is also used in the treatment of CAD via a procedure known as percutaneous transluminal angioplasty (PCTA) (see Chapter 5).

The treatment of angina (discussed in Chapter 5) is directed toward symptom relief and arresting the progress of the disease with medications, surgical procedures, and appropriate life-style modification. Chronic angina is treated pharmacologically with nitrates and calcium channel blockers, specifically nifedipine.

In CAD, the degree of stenosis (structural change) does not always correlate well with the functional impact of the disease because of individual variations in oxygen demand and workload tolerance. Predicting the extent of the coronary artery disease based on the anginal symptoms alone is difficult.[7]

Myocardial Infarction

Myocardial infarction (MI), the second manifestation of CAD, is the death or necrosis of some portion of the cardiac muscle secondary to sustained myocardial ischemia. Reduced coronary artery blood flow is most often caused by acute occlusion of coronary arteries at the site where atherosclerotic plaques have significantly compromised the coronary circulation. The acute occlusions may be the result of a coronary artery thrombus or a coronary artery spasm.[5,7] Decreased blood flow associated with hemorrhage or profound shock (hypovolemia) may also result in infarction.

Because the underlying pathology of angina and MI is similar, the initial clinical presentation may also be similar. The classic presenting symptom of MI is "vise-like" tightening of the chest retrosternally. The tightening becomes progressively intense over a period of hours to days until the pain becomes absolutely unbearable. The pain typically radiates to any number of areas with the most common being the jaw, upper back, and down the inner aspects of both arms. The pain of the myocardial infarction usually begins at rest and is unrelieved by nitrates, rest, or any other method the individual typically uses to relieve anginal pain.[34]

ASSESSMENT AND DIAGNOSIS

The medical diagnosis of MI is based on the individual's history, current symptoms, serum enzymes, and ECG changes. Positive findings in any two of these three diagnostic parameters are unequivocal evidence of MI.[7,24] However, because of the vulnerability of the myocardium, even suspect MIs are treated as MIs until the diagnosis is ruled out.

HISTORY AND CURRENT SYMPTOMS

Patients with suspect MIs often have histories of angina pectoris. However, a considerable number of patients experience an acute infarct as the first indication of cardiovascular problems.[18,27] Other individuals, about 15 percent of those who have MIs, may experience no discomfort at all ("silent MI").[18,28,29]

The typical patient presents with complaints of severe substernal pressure or pain. They may appear to be in acute distress: dyspneic, diaphoretic, with pale, cool, and clammy skin and associated complaints of nausea and vomiting. Extreme weakness and an overwhelming feeling of impending doom may also be expressed.

On examination an S_3 gallop, indicating decreased compliance of the myocardium, or a mitral murmur, indicating an ischemic papillary muscle, may be auscultated. The blood pressure may be elevated (partially in response to the pain) or may be very low, if the left ventricular function is severely compromised, resulting in a decreased cardiac output. The pulse may be very rapid and feeble. Arrhythmias are very common. They may include premature ventricular contractions, atrial fibrillation or flutter, conduction blocks, ventricular tachycardia and fibrillation.

There are two particularly vulnerable periods when fibrillation is most likely to occur: within the first 10 minutes following the infarction, and during a second period of cardiac irritability beginning 3 to 5 hours after the infarct and lasting for several days. Multiple arrhythmias are often observed.[5]

ECG CHANGES

Typical ECG changes are observed in 88 percent of individuals having MIs.[15,29,34] The ECG reflects change in myocardial electrical conduction in the area of the myocardial injury. Ischemia causes the T wave to become enlarged and symmetrically inverted owing to late repolarization. With injury, cells depolarize normally but repolarize more rapidly, resulting in ST-segment elevation. An absence of current flow through the infarcted cells and opposing currents from other parts of the heart cause a permanent Q wave (Figure 4 – 2).[35] However, if the infarction is small, an abnormal Q wave may not appear. Approximately 30 percent of abnormal Q waves disappear or revert to borderline significance within 18 months after infarction.[27]

In the MI, the infarcted area is surrounded by a zone of injury, which in turn is surrounded by a zone of ischemia. As the areas of ischemia and injury resolve (usually within 1 to 2 weeks of the MI), the ECG changes associated with them return to normal. The area of infarction is permanent and therefore so is the Q wave.[7,35]

SERUM ENZYMES AND ISOENZYMES

Enzymes are groups of proteins found in all cells. The major cardiac enzymes are creatine kinase (CK), lactate dehydrogenase (LDH), and serum glutamic-oxaloacetic transaminase (SGOT). These particular enzymes are found in all cells, but specific forms of each of these enzymes, their isoenzymes, are found only in cardiac cells. With cellular ischemia and death, the enzymes and isoenzymes are released into the serum in a characteristic pattern over the ensuing hours to days following the infarct. Each enzyme has an individual pattern of rise and fall. Serial blood samples can reveal patterns that are diagnostic of acute myocardial infarction (Figure 4 – 3).[7,11,26,27] Enzyme elevation patterns may also be indicators of the prognosis following myocardial infarction. Laboratory studies for these specific enzymes (LDH, CK, and SGOT) are sensitive but may have a false-positive rate as high as 15 percent.[27] More accurate identification of the enzyme activity indicative of myocardial necrosis can be made from the separation of the total enzyme activity into subunits, isoenzymes. This separation is done by electrophoresis.

CK is found in high concentrations in skeletal muscle, brain, and myocardium.

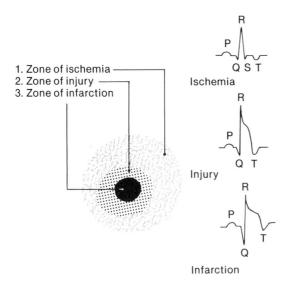

1. Zone of ischemia
2. Zone of injury
3. Zone of infarction

R
P
Q S T
Ischemia

R
P
Q T
Injury

R
P
T
Q
Infarction

FIGURE 4–2. ECG changes of infarction, injury, and ischemia as they correspond to the zones of infarction. 1) Ischemia causes inversion of T wave. 2) Injury causes ST-segment elevation. 3) Infarction causes permanent Q waves. (From Underhill, SL et al: Cardiac Nursing. JB Lippincott, Philadelphia, 1983, p 206, with permission.)

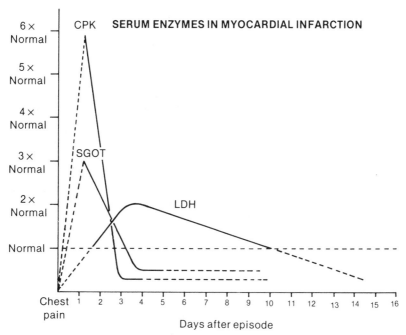

FIGURE 4–3. Serum enzymes in myocardial infarction. (From Vinsant, MO and Spence, MI: Commonsense Approach to Coronary Care. CV Mosby, St Louis, 1985, p 166, with permission.)

Trauma to any of these tissues will cause an elevation in the total CK. The isoenzymes, subunits of CK, are tissue specific. Therefore, elevations in isoenzymes identify the tissue that has been injured. CK-MM is predominant in skeletal muscle, and CK-BB is predominant in brain tissue. Myocardial tissue is the only human tissue containing substantial amounts of CK-MB. Elevation in CK-MB is highly specific for myocardial necrosis. The level begins to rise 2 to 4 hours after the infarct, with an increase greater than 5 percent considered abnormal. Serial CK-MB levels have been correlated with infarct size, arrhythmic complications, and prognosis. CK-MB may also be elevated after cardiac surgery or cardiopulmonary resuscitation and in individuals with muscular dystrophy.[7,27]

LDH can be separated into five separate isoenzymes by electrophoresis. Cardiac tissue is rich in LDH_1 and LDH_2. Normally, LDH_2 exceeds LDH_1 activity. Myocardial infarction results in LDH_1 activity exceeding LDH_2. This is referred to as a flipped LDH pattern. Elevated LDH_1 activity is usually seen within 24 hours and returns to normal in 7 to 10 days. An increase in LDH_1 activity is seen with hemolytic anemias, hemolysis of blood specimens, renal infarction, hyperthyroidism, and cancer of the stomach.

The flipped LDH pattern in combination with at least a 5 percent elevation of CK-MB provide objective evidence of myocardial necrosis.[7,27]

INFARCTION SITES AND MUSCULAR INVOLVEMENT

Myocardial infarcts are identified by their anatomic location and the layers of the myocardium involved in the infarct. The location is identified by the surface or combination of surfaces of the ventricle that is infarcted: lateral, inferior, posterior and anterior, septal or anteroseptal, inferoposterior, and so forth. The location of the infarction depends on which coronary artery is occluded and the location of the occlusion within the arterial tree. Occlusions that occur in the large branches of the coronary circulation result in more extensive damage than those occurring in smaller arteries. (Table 4–1 summarizes the areas of the heart that are supplied by the left and right coronary arteries.) It is important to note that 75 to 80 percent of the vessel must be occluded before the myocardial blood flow is diminished.[19] Therefore, significant disease is usually present when symptoms begin to appear. Additional information on myocardial blood supply and MI location can be found in references[7,11,26,27] at the end of this chapter.

The myocardial infarction is also identified by the layers of myocardium involved. Transmural infarcts, those that extend from the endocardium to the epicardium are most commonly diagnosed.[7] Infarcts may be limited to the layers of muscle below the epicardium (subepicardial), in the middle of the heart muscle (intracardial), or the muscle below the endocardium (subendocardial). Because of its poor blood supply and greater ventricular wall pressure, the subendocardial layer is the most vulnerable to ischemia.[5,7,11]

The location, size, and degree of myocardial involvement are determined by the patterns of ECG changes revealed in the various leads of the 12-lead ECG. Knowledge of the location and amount of muscular damage enables health-care providers to anticipate the clinical course, complications, and prognosis following the infarction.[26]

TREATMENT GOALS

The immediate goals of treatment for the individual who has experienced a myocardial infarction are:

1. Rapid management of myocardial ischemia/infarction and related symptoms (pain, dyspnea, nausea/vomiting)
2. Prevention or early detection and treatment of arrhythmias
3. Prevention of complications (see Complications of MI, p. 55.)

CLINICAL COURSE

Uncomplicated MI. An uncomplicated MI is one in which the infarction is small and no complications arise during recovery.

TABLE 4–1. Comparison of Right and Left Coronary Distribution

Right Coronary Artery Supplies	Left Coronary Artery Supplies
1. SA node (55%)	1. SA node (45%)
2. AV node	2. Anterosuperior division of left bundle
3. Bundle of His (a portion)	3. Right bundle branch (major portion)
4. Posterior one third of septum	4. Anterior two thirds of septum
5. Posteroinferior division of left bundle (a portion)	5. Posteroinferior division of left bundle (a portion)
6. Inferoposterior surface of left ventricle	6. Anterolateral surface of left ventricle

(From Vinsant and Spence,[7] p. 24, with permission.)

Initially, the individual is treated in the coronary care unit, where he or she is allowed minimal activity. All efforts are directed toward decreasing myocardial workload and myocardial oxygen demand.[5] The patient is treated symptomatically. Oxygen, nitroglycerin, and/or morphine sulfate are given to reduce ischemic pain. Antihypertensives (although many people are hypotensive after an MI[18]) are administered for hypertension. Other drugs like beta blockers or calcium channel blockers are given as necessary (see Chapter 5). Beta blockers reduce myocardial oxygen demand by decreasing the heart rate and contractility. Calcium channel blockers decrease the heart rate and also decrease the workload of the heart by systemic vasodilation (decreased afterload).

Cardiac rhythm is observed for arrhythmias. Ninety percent of all people who experience MIs have some type of arrhythmia. Early detection and treatment with appropriate pharmacologic agents have significantly reduced inhospital mortality.[5,27,34]

The individual typically remains in the coronary care unit 3 to 5 days postinfarction and remains in the hospital an additional week. During this time, activity is gradually increased, and the patient is monitored for signs and symptoms of repeat ischemia. The rehabilitation process, which begins in intensive care with low intensity exercise to prevent complications of bed rest, continues. Education of the individual and his or her family centers on understanding the coronary artery disease process, life-style modification, and risk factor adjustment.

Complications of Myocardial Infarct. Myocardial infarction has four major complications: arrhythmias, heart failure, thrombolytic complications, and damage to the heart structures.

Arrhythmias. Arrhythmias of some type occur in 90 percent of the individuals who have MIs. Although some arrhythmias may be benign, others are potentially life-threatening and require immediate treatment (see Chapter 6). The types of arrhythmias seen as a result of MIs vary with the surface of the heart infarcted and the point on the conduction pathway where the tissue is ischemic or infarcted.

Ischemia of a myocardial cell causes an alteration in the initiation and conduction of impulses throughout that area. Infarcted cells are electrically silent and neither initiate nor conduct impulses. Abnormalities in conduction may also result from the elongation of conduction pathways secondary to dilation of the infarcted ventricle.

Heart Failure. Heart failure is a syndrome characterized by the inability of the heart to maintain a cardiac output sufficient to meet the oxygen and nutritional needs of the tissues. Heart failure manifests itself in two ways. First, in an ischemic state the myocardial muscle does not contract normally, and the infarcted myocardium does not contract at all. This results in asynchronous contraction and a low cardiac output. The second way heart failure is manifested is congestive heart failure, which is characterized by hypotension and resultant retention of water and sodium secondary to decreased renal perfusion and by the damming of blood in either the pulmonary or systemic venous beds.

Acutely, following an infarct, the cardiac output may be greatly reduced. Sympathetic stimulation increases the heart rate and the contractility within seconds of the infarct in an attempt to maintain cardiac output. (Cardiac output equals stroke volume times heart rate: $CO = SV \times HR$.) These compensatory mechanisms may be adequate to regain a normal cardiac output. If they are not, the kidneys, sensing the decreased renal blood flow, retain water and sodium in an attempt to increase the circulatory volume and venous return to the heart. If the heart is not damaged severely, these changes may be enough to compensate for the diminished pumping ability (even when it is as low as 30 to 50 percent of normal) and bring the cardiac output back to normal.[36] If the heart is severely damaged and neither compensatory mechanisms nor medical intervention can return the cardiac output to normal, the patient deteriorates. When more than 40 percent of the left ventricle is infarcted, cardiogenic shock (low output failure) develops. This condition is associated with an 80 to 90 percent mortality rate. Chronic congestive heart failure, which develops as a result of an MI, may require continued treatment or may eventually be resolved. As the myocardium heals, the scar contracts and becomes smaller. This allows progressively less systolic bulge at the sight of the scar. Systolic bulge is a ballooning of the infarcted area of myocardium when left ventricular pressure increases during systole. Over time, the normal areas of the heart hypertrophy to compensate, at least partially, for the scarred musculature, and the heart at rest may have a normal cardiac output.[5,29]

Thrombolytic Complications. Two types of thrombus formation, venous and mural thrombi, may occur after myocardial infarction. Both are primarily triggered by venous stasis (stoppage of the flow of blood).

Deep vein thrombi usually form in the calf as a result of circulatory stasis imposed by activity restrictions. Mural thrombi form on the areas of relative stasis that are present after infarction in the ventricular wall. Both have the potential for embolism.

Emboli from a venous thrombus may result in a pulmonary embolism. Pulmonary embolism, once a major complication and cause of death after myocardial infarction, now accounts for less than 1 percent of total deaths.[27] Early ambulation for individuals with uncomplicated MIs and in-bed exercises for patients who are confined to bed have decreased the incidence of deep vein thrombus.

Emboli from a mural wall thrombus may lodge in visceral arteries and result in an infarction of the brain, kidney, spleen, or intestine, or lodge in an extremity and cause sudden pain, numbness, and coldness in the affected extremity. Embolectomies successfully remove the obstruction to the blood flow in extremities.

Heart Structural Damage. Damage to the heart structures as a result of ischemia or infarction is a fourth major complication of myocardial infarction. Structural damage includes ventricular aneurysm formation, papillary muscle rupture, ventricular free wall rupture, and intraventricular septal rupture. Ventricular aneurysms, the bulging of the wall in the weakened area, occur in transmural infarcts. Papillary muscle dysfunction or rupture occurs with papillary muscle ischemia or infarction. It results in mitral valve insufficiency. Ventricular free wall rupture is common in the second week post-MI when the scar is forming. The site is weakened because phagocytosis occurs earlier than collagen tissue formation. Rupture of the intraventricular septum, although rare, may also occur as a result of necrosis and the inability of the infarcted area to withstand the repeated pressure generated by the left ventricle in systole.[27,29] The "rupture" is usually a tunnel-like lesion through the septum. Any one of these structural problems may be fatal or result in mild to severe heart failure. Surgical intervention may be required to repair the damage.

Pericarditis, an inflammation of the pericardium, may also occur post-MI. The characteristic symptom is pain over the precordium, which is aggravated by breathing and relieved by sitting up. Pericarditis accompanied by the accumulation of fluid in the pericardial sac is known as pericardial effusion. The accumulation of fluid may be sufficiently slow that the pericardium stretches and accommodates the fluid without interfering with cardiac performance. However, if the onset is abrupt and the fluid accumulates rapidly, the heart is compressed and tamponade results. Cardiac tamponade is a life-threatening complication of pericarditis. The increased pressure restricts diastolic filling and results in reduced ventricular volume, elevated ventricular diastolic pressure, and reduced ventricular diastolic compliance. The cardiac output is decreased, as is the arterial blood pressure. Tachycardia is often insufficient to maintain cardiac output even at rest.

The decreased cardiac output is not a result of mechanical pump failure but of the external restraint to cardiac filling and inadequate ventricular preload. Treatment is by pericardial aspiration. The accumulated fluid is removed to relieve the tamponade. Heart function returns to normal. Further treatment with analgesics, steroids, and antibiotics may be indicated.

PROGNOSIS POST–MYOCARDIAL INFARCTION

Occasionally, after the MI, the heart returns to its full functional capacity. More often, the functional capacity is decreased.[36]

The prognosis depends on many factors. The most important factors include the extent of ventricular damage, the remaining cardiac reserve (the ability to respond to increased metabolic demands), and the severity of the CAD.

The medical and surgical management of the individual post-infarct is directed toward maximizing the cardiac function and minimizing any residual effects of the infarct. Cardiac rehabilitation programs, through education, exercise, diet, and risk factor reduction, facilitate life-style modifications that may reduce the risk of future infarctions.

Sudden Cardiac Death

In addition to the previously discussed clinical syndromes of angina and myocardial infarction, a third clinical manifestation of CAD is sudden cardiac death. Sudden cardiac death (SCD) is commonly defined as an unexpected cardiac death occurring in apparently healthy individuals engaged in their normal activities of daily living, without prior symptoms or with symptoms of less than an hour's duration.[27] The American Heart Association estimated that in 1984 one of every three individuals who had a myocardial infarction died. Sixty percent of these died before they reached the hospital.[1,5,26]

Sudden occlusion of one of the major coronary arteries is a likely cause of ventricular fibrillation, which may result in sudden cardiac death. Ventricular fibrillation is a rapid and chaotic heart rhythm due to myocardial hypoxia. The ventricle quivers rather than contracts. There is no effective cardiac output. If sustained, death may result within 4 minutes.[5] Prompt initiation of cardiopulmonary resuscitation is the only proven means of preventing SCD.

Most victims of SCD are males about 60 years of age. Four characteristics are associated with an increased risk of SCD: ventricular electrical instability, extensive coronary artery narrowing, abnormal left ventricular function, and electrocardiographic conduction and repolarization abnormalities.

Four conditions contribute to the heart's tendency to fibrillate. Ischemia of the muscle cells causes the release of potassium into the extracellular fluid and may increase myocardial irritability. Ischemic muscle remains negatively charged and can elicit abnormal impulses that may cause fibrillation. Sympathetic stimulation resulting from the low cardiac output may increase myocardial irritability. The myocardial infarction itself may, by dilating the ventricle, cause stretching of the conduction pathways or cause routing of impulses along abnormal pathways around the infarcted site. This final factor allows for a cyclic state of myocardial cell excitation. In this situation, impulses re-enter muscle during the relative refractory period and set up a cycle of excitation that overrides the normal depolarization-repolarization cycle allowing the heart to fibrillate.[5,11,27]

Congestive Heart Failure

Congestive heart failure (CHF) is a fourth manifestation of coronary artery disease. This syndrome is characterized by the inability of the heart to maintain an adequate cardiac output. CHF may result in diminished blood flow to the tissues, abnormal retention of sodium and water, and congestion in the pulmonary and systemic circulation. The most common etiology is ischemic heart disease secondary to CAD. CHF may also be associated with hypertension, valvular disease, or congenital heart disease.[5]

The ability of the heart to maintain an adequate cardiac output depends on the heart rate and the stroke volume. The stroke volume is a function of: preload, the end-diastolic volume in the left ventricle; afterload, the systemic vascular resistance or the force against which the heart must pump; and contractility, the force of the contraction generated by the myocardium. Alterations in any one of these three factors result in decreased cardiac output. Changes in myocardial contractility are the most frequent cause of heart failure.[5,27]

In the person with CAD, decreases in normal coronary blood flow cause hypoxia and acidosis of the myocardial cells. Contractility is altered by such changes in the cellular environment. Whether the change is gradual or acute, as in myocardial infarction, there is a resultant change in the cardiac output.

When a reduction in cardiac output occurs, the body immediately brings compensatory mechanisms into play to restore the balance. Compensatory mechanisms are physiologic alterations in the body's functioning that maintain homeostasis or, in this case, cardiac output. These mechanisms include: increased sympathetic nervous system stimulation, increased sodium and water retention by the kidneys, increased dilation of the cardiac muscle fibers to accommodate the increased volume, and ventricular hypertrophy. Increased sympathetic activity occurs immediately and causes increased heart rate and contractility. It also increases vascular tone, augmenting both venus return(preload) and systemic vascular resistance (afterload). The second compensatory mechanism is retention of water and sodium, triggered by a drop in kidney perfusion. Initially the increased circulating volume augments preload, afterload, and contractility. The heart may also dilate or hypertrophy, increase its muscle mass, in response to the increased workload.[26,36] These mechanisms may be successful to maintain a normal cardiac output for some period of time, but they all increase myocardial oxygen consumption. They may not be able to sustain the cardiac output if the pump function does not improve or if it deteriorates.

TYPES OF HEART FAILURE

There are several types of heart failure. Each is described briefly below.

Acute Versus Chronic Failure. Acute heart failure may identify the initial manifestation of heart disease, or it may be acute exacerbation of a chronic cardiac condition. The events that precipitate the symptoms of acute heart failure occur rapidly. The rapid failure of the pump may result in an acute shift of blood from the systemic circulation to the pulmonary circulation before the compensatory mechanisms can be effective. The patient may experience a symptomatic fall in cardiac output and rapid onset of the associated symptoms.[7]

Chronic heart failure develops gradually and is associated with the chronic retention of fluid and salt by the kidneys and other compensatory mechanisms. With time, the chronic overstimulation of compensatory mechanisms may lead to end organ failure.

Compensated Versus Uncompensated Failure. In compensated failure, the heart has been able to maintain adequate cardiac output by means of the compensatory mechanisms described previously. Sympathetic stimulation and renal retention of water and sodium have maintained the cardiac output at normal levels, except for a mild to moderately elevated right atrial pressure (+4 mmHg to +6 mmHg). Cardiac function at rest appears normal.[5] Symptoms appear when myocardial oxygen demand increases. A rapid heart rate, pallor, and diaphoresis all indicate that the cardiac output cannot meet the increased demand.

Uncompensated failure occurs when a severely damaged heart cannot regain normal cardiac output. Although compensatory mechanisms are at work, normal cardiac output is not attained. Fluid retention worsens because inadequate renal perfusion persists. Gradually the heart is stretched until it is unable to pump even moderate quantities of blood. The heart may fail completely. The patient may die of uncompensated cardiac failure. Often this progression can be halted or slowed by appropriate pharmacologic therapy. Diuretics and fluid and salt restriction may control circulating volume while cardiac glycosides (for example, digitalis) are given to improve the contractility. In this way an adequate cardiac output may be maintained. Although digitalis has little effect on the contractility of the normal myocardium, in the failing heart it may double the strength of contraction.[5]

Intractable Heart Failure. Intractable heart failure persists despite application of all therapies. Pulmonary and systemic congestion and a low cardiac output exist even at rest.[27]

Left Ventricular Failure Versus Right Ventricular Failure. The left and right sides of the heart may fail separately or together. Left-sided failure is more common than right-sided failure and frequently leads to right-sided failure.[5,36,39]

Left-sided failure is most frequently seen after myocardial infarct. When the heart is damaged, it may not pump effectively and blood can back up in the left ventricle. As the pressure from the increased volume builds, it is communicated in a retrograde fashion to the left atrium and on through the pulmonary capillary beds. Pulmonary capillary pressure builds. The fluid is forced from the capillaries into the interstitial spaces and then into the alveoli. The presence of fluid in the interstitial spaces and the alveoli produces edema, which interferes with the diffusion of gases. Clinically, the patient is dyspneic at rest even when sitting upright. As pulmonary congestion increases, the lungs become stiff and less compliant and dyspnea worsens. The cough produces frothy pink (blood-tinged) sputum, and rales (abnormal breath sounds from the movement of air through fluid in the alveoli) are audible over the lungs. Signs and symptoms of left ventricular failure are included in Table 4–2.

Right ventricular failure may occur unilaterally. It can result from congenital heart problems or chronic obstructive pulmonary disease (COPD). In the latter, lung compli-

TABLE 4–2. Signs and Symptoms of Cardiac Failure

	Left Ventricular Failure	Right Ventricular Failure
Subjective	Dyspnea	Abdominal pain
	Orthopnea	Anorexia/nausea
	Paroxysmal nocturnal dyspnea	Bloating
	Cough	Fatigue
	Fatigue	Ankle swelling (bilateral)
Objective	Rales	Distended neck veins
	S₃ gallop	Hepatojugular reflux
	Pleural effusion	Hepatomegaly/splenomegaly
	Peripheral cyanosis	Ascites
	Increased respiratory rate	Elevated CVP, right atrial pressure
	Cheyne-Stokes respirations	S₄ gallop
	Decreased urine output	Peripheral edema
	Pink frothy sputum	Decreased urine output

(From Patrick, Woods, Craven, and Rokosky,[29] p. 548, with permission.)

ance decreases significantly, and pulmonary vascular resistance increases signficantly. The most common cause of right ventricular failure, however, is left ventricular failure.[5,27,56] Right ventricular failure follows left ventricular failure when the increase of pressure through the pulmonary circulation overloads the right ventricle (Figure 4–4). The first sign of right ventricular failure is elevated central venous pressure (CVP) and neck vein distention. Liver engorgement, ascites, and peripheral edema of the dependent portion of the body (feet and ankles) are also observed.

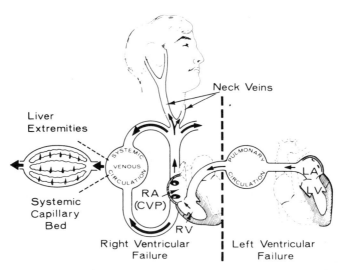

FIGURE 4–4. Retrograde failure of right ventricle from left ventricular failure. (From Vinsant, MO and Spence, MI: Commonsense Approach to Coronary Care. CV Mosby, St Louis, 1985, p 350, with permission.)

Individuals with heart failure all complain of fatigue and a decreased tolerance for activity. Treatment of the acute episode is directed toward decreasing circulatory overload, decreasing myocardial workload and oxygen demand, and increasing myocardial contractility. These goals may be accomplished with the judicious use of diuretics, water and sodium restrictions, cardiac glycosides (to increase myocardial contractility), and oxygen therapy as necessary.

CHF is usually a recurring phenomenon characterized by repeated exacerbations of symptoms increasing in frequency and severity as the myocardial muscle becomes progressively weaker and distended.[11,27] Chronic management attempts to decrease the frequency and severity of the symptoms.

PHYSIOLOGIC CHANGES IN INDIVIDUALS WITH CORONARY ARTERY DISEASE IN RESPONSE TO PHYSICAL CONDITIONING

The role of exercise in preventing or reversing CAD is undefined. The World Health Organization has concluded that regular vigorous exercise can enhance approaches to treatment and modify risk factors in patients with CAD.[41] There are, however, definite physiologic responses to physical conditioning in the individual with CAD (see Chapter 3). The most beneficial physiologic change is an improvement in functional capacity, attributable to an increase in myocardial oxygen supply and a decrease in myocardial oxygen demand. This allows the individual to perform higher workloads for longer periods of time without reaching his or her ischemic threshold.[47] The workload can be expressed as the product of the heart rate (HR) and the systolic arterial blood pressure (SBP); this is known as the rate pressure product (RPP) or double product (HR $\times$ SBP = RPP; for example, $70 \times 100 = 7000$ or 70×10^2) (see Chapter 7). Both the heart rate and arterial BP are major determinants of the myocardial oxygen consumption during exercise. As they increase, so does the RPP. In the physically conditioned individual with CAD, heart rate and blood pressure are decreased at rest and with submaximal exercise. Therefore, the RPP, the myocardial oxygen demand, and myocardial oxygen consumption are all lower.

Another benefit of training is the increased efficiency with which the peripheral muscles use oxygen.[43] This efficiency has not been documented in the heart as yet,[41,43] but the increased efficiency in the periphery decreases myocardial oxygen demand for any given level of exercise.

Physical conditioning also results in a swifter return to the resting heart rate after exercise. To date, physical conditioning has not been shown to facilitate the development of collateral coronary circulation,[46,47] but in a recent cumulative analysis by Shephard,[44] the data show that individuals who had undergone physical conditioning not only experienced fewer repeat myocardial infarcts but also had a smaller percentage of these events with a fatal outcome.[44,47]

In addition to the physiologic response to exercise, the psychological satisfaction, the improved sense of well-being, and the decrease in cardiac risk factors that occur as a result of physical conditioning are of great benefit to the individual with CAD.

SUMMARY

In presenting the pathophysiology of coronary artery disease, particular attention was given to atherosclerosis and to the ischemia-infarction process that is the basis for all the related clinical manifestations of CAD.

The clinical manifestations of CAD, including angina, myocardial infarction, sudden cardiac death, and cardiac failure, were discussed in relation to the pathophysiology and the progression of CAD, their presenting symptoms, and their major complications.

The major physiologic changes in relation to training and physical conditioning of individuals with CAD were found to be improvement in functional capacity and the increased efficiency with which peripheral muscles use oxygen.

REFERENCES

1. Heart Facts, 1984. American Heart Association, Dallas, 1984.
2. Years of Life Lost From Cardiovascular Disease. Morbidity and Mortality Weekly Report, Massachusetts Medical Society 35:42, 1986.
3. Atherosclerosis; Arteriosclerosis. In Holvey, DG (ed): Merck Manual, ed 12. Merck, Sharp, and Dohme, Rahway, NJ, 1972.
4. Cowan, MJ: Pathogenesis of Atherosclerosis. In Underhill, SL, et al (eds): Cardiac Nursing. JB Lippincott, Philadelphia, 1982.
5. Guyton, AC: Textbook of Medical Physiology, ed 6. WB Saunders, Philadelphia.
6. Underhill, SL: Assessment of Cardiovascular Function. In Brunner, LS and Suddarth, DS: Textbook of Medical-Surgical Nursing. JB Lippincott, Philadelphia, 1984.
7. Vinsant, MO and Spence, MI: Commonsense Approach to Coronary Care. CV Mosby, St Louis, 1985, pp 160–243.
8. Chaffee, EE and Greisheimer, EM: Basic Physiology and Anatomy, ed 2. JB Lippincott, Philadelphia, 1969, pp 343–91.
9. Cowan M: Atherosclerosis. In Patrick, MG, et al (eds): Medical Surgical Nursing: Pathophysiological Concepts. JB Lippincott, Philadelphia, 1986.
10. Schwartz, CJ: Gross Aortic Sudanophilia and Hemosideria Deposition. A Study of Infants, Children, and Young Adults. Archives of Pathology 83:325, 1967.
11. Fowler, NO (ed): Cardiac Diagnosis and Treatment, ed 3. Harper & Row, Hagerstown, MD, 1980.
12. Ross, R and Glosmet, JA: The Pathogenesis of Atherosclerosis, Part I. N Eng J Med 295:369, 1976.
13. Ross, R and Glosmet, JA: The Pathogenesis of Atherosclerosis, Part II. N Eng J Med 295:426, 1976.
14. Benditt, E: The Origin of Atherosclerosis. Scientific American 236:74, 1977.
15. Sokolow, M and McIlroy, MB: Clinical Cardiology. Lange Medical Publications, Los Altos, CA, 1986.
16. Wolff, R: Coronary Heart Disease. Medical Clinics in North America 57:1, 1973.
17. Glasgov, S: Mechanical Stress on Vessels and the Non-Uniform Distribution of Atherosclerosis. Medical Clinics in North America 57:1, 1973.
18. Coronary Artery Disease. In Holvey, DH (ed): Merck Manual, ed 12. Merck, Sharp, and Dohme, Rahway, NJ, 1972.
19. Zak, R and Rabinowitz, M: Metabolism of the Ischemic Heart. Medical Clinics in North America 57:1, 1973.
20. Solack, SD: Pathophysiology of Myocardial Ischemia and Infarction. In Underhill, SL, et al (eds): Cardiac Nursing. JB Lippincott, Philadelphia, 1982.
21. Tannenbaum, RP, Sohn, CA, Cantwell, R, and Rogers, M: Angina Pectoris: How to Recognize; How to Manage It. Nursing 81 11:9, 1981.
22. Rokosky, JS: Ischemia and Infarction. In Patrick, SL, et al (eds): Medical-Surgical Nursing: Pathophysiological Concepts. JB Lippincott, Philadelphia, 1986.
23. Riseman, JEF: Diagnosis of Angina Pectoris at the Present Time. Medical Clinics in North America 58:2, 1974.
24. Altschule, MD: Physiology in Acute Myocardial Infarction. Medical Clinics in North America 58:2, 1974.
25. Texon, M: Atherosclerosis: Its Hemodynamic Basis and Implications. Medical Clinics in North America 58:2, 1974.
26. Braunwald, E: Heart Disease, ed 2. WB Saunders, Philadelphia, 1984.

27. Hurst, J, et al (eds): The Heart, Arteries, and Veins, ed 5. McGraw-Hill, New York, 1982.
28. Underhill, SL: Diagnosis and Treatment of the Patient with Coronary Artery Disease and Myocardial Ischemia. In Underhill, SL, et al (eds): Cardiac Nursing. JB Lippincott, Philadelphia, 1982.
29. Woods, SL, and Underhill, SL: Coronary Heart Disease: Myocardial Ischemia and Infarction. In Patrick, ML, et al (eds): Medical Surgical Nursing: Pathophysiological Nursing. JB Lippincott, Philadelphia, 1986.
30. Heupler, FA, and Proudfit, WL: Nifedipine Therapy for Refractory Coronary Artery Spasm. American J Cardiology 44, October, 1979.
31. Kannel, WB: Update on the Role of Cigarette Smoking in Coronary Artery Disease. American Heart J 101, 1981.
32. Forman, MB, et al: Increased Adventitial Mast Cells in a Patient with Coronary Spasm. N Eng J Med 313:18.
33. Spittle, L: Management of Patients with Cardiovascular Disorders. In Brunner, LS and Suddarth, DS: Textbook of Medical-Surgical Nursing, ed. 5. JB Lippincott, Philadelphia, 1984.
34. Woods, SL: Diagnosis and Treatment of the Patient with an Uncomplicated Myocardial Infarction. In Underhill, SL, et al (eds): Cardiac Nursing. JB Lippincott, Philadelphia, 1982.
35. Woods, SL: Electrocardiography, Vectorcardiography, and Polarcardiography. In Underhill, SL, et al (eds): Cardiac Nursing. JB Lippincott, Philadelphia, 1982.
36. Mechanical Complications in Coronary Heart Disease: Heart Failure and Shock. In Vinsant, MO and Spence, MI: Commonsense Approach to Coronary Care. CV Mosby, St Louis, 1985.
37. Bopp, DL: Heart Failure. In Patrick, ML, et al (eds): Medical Surgical Nursing: Pathophysiological Nursing. JB Lippincott, Philadelphia, 1983.
38. Niles, NA and Wills, RE: Heart Failure. In Underhill, SL, et al (eds): Cardiac Nursing. JB Lippincott, Philadelphia, 1982.
39. Niles, NA and Wills, RE: Heart Failure. In Underhill, SL, et al (eds): Cardiac Nursing. JB Lippincott, Philadelphia, 1982.
40. Sivarajan, ES: Cardiac/Rehabilitation Activity and Exercise Program. In Underhill, SL, et al (eds): Cardiac Nursing. JB Lippincott, Philadelphia, 1982.
41. Oberman, A: Exercise and the Primary Prevention of Cardiovascular Disease. American J Cardiology 55:100, 1985.
42. Sami, M, et al: Significance of Exercise Induced Ventricular Arrhythmias in Stable Coronary Artery Disease. American J Cardiology 54:1182, 1984.
43. Wenger, N and Fletcher, GF: Rehabilitation of the Patient with Atherosclerotic Coronary Heart Disease. In Hurst, J, et al (eds): The Heart, Arteries and Veins, ed 5. McGraw-Hill, New York, 1982.
44. Shephard, RJ: The Value of Exercise in Ischemic Heart Disease: A Cumulative Analysis. J Cardiac Rehabilitation 3:294, 1983.
45. Stern, MJ and Cleary, P: National Exercise and Heart Disease Project. Psychosocial Changes Observed During Low Level Exercise Programs. Archives of Internal Medicine 141:1463, 1981.
46. Wenger, NK: Rehabilitation of the Patient with Symptomatic Coronary Atherosclerotic Heart Disease: Part II. In McIntosh, HD (ed): Cardiology Series, Vol 3, No 3. Parke-Davis, Morris Plains, NJ, 1980.
47. Dehn, MM: Rehabilitation of the Cardiac Patient: The Effects of Exercise. American J Nursing 80:435, 1980.

CHAPTER 5

The Medical and Surgical Management of Coronary Artery Disease

The medical and surgical management methods for coronary artery disease (CAD) are as diverse as the symptoms displayed by individuals with the disease. Each year, as surgical techniques are more finely perfected and new pharmacologic agents are developed and tested, the outlook becomes brighter for these individuals. In all cases, treatment is aimed at relieving symptoms and slowing the progression of the disease. Many individuals have had their symptoms managed by a variety of therapies with appropriate modifications to maintain an optimal level of well-being.

In this chapter, the pharmacologic agents commonly used in the medical management of acute and chronic CAD are reviewed. Surgical interventions, including myocardial revascularization and percutaneous transluminal angioplasty, are discussed. The identification of cardiac rehabilitation as an important adjunct to therapy is addressed.

MEDICAL MANAGEMENT

The main thrust of the medical management of CAD concerns the various pharmacologic agents specifically used in the long-term treatment of CAD and its symptoms: nitrates, beta blocking agents, antiarrhythmics, cardiac glycosides, calcium channel blockers, and antihypertensives. Treatment is directed toward preventing myocardial ischemia and infarction while maximizing and improving the existing cardiac function.

Nitrates

Nitrates are classified in two groups, those that act rapidly to eliminate acute anginal attacks and those that are of prolonged duration to prevent anginal attacks. Table 5–1 outlines various preparations of nitrates.

ACTIONS AND USES

Nitrates are vasodilators used in the first-line management of all types of angina. By acting directly on the smooth muscles of the vessel walls, nitrates cause general vasodilation throughout the body. This peripheral vasodilation results in venous pooling, decreased blood return to the heart, decreased left ventricular dimensions, and decreased diastolic filling pressure. The decreased preload, together with decreased afterload (a result of decreased arterial wall tone), significantly reduces the myocardial oxygen demand and may relieve angina or delay its onset. Nitrates may also dilate normal coronary arteries and cause redistribution of blood flow to ischemic areas.[2]

CONTRAINDICATIONS AND SIDE EFFECTS

The side effects of nitrates include tachycardia, hypotension, flushing, and headache, all related to generalized vasodilation.

EFFECTS ON EXERCISE IN INDIVIDUALS WITH CAD

Anginal pain, often experienced at low levels of exercise by individuals with CAD, results from inadequate cardiac reserve. The heart cannot meet the increased oxygen demand of exercise. Nitrates, given prior to exercise or administered chronically, reduce cardiac workload and improve exercise performance. This is evidenced by an increased tolerance for activity before the onset of anginal pain and/or ischemic electrocardiographic changes.

NITRATE THERAPY MANAGEMENT

Careful consideration should be given to the following:

1. Administer sublingual nitrate, if prescribed, at the onset of chest pain.
2. Monitor blood pressure. Observe for symptoms of hypotension (light-headedness, dizziness, decreased urine output).
3. If pain is unrelieved by three doses of nitroglycerin (one tablet every 5 min), institute the appropriate procedure for obtaining emergency medical care.

Beta Blocking Agents

ACTIONS AND USES

Beta blocking agents (Table 5–2) reduce myocardial oxygen demand by decreasing the heart rate and depressing contractility. They increase diastolic fill time (increasing blood supply) as a result of decreasing the heart rate. Competing with epinephrine for available

TABLE 5-1. Nitrates: Acute and Chronic Management[1,2,5,25]

Generic Name (Trade Name)	Mode of Administration and Dosage	a. Onset b. Peak Action	Duration of Action	Implications for the Individual with CAD
Acute Management				
Nitroglycerin (Nitrostat)	Sublingual: 1/100 – 1/400 gr prn (for acute anginal pain)	a. 2 min b. 5 min	10 – 15 min	Nitroglycerin should be taken with onset of chest pain and repeated every 5 min × 3 doses. Additional medical attention should be obtained if pain not relieved after 15 min.
	IV dosage titrated to relieve pain	a. immediate	10 min	
Isosorbide dinitrate (Isordil)	Sublingual/ chewable: 2.5 – 5.0 mg	a. 3 – 5 min b. 15 – 30 min	1 – 2 hr	Individual should be seated to prevent light-headedness. Keep nitroglycerin in dark glass bottle.
Chronic Management				
Isosorbide dinitrate (Isordil, Sorbitrate)	po: 5 – 30 mg QID	a. 20 min b. 30 – 45 min	1/2 – 2 hr	Tolerance may develop.
Nitroglycerin (Sustained-Release) (Nitro-Bid, Nitrospan)	po: 2.5 – 6.5 mg tablet q 8 – 12 hr	a. 30 min b. 3 – 4 hr	8 – 12 hr	
Nitroglycerin (Topical) (Nitro-Bid, Nitrol)	Topical: 1/2 – 4 in ribbon of ointment	a. 30 min	3 – 4 hr	Ointment may be placed on any body part. Ointment should be covered with a plastic-coated paper for better absorption.
Nitroglycerin transdermal patches (Nitro-Dur, Transderm)	Topical patch: QD 26 – 154 mg	a. 30 min	24 hr	Ease of administration may increase compliance.

TABLE 5–2. Beta Blocking Agents[1,3–6]

Generic Name (Trade Name)	Dosage	Therapeutic Uses	Implications
Propranolol hydrochloride (Inderal)	10–12 mg BID to QID. Extremely variable dosages and varied uses.	Hypertension, angina, some arrhythmias (PAT). Post infarct to prevent reinfarction. Migraine headaches.	Limit smoking as it may result in elevated blood pressure.[3] Caution patient that sudden cessation of drugs may cause an exacerbation of angina.
Metoprolol (Lopressor)	100–450 mg/day single dose or TID. Cardioselective at lower doses.[1]	Hypertension, angina, some arrhythmias	Cardioselective beta blockers should be administered to individuals with lung disease.
Nadolol (Corgard)	40–320 mg/day single dose or TID	Hypertension, angina, some arrhythmias	
Timolol (Blocadren)	10 mg BID. Ophthalmic— 0.25% solution	Hypertension, angina. Post infarction to prevent reinfarction. To decrease intraocular pressure	
Atenolol (Tenormin)	50–100 mg/day single dose. Cardioselective at low doses	Hypertension, angina	
Pindolol (Visken)	10–60 mg TID or QID	Hypertension, some arrhythmias	This new beta blocker possesses some intrinsic sympathetic activity (ISA), which is most apparent at rest, producing less resting bradycardia.[1]

beta-receptor sites in the heart and other tissues, beta blockers inhibit the normal response to adrenergic stimuli. Drugs that block the beat receptors of the sympathetic nervous system decrease the heart rate, AV conduction, contractility, and automaticity in the heart and cause bronchoconstriction in the lungs. There are $beta_1$ and $beta_2$ receptor sites. $Beta_1$ sites are primarily in the heart, and $beta_2$ sites are in the lungs and throughout the body. Beta blockers that work specifically on $beta_1$ sites are referred to as cardioselective.

Beta blockers are used in combination with nitrates for the treatment of chest pain in effort angina. They relieve chest pain by decreasing oxygen demand and restoring the balance of oxygen demand and supply.

Beta blockers are contraindicated in Prinzmetal angina and coronary artery spasm because they allow alpha-adrenergic activity (vasoconstriction) to predominate. They are used in the treatment of mild hypertension and cardiac arrhythmias because they decrease SA-node automaticity and slow conduction through the AV node. Following an acute myocardial infarction, beta blockers can be used to salvage ischemic myocardium by decreasing myocardial oxygen demand.

The six beta blockers currently available are listed in Table 5–2. Pindolol (Visken), one of the newest beta blocking agents, possesses some intrinsic sympathetic activity (ISA). Beta blockers with ISA may be advantageous in that little, if any, slowing of the heart rate, depression of contractility, or slowing of AV conduction occurs at rest when sympathetic activity is low. The effects of beta blockers with ISA are similar to the effects of other beta blockers during exercise.[1] The slightly higher than anticipated resting heart rate in individuals taking pindolol reflects this intrinsic sympathetic activity.[1]

CONTRAINDICATIONS AND SIDE EFFECTS

Beta blockers must be used cautiously in patients with chronic lung disease because blockade of beta$_2$ receptor sites in the lung may cause bronchospasm. Beta blockers should also be used cautiously in patients with hyperglycemia and in patients with severe congestive heart failure. In the latter individuals, beta blockers further decrease contractility and the cardiac output and, therefore, further increase the failure.

Side effects of beta blockers include bronchospasm, hypotension, drug fever, gastrointestinal disturbances, transient thrombocytopenia, fatigue, and sleep disorders. Abrupt cessation of beta blockers may bring on a recurrence of anginal pain, arrhythmias, or sudden death. Individuals should be cautioned about the importance of titrating the drug when it is to be discontinued, as abrupt withdrawal exacerbates angina.

EFFECTS ON EXERCISE IN INDIVIDUALS WITH CAD

Therapy with beta blockers results in increased exercise tolerance and increased aerobic capacity.[9] The individual taking beta blockers experiences a decrease in both resting and submaximal heart rate and blood pressure. Therefore, there is a decrease in the rate pressure product (the cardiac workload) and myocardial oxygen demand. Higher levels of activity are attained before the individual's ischemic threshold is reached and anginal pain or ECG changes occur.

BETA-ADRENERGIC BLOCKADE THERAPY MANAGEMENT

Careful consideration should be given to the following:

1. Individuals should be cautioned never to abruptly stop taking beta blockers.
2. Increases in heart rate normally seen with exercise are lower in individuals on beta blockers.

3. Changes in beta blockade therapy necessitate a repeat graded exercise test and reassessment of the exercise prescription.

Calcium Channel Blockers

Calcium channel blockers inhibit the flow of calcium ions across the membranes of myocardial and vascular smooth muscle cells. Calcium plays an important role in myocardial contractility, vasomotor tone, and cardiac electrical activity (see Chapter 2).

There are three calcium channel blockers, verapamil (Isopton, Calan), nifedipine (Procardia), and diltiazem (Cardizem). All are effective in the treatment of angina, but they work via different mechanisms (Table 5–3).

Verapamil decreases myocardial oxygen demand in three ways. It decreases afterload by peripheral vasodilation, and it decreases heart rate (negative chronotropic effect) and contractility (negative inotropic effect). Verapamil is used in the treatment of arrhythmias, specifically supraventricular tachycardias. Diltiazem acts through these same mechanisms but the effects are not as strong with verapamil.

Nifedipine is a strong peripheral vasodilator. It decreases myocardial oxygen demand by that mechanism. However, it has no direct effect on heart rate or contractility. It may

TABLE 5–3. Calcium Channel Blockers[1,3,5,8]

Generic Name (Trade Name)	Dosage	Therapeutic Uses	Effects on Cardiovascular System
Diltiazem (Cardizem)	30 mg TID to QID (to maximum of 240 mg/24 hrs)[5]	Angina and hypertension, some arrhythmias	Dilates coronary arteries. Antiarrhythmic action. Some decrease in contractility.
Nifedipine (Procardia)	Initially 10 mg TID. Maintenance 10–30 mg TID or QID	Angina, hypertension	Potent peripheral vasodilator. Dilates coronary arteries.
Verapamil (Calan, Isopton)	Initially 80 mg q 6–8 hrs. 320–480 mg in divided doses	Angina, tachyarrhythmias	Slows AV conduction (negative chronotropic* effect; negative inotropic* effect), some peripheral and coronary dilation.

*The effects of autonomic stimulation on the heart may be classified as (1) chronotropic—affecting heart rate and (2) inotropic—affecting contractility. Positive and negative are used to describe the responses of the heart to a drug (for example, a drug that increases contractility has a positive inotropic effect).[7]

cause a reflex increase in heart rate in response to vasodilation. Nifedipine is the calcium channel blocker most safely used in individuals with CHF and is a preferred therapy in the treatment of variant angina.

Calcium channel blockers are also used in the treatment of hypertension. They can be used in combination with nitrates to treat effort angina and the angina of coronary artery spasm. They may also be used in combination with beta blockers in the treatment of effort angina, because they permit the use of lower doses of the beta blockers and avoid the undesirable effects of beta blockade.[1] Calcium channel blockers neither constrict the bronchial tree nor aggravate coronary and peripheral vascular spasm, characteristics making them more desirable than some beta blockers. Calcium channel blockade therapy results in decreased myocardial contractility, vasomotor tone, peripheral vascular resistance, and heart rate. The latter is a result of slower impulse conduction. The outcome is a decrease in myocardial oxygen demand.

CONTRAINDICATIONS AND SIDE EFFECTS

Calcium channel blockers are contraindicated in moderate to severe CHF, significant hypotension, aortic stenosis, and sick sinus syndrome.

Side effects, occurring in approximately 17 percent of individuals on calcium channel blockade therapy,[3] include hypotension, reflex tachycardia, peripheral edema, and headache. Central nervous system side effects include tremors, mood changes, and fatigue. Gastrointestinal distress and skin reactions have also been reported. Nifedipine can cause significant noncardiac pedal edema.

EFFECTS OF EXERCISE IN THE INDIVIDUAL WITH CAD

The decreased myocardial oxygen demand and improved myocardial blood supply may improve an individual's tolerance for activity.

CALCIUM CHANNEL BLOCKADE THERAPY MANAGEMENT

Careful consideration should be given to the following:

1. Observe the individual for symptoms of postural hypotension (light-headedness upon arising, tachycardia, and pallor).
2. Monitor blood pressure (poorly tolerated hypotension has occurred during initial titration or at the time of subsequent upward dosage adjustment and may be more likely to occur in individuals on concomitant beta blockers).

CARDIAC GLYCOSIDES

The most common cardiac glycosides include digitalis, digitoxin, digoxin (Lanoxin) and Quabain.

ACTIONS AND USES

The exact mechanism of action of cardiac glycosides is unknown. They are believed to increase the influx of calcium ions into the myocardial cell. They also alter the electrochemical properties of the cell by their effect on the active transport of sodium and potassium.

Cardiac glycosides have both a positive inotropic effect (increasing the contractility) and a negative chronotropic effect (decreasing the heart rate). The associated decreased heart rate may result from the vagal stimulation initiated by carotid baroreceptors when increased systolic pressure is sensed.[5] Although these effects are seen in the healthy heart, they are more significant in the failing heart.[3] Increased contractility increases the cardiac output and decreases preload, cardiac workload, and myocardial oxygen demand. This, in turn, reduces congestive heart failure.

Cardiac glycosides act directly on the heart rate by increasing the refractory period of the AV node and Purkinje fibers. They also increase the excitability of the Purkinje fibers but have only a variable effect on the excitability of the ventricles and no effect on the excitability of the atrium. Cardiac glycosides have little effect on the pacemaker automaticity of the SA node, but they increase the automaticity of the Purkinje fibers.

Cardiac glycosides are the drugs of choice in the treatment and control of congestive heart failure. The increased contractility improves oxygen delivery to all tissues. Increased renal perfusion results in a diuretic effect, decreasing circulating blood volume. Circulatory volume is further decreased by diuretic therapy administered in conjunction with the cardiac glycosides in the treatment of heart failure. Although they relieve the symptoms of CHF, cardiac glycosides do not relieve the cause.

Cardiac glycosides are also used to treat and control certain arrhythmias, including atrial fibrillation, atrial flutter, and atrial tachycardia. Digoxin (Lanoxin) is the most commonly prescribed cardiac glycoside.

CONTRAINDICATIONS AND SIDE EFFECTS

In general, these drugs have a relatively narrow margin of safety between therapeutic range and toxic range. Levels near or in the toxic range may be very poorly tolerated. Toxicity is assessed on the basis of blood levels. Characteristic ECG changes associated with toxicity include bradycardia, prolongation of the P-R interval (first-degree heart block), and a shortening of the Q-T interval. Other arrhythmias may be observed as the conduction blockade at the AV node increases. Premature ventricular contractions, ventricular tachycardia, and supraventricular tachycardia may all be caused by the alteration in conduction in digitalis toxicity. Other side effects include nausea, vomiting, anorexia, drowsiness, fatigue, and confusion. Visual disturbances, like seeing yellow or green dots and experiencing double vision, are common.[3] Toxicity is facilitated by electrolyte imbalances, particularly hypokalemia.

Cardiac glycoside therapy is contraindicated in individuals with idiopathic hypertrophic subaortic stenosis (IHSS), diffuse cardiomyopathies, and constrictive pericarditis. Cardiac glycosides are contraindicated in pre-existing AV block. They are also contraindicated in individuals with increased cardiac automaticity, in which increased AV conduction time may precipitate tachyarrhythmias. In acute myocardial infarction, cardiac glycoside therapy is also contraindicated because the increased contractility increases myocardial oxygen demand and may extend an infarction.

EFFECTS ON EXERCISE IN THE INDIVIDUAL WITH CAD

The individual with CHF receiving cardiac glycoside therapy will demonstrate increased exercise tolerance because of the increased efficiency of the ventricular function and oxygen utilization. The ST and T-wave changes associated with cardiac glycoside therapy may mimic the ECG changes of ischemia. Evaluation of the individual's rhythm strip or 12-lead ECG at rest and exercise will permit definitive diagnosis.

CARDIAC GLYCOSIDES THERAPY MANAGEMENT

Careful consideration should be given to the following:

1. Familiarity with the effect of cardiac glycosides on the ECG is essential. The sagging ST segment may be mistaken for the ST depression seen in ischemia.
2. Arrhythmias associated with cardiac glycosides may be precipitated by exercise, especially if the patient is hypokalemic.
3. Individuals should learn to check their peripheral pulse daily and report brady-cardia or sustained tachycardia.
4. Nausea and vomiting are classic signs of digoxin toxicity (hypokalemia from persistent vomiting may precipitate toxicity).
5. Maintenance doses of digoxin, the most commonly prescribed cardiac glycoside, are 0.125 mg to 0.25 mg QD. Elderly individuals usually require smaller doses.
6. Caution should be taken during exercise because of potential visual disturbances with cardiac glycosides.

Antiarrhythmics

Antiarrhythmic drugs alter the conductivity and automaticity of the myocardium to correct abnormalities in electrical activity. Generally they suppress ectopic (impulses arising outside of the sinoatrial node, the normal pacemaker of the heart) stimuli, slow the rate of impulse generation and conduction, and decrease myocardial irritability.

There are five recognized classes of antiarrhythmics (Table 5–4). They are classified according to their mechanism of action:[3]

Class I agents: Suppress sodium (Na^+) channels and reduce conduction velocity
Class II agents: Cause increased potassium (K^+) conductance, decrease conduction velocity, and depress Na^+ conductance in ischemic tissue
Class III agents: Block sympathetic receptors or chemicals (beta blockers)
Class IV agents: Act selectively on repolarization and re-entry circuits and are most effective in abolishing ventricular fibrillation
Class V agents: Depress calcium (Ca^{++}) channels (calcium channel blockers)

TABLE 5–4. Common Antiarrhythmics

Generic Name (Trade Name)	Dosage	Class	ECG Changes	Implications/ Side Effects
Quinidine sulfate (Quinidex)	200–400 mg q 4–6 hr	I	Prolonged QT interval.	Severe nausea and diarrhea may make it intolerable. Observe ECG for prolonged QT interval of greater than 25%.
Quinidine gluconate (Quinaglute)	324 mg q 6 hr	I	Widened QRS complex.	
Procainamide hydrochloride (Pronestyl)	250–500 mg q 3–4 hr	I	Prolonged QT interval. Does increase AV conduction.	Use cautiously in digoxin toxicity, CHF.
Sustained-release (Procan SR)	500–1000 mg q 6hr	I		IV injection can cause severe hypotension. Systemic lupus erythematosus syndrome may develop.
Disopyramide (Norpace)	400–800 mg/day in divided doses	I	Significant widening of QRS. May cause second- or third-degree heart block.	Use cautiously with urinary retention or glaucoma. Specific for ventricular arrhythmias. May cause cardiac decompensation.
Lidocaine (Xylocaine)	50–100 mg IV rapidly. Repeat if necessary, followed by continuous drip intravenously titrated to control PVCs	II	Negligible ECG effects. Decrease or elimination of ventricular ectopy.	May cause disorientation, seizures. IM injection may be used to control PVCs (for 1 hr) until emergency center is reached.[3] May cause hypotension.
Propranolol (Inderal)	10–30 mg TID or QID	III	Increases PR interval. Slight decrease in the QT interval.	High doses may be necessary to control SVT. Observe for hypotension. Increases in heart rate with exercise will be less than in individual not on beta blockade.

(continued)

TABLE 5-4. Common Antiarrhythmics *Continued*

Generic Name (Trade Name)	Dosage	Class	ECG Changes	Implications/ Side Effects
Bretylium (Bretylol)	5-10 mg/kg IV over 30 min (Acute care setting only)	IV	May potentiate digitalis toxicity. Observe for prolonged PR interval. Resolution of ventricular arrhythmias.	Used in the acute care setting to treat refractory VT and VF. Hypotension is common. Nausea/vomiting may occur with rapid infusion; relieved by decreasing rate of infusion.
Verapamil (Calan, Isopton)	IV 0.1 to 0.15 mg/kg to treat SVT initially; maintenance oral dose 40-160 mg q 8 hr	V	Decreased heart rate. Control of SVT. Increased PR interval.	Observe for hypotension (infrequent). Contraindicated in CHF, cardiogenic shock, hypotension. Observe for reflux increase in heart rate with decreased cardiac output. Superior to digoxin in controlling atrial fibrillation.[3]

Generally, antiarrhythmics are beneficial hemodynamically because they restore normal heart rhythm and allow the heart to work efficiently. By restoring the normal rhythm, antiarrhythmics improve an individual's exercise tolerance.

CLASS I

Class I drugs are effective in the treatment of both atrial and ventricular arrhythmias, including atrial fibrillation, premature ventricular contractions, and ventricular tachycardia. Because they have little or no effect on the SA node, they are not effective against disturbances in SA node function. They cause a prolongation of the relative refractory period and a dose-related slowing of the AV junctional and interventricular conduction.

Two marked ECG changes seen with class I antiarrhythmics are a 25 to 50 percent elongation of the QRS complex and the QT interval. Therapy with these antiarrhythmics should be discontinued if ECG changes are observed because the increase in the vulnerable period of the ventricle can lead to the development of polymorphous ventricular tachycardia (VT), or torsade de pointes. Characterized by bursts of VT and an undulating QRS axis that cannot be converted by conventional antiarrhythmics, torsade de pointes is usually associated with bradycardia, prolongation of the QT interval, and hypokalemia. Progression to ventricular fibrillation is common and life-threatening.[47] Class I antiarrhythmics are administered with caution to patients with congestive heart failure. Table 5-4 includes some of the common class I antiarrhythmics.

Quinidine is one of the best-known class I antiarrhythmics. It is specific to atrial arrhythmias, although it is also effective for ventricular arrhythmias.

Quinidine is contraindicated in patients who are hypersensitive to it or who have conduction defects of the AV node, digitalis toxicity, or potassium imbalance. The most common side effects are severe nausea, diarrhea, and arrhythmias, including torsade de pointes. Quinidine is now used less often because of its significant side effects and the development of other drugs equally effective in the treatment of certain arrhythmias.

Procainamide is another class I antiarrhythmic commonly used in the treatment of both atrial and ventricular arrhythmias. It is, however, more specific to ventricular arrhythmias. Procainamide controls cardiac arrhythmias by decreasing myocardial automaticity, decreasing conduction velocity, and increasing the relative refractory period of the myocardial cells. It does not cause a change in myocardial oxygen demand during dynamic exercise but may mask ST depression. Gastrointestinal disturbances and fatigue are common side effects. Chronic therapy may result in systemic lupus erythematosus syndrome (SLE).

Class I Antiarrhythmic Management

Careful consideration should be given to the following:

1. Observe the ECG for prolongation of the QRS or QT interval.
2. Observe ECG for the development of new or recurrent arrhythmias.
3. With quinidine, observe for symptoms of CHF. It may reduce the risk of exercise-induced arrhythmias but may result in exertional ST-segment depression.
4. With procainamide, arthritic-like joint pains may be the first sign of SLE syndrome.

CLASS II

Class II antiarrhythmics are used in the treatment and control of both acute and chronic ventricular arrhythmias. They are generally ineffective in the treatment of atrial arrhythmias. They do not decrease conduction velocity and may actually increase the speed of propagation, which may prevent re-entry arrhythmias. They do not cause AV conduction blocks and cause negligible effects on ECG.[47]

Class II antiarrhythmics are contraindicated in individuals who show hypersensitivity to them.

Lidocaine, a class II antiarrhythmic, is the most frequently used antiarrhythmic in the treatment of acute ventricular arrhythmias associated with acute myocardial infarction, cardiac surgery, and other life-threatening situations. It is usually given intravenously and acts immediately to decrease ventricular irritability.

Lidocaine is contraindicated in individuals with a hypersensitivity to it and in those with a pre-existing bundle branch block. Its most common side effects are related to its anesthetic effects on the central nervous system. Agitation, disorientation, twitching, and seizures may occur, which are reversed with cessation of the drug (Table 5–4).

Phenytoin (Dilantin) is also a common class II antiarrhythmic used in the management of ventricular arrhythmias. Tocainide and ecainide are experimental class II drugs currently being investigated.[3]

Class II Antiarrhythmic Therapy Management
Particular attention should be given to the following:

1. Observe for change in mental status.
2. There are minimal ECG changes with class II antiarrhythmics.
3. In the acute care setting, lidocaine is administered when there is a new onset of greater than six PVCs per minute, multifocal PVCs, or ventricular tachycardia. In the cardiac rehabilitation setting, this may be an expected arrhythmia and handled according to what is "normal" for that individual.

CLASS III

Antiarrhythmics in class III are beta blockers. They block sympathetic stimulation at the SA node, increase the effective refractory period of the AV node, and reduce automaticity in the Purkinje fibers. Propranolol (Inderal) is currently the only beta blocker approved by the Food and Drug Administration (FDA) for use as an antiarrhythmic.[3]

Propranolol effectively slows ventricular response in individuals with supraventricular tachycardias (SVT). It is effective in the treatment of SVT precipitated by coronary artery disease or exercise.

Contraindications include heart block, CHF, and bradyarrhythmias due to the negative inotropic effect of propranolol. It is given with caution to diabetic patients because their sympathetic response to hypoglycemia may be masked.

Side effects include an exacerbation of congestive heart failure secondary to the negative inotropic effects and all other side effects previously identified for beta blockers.

Class III Antiarrhythmic Therapy Management
Particular attention should be given to the following:

1. An abrupt cessation of propranolol may exacerbate anginal pain in individuals with CAD.
2. Observe ECG for bradyarrhythmias and heart block associated with beta blockade therapy.
3. There is a decrease in resting and submaximal heart rate and blood pressure with beta blockers.
4. Decreased contractility and preload result in decreased myocardial oxygen demand and an increased tolerance for activity.

CLASS IV

The only class IV drug currently available is bretylium tosylate. A sympathetic blocking agent, it is used in the emergency treatment of ventricular arrhythmias refractory to treatment with other antiarrhythmics. Bretylium may potentiate digitalis toxicity (cardiac glycoside) because it causes a transient increase in norepinephrine release. Therefore, it should be administered with caution to individuals receiving digitalis. Side effects include hypotension and the related symptoms of light-headedness, dizziness, and vertigo.

Another drug, amiodarone (Cordarone), is currently being tested. With a slow onset of action (4 to 10 days), it may be useful for the long-term management of a variety of arrhythmias. Amiodarone prolongs the refractory period throughout the entire conduction system, reducing heart rate and decreasing myocardial oxygen demands. Currently, amiodarone is associated with several severe but reversible side effects.[3,10]

Class IV Antiarrhythmic Therapy Management
Careful attention should be given to the following: Currently bretylium is used only in the acute setting for emergency treatment of refractory ventricular arrhythmias.

CLASS V

Class V antiarrhythmics are the calcium channel blockers, of which only verapamil and diltiazem have significant electrophysiological effects. Verapamil, accepted for use as an antiarrhythmic, blocks the flow of extracellular calcium into cardiovascular cells in the SA and AV node. This prolongs SA and AV node refractory periods and conduction time. It effectively decreases ventricular response in supraventricular tachycardias. Verapamil also decreases myocardial contractility and is, therefore, contraindicated in CHF, severe hypotension, and cardiogenic shock. Side effects include hypotension, a reflex increase in heart rate, constipation, vertigo, and tremors.

Class V Antiarrhythmic Therapy Management
Careful attention should be given to the following:

1. Observe for signs of hypotension: light-headedness, dizziness, fatigue.
2. Monitor blood pressure.
3. Observe for symptoms of CHF (dyspnea, cough, decreased activity tolerance, peripheral edema).

Antihypertensives

There are a wide variety of medications used for the treatment of hypertension in the individual with CAD. Many of those drugs, including calcium channel blockers and beta blockers, have been discussed previously.

The goal of antihypertensive therapy is to obtain and maintain a diastolic pressure of less than 90 mmHg, without producing intolerable side effects.[3] The antihypertensive medications lower the blood pressure, decrease myocardial workload, and control some of the complications of hypertension. There are four types of antihypertensives, categorized by mechanism of action. The four types are centrally or peripherally acting sympathetic nervous symptom inhibitors, peripheral vasodilators, inhibitors of the renin-angiotensin mechanism of the kidney, and diuretics. The reader is referred to listed references for further information on specific antihypertensive agents.[1,3,5,6,12,23,34,36,40]

Additional Medications

Many other medications, either over-the-counter or prescription drugs, may impact cardiac function and exercise tolerance. These include caffeine, nicotine, psychotropic drugs (phenothiazines and tricyclic antidepressants), and alcohol. Because of the actions and interactions of many of these drugs, it is important that cardiac rehabilitation personnel monitor medication changes and make appropriate modifications in exercise prescriptions in relation to those changes.

Streptokinase

Streptokinase is a thrombolytic enzyme effective in dissolving thrombi and restoring patency to an occluded coronary artery during the early hours of an acute myocardial infarction. It can be administered indirectly by the intravenous route or directly by cardiac catheterization. Streptokinase therapy promotes the lysis of fibrin and circulating fibrinogen.[40] In coronary artery occlusion, the goal of streptokinase therapy is to restore coronary perfusion and minimize the size of the myocardial infarction. Most guidelines suggest that to be effective it should be initiated within 3 to 6 hours after the onset of chest pain.[42,44] A delay in therapy decreases the potential to salvage the myocardium. Streptokinase effectively lyses new clots for approximately 14 hours. The effect of this therapy is evaluated within 30 to 60 minutes after the start of therapy. Criteria for effectiveness include: abrupt abatement of chest pain, resolution of ST-segment elevation and T-wave changes, and abrupt and rapid increase in the release of creatine kinase (CK) into the blood.[44]

Randomized studies of intravenous and intracoronary streptokinase therapy have shown a reperfusion rate (re-establishing perfusion of the obstructed vessel) of 80 to 90 percent,[46] and others report results of 40 to 60 percent for intravenous streptokinase alone.[40] The clinical impact of this therapy depends specifically on how soon after the occlusion reperfusion is achieved.

There are several contraindications to streptokinase therapy: individuals with a predisposition to intracranial hemorrhage, infective endocarditis or known left ventricular thrombus, tuberculosis or bronchopleural fistula, recent surgery, severe liver impairment, and previous streptokinase infusion in greater than 5 days and less than 6 months. Streptokinase stimulates an immunological response and an increased titer of neutralizing antistreptokinase for up to 6 months; therefore, additional therapy with streptokinase may be ineffective.

The major side effects of streptokinase therapy include hemorrhage, arrhythmias, recurrent thrombosis, severe hypotension, and allergic reaction. Arrhythmias are a result of a reperfusion phenomenon from the alteration in electrical conduction in ischemic cells.

Currently, tissue plasminogen activator (t-PA) is being investigated as an alternative to IV streptokinase. It is clot specific and does not produce a systemic lytic state.[40]

THERAPEUTIC PROCEDURES AND SURGICAL INTERVENTION IN CORONARY ARTERY DISEASE

Surgical intervention and therapeutic procedures in coronary artery disease do not alter the atherosclerotic disease process. They improve the quality of life by relieving the symptoms of coronary artery disease (angina) and restoring myocardial perfusion. Both types of intervention contribute to improving the individual's tolerance for activity. Coronary disease is treated surgically with myocardial revascularization with coronary artery bypass grafting and by heart transplant. A special therapeutic technique used both acutely and electively to alter structural changes contributing to coronary stenosis is percutaneous transluminal coronary angioplasty (PTCA).

Coronary Artery Bypass Grafting

Coronary artery bypass grafting (CABG) is surgical revascularization of the myocardium (Fig. 5–1). It is accomplished by one or both of the following methods: (1) anastomosing grafts, usually the individual's own saphenous vein (SVG), to the aortic root and to the coronary artery distal to the stenosis and/or (2) direct revascularization by anastomosing the distal end of the internal mammary artery (IMA) to the coronary artery distal to the lesion. The use of the IMA graft is becoming more popular as studies indicate that the IMA conduit has an 85 to 95 percent patency rate 7 to 10 years post-bypass as opposed to the SVG rate of 52 percent.[19,22]

Postoperatively, the SVG conduits show progressive intimal proliferation and atherosclerotic plaque development and atherosclerosis is rarely observed in IMA conduits.[15, 22] Loop and others[19] found that individuals with IMA grafts over the first 10 years postsurgery had not only a higher graft patency rate, but also a lesser incidence of late

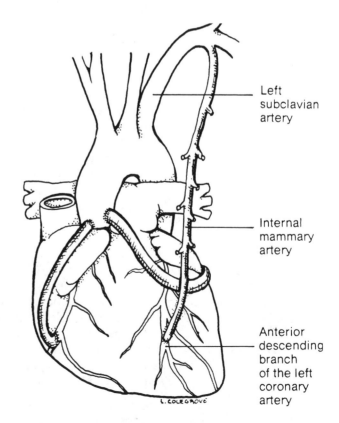

Left
subclavian
artery

Internal
mammary
artery

Anterior
descending
branch
of the left
coronary
artery

FIGURE 5–1. Coronary artery bypass graft using the SVG and IMA.

L. COLEGROVE

myocardial infarction, reoperation, and death than those who had only SVG conduits. The IMA is, however, limited by its length and anatomical position. It may be used to revascularize only the anterior portion of the heart and must be grafted to the left anterior descending coronary artery. In addition, the IMA is more difficult to dissect from the chest wall and may extend the length of the surgery up to an hour.[19] In dissecting the IMA, most often the pleural space must be entered to ensure appropriate dissection, although no increase in the incidence of postoperative pulmonary complications has been documented.[22]

Use of the IMA is contraindicated in patients with severe vascular disease of the upper extremities and in individuals who are unstable in surgery in which the extra time necessary for an IMA dissection and anastomosis would be detrimental.[19,20,22] Overall, the improved long-term results, primarily due to minimal graft atherosclerosis in the IMA conduit, may lead to more widespread use of the IMA graft.[24]

There are many indications for CABG surgery and the criteria for patient selection vary among institutions. The use of CABG surgery is changing as percutaneous transluminal coronary angioplasty (PTCA) has become increasingly more popular as an alternative. PTCA allows patients with single or multiple high-grade lesions to undergo a less traumatic procedure to relieve coronary artery occlusion. The criteria for patient selection for CABG generally include:

1. Stable angina with a high grade left main trunk (LMT) lesion.
2. Stable angina with triple vessel CAD.
3. Unstable angina with triple vessel CAD or severe two vessel disease.
4. Recent myocardial infarction with continued angina and
5. Ischemic heart failure with shock.[15]

The location and degree of stenosis caused by the lesion, the amount of myocardium served by the affected artery, and whether the individual has had a previous myocardial infarction are all considered when evaluating the need for surgical intervention. Usually a lesion of greater than 70 percent occlusion of the coronary artery is cause for consideration of surgical intervention. When the occlusion is in the LMT, surgery is considered earlier in the course of CAD. Surgery unquestionably enhances survival when a 50 percent or greater occlusion of the LMT is present.[13,17] In most individuals the LMT and its branches deliver 80 percent of the blood supply to the left ventricle and therefore, with a high-grade lesion, the risk of death from coronary artery occlusion is greater than the risk of surgery.[14,17]

Individuals are evaluated for surgery on the basis of their presenting symptoms, the coexistence of other chronic disease, and a battery of medical tests. The tests include blood studies, pulmonary function studies, electrocardiograms, and, most importantly, coronary arteriography and a left ventriculogram. Arteriography, performed under fluoroscopy, allows direct visualization of the extent and location of lesions and the status of the coronary circulation distal to the obstruction. This visualization allows the surgeon to determine, to a great extent, if bypassing the lesion will permit effective revascularization or if the disease process is so diffuse that the grafting would have little value. The ventriculogram allows for visualization of the left ventricular muscle function, identification of hypokinetic, poorly moving, or akinetic, immobile segments, and the measurement of pressures in the heart chambers, all of which provide vital information regarding the heart's effectiveness as a pump.

In CABG surgery, with the patient under anesthesia, a median sternotomy is performed. This allows direct visualization of the heart. The circulation is supported by means of an extracorporeal oxygenation pump (cardiopulmonary bypass pump) that allows the blood to bypass the heart, become oxygenated, and then flow to the systemic circulation. The heart is paralyzed by administration of a cold, hyperkalemic solution (cardioplegia) instilled into the coronary arteries.[18] The motionless heart allows the surgery to be performed more easily. From one to seven grafts are placed, using the SVG or the IMA as conduits. Four is the average number of grafts.[24] Following the procedure, the heart is rewarmed and the blood is again circulated through it. The heart beat either begins spontaneously or is initiated by means of internal defibrillation with a 5 watt-second stimulus.

Improvements in surgical techniques, coronary bypass pumps, cardioplegia, and myocardial preservation have decreased perioperative morbidity and mortality. These same improvements have safely allowed extended operative time to do more complete revascularizations.[24]

Operative mortality is 3 percent nationally,[24] with perioperative infarction and neurological incidents (secondary to some type of embolic episode) the greatest complications of CABG surgery.

Following uncomplicated CABG surgery, individuals progress rapidly. They are usually out of bed within 24 to 48 hours, ambulating from the hospital on the seventh to tenth day. Activities, particularly lifting, are restricted for 6 weeks to 3 months. Return to work is usually dictated by the patient's occupation, rate of recuperation, and duration of unemployment prior to surgery. Statistics indicate that the longer the individual is unemployed prior to surgery, the less likely the individual is to return to work.[13]

Postoperative recurrence of angina has also delayed the return to work for some individuals.[13] The improved myocardial blood supply due to the revascularization is intended to provide for improved left ventricular function, decreased incidence of myocardial infarction, and thus an increase in life expectancy.[25]

The most direct explanation for the "relief" of anginal pain is successful coronary revascularization and elimination of myocardial ischemia. There is excellent correlation between anginal relief and graft patency, but other mechanisms, including the infarction of angina-producing myocardium, the transection of afferent cardiac nerves during the procedure, and the placebo effect of surgery itself, are all offered as explanations for the 70 to 80 percent success rate for relief of angina with CABG.[14,15,24,25] Improved exercise tolerance has also been associated with complete revascularization.

Ten-year survival (excluding deaths within the postoperative hospital stay) has been found to be 86 percent with IMA grafts and 76 percent with SVG grafts. Graft patency observed in postoperative arteriography is the crucial determinant of longevity and freedom from other cardiac events.[14]

Again it should be emphasized that revascularization is not a cure for the atherosclerotic process. As evidenced by postsurgical coronary arteriography, atherosclerosis of the native vessels and of the grafts continues.[24,25] Life-style modifications to reduce CAD risk factors are an important adjunct to surgery for the CAD patient.

Percutaneous Transluminal Coronary Angioplasty

Percutaneous transluminal coronary angioplasty (PTCA), a procedure similar to cardiac catheterization, is being used with increasing frequency as an alternative to CABG surgery and the medical management of CAD (Fig. 5–2). Under fluoroscopy, a small balloon-tip catheter is inserted via the femoral artery and advanced in a retrograde fashion to the coronary arteries. The catheter is advanced across the stenotic area, and the balloon is intermittently inflated. The soft, noncalcified plaque is compressed into the intima of the coronary artery, thereby decreasing the stenosis. Pressure differences proximal and distal to the lesion are measured prior to and following the procedure. These values (gradients) are compared to determine the success of the dilation. Repeat arteriography with contrast media confirms the reduction of the stenosis, which permits significant improvement in myocardial blood flow.[17,18,30]

Criteria for patient selection include: single or multiple lesions in the proximal coronary arteries, anginal symptoms of less than one year, absence of diffuse disease distal to the primary lesion, and adequate left ventricular function. PTCA is usually done as an elective procedure but is also done in conjunction with streptokinase in the management of acute myocardial ischemia. The criteria are currently changing as success and continued experience allow the use of PTCA to be greatly expanded.[30]

Complications of PTCA include: acute occlusion of the coronary artery by spasm, clot, or collapse, coronary artery dissection or rupture, or myocardial infarction. A surgical team stands by to perform emergency CABG surgery, should the artery be ruptured by the attempt to dilate the vessel.[17,33]

Postprocedure, the individual is observed in the coronary care unit for 24 to 48 hours for any sign of arterial reocclusion. Upon discharge, generally patients have minimal activity restrictions and some individuals may return to work within a week. Initial research has shown that because of the minimal disability suffered with PTCA there is a correspondingly lower incidence of psychological problems in PTCA individuals as compared to individuals who undergo CABG.[31]

The long-term effectiveness of PTCA has not yet been determined. Many questions concerning the extent of the endothelial damage and the effect of the interaction between the balloon catheter and the vessel are not yet answered. It is known, however, that PTCA has resulted in improved myocardial blood flow, and individuals have reported immediate relief of their anginal pain while experiencing minimal surgical discomfort.[30] It should

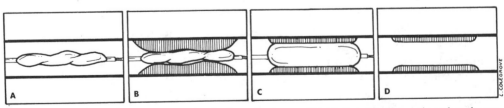

FIGURE 5–2. Percutaneous transluminal angioplasty. (A) Deflated balloon-tipped catheter. (B) Balloon-tipped catheter positioned within the atherosclerotic lesion. (C) With controlled pressure, the balloon is rapidly inflated and deflated to compress the soft plaque into the vessel walls. (D) After the balloon-tipped catheter is removed, the artery has improved patency.

also be emphasized that PTCA does not change or arrest the atherosclerotic process and that appropriate risk reduction techniques must be encouraged.

Heart Transplantation

Heart transplantation is performed in end-stage myocardial disease when the heart is too weak to maintain any appreciable cardiac output, and there is no expectation of recovery. These characteristics occur in idiopathic cardiomyopathy and end-stage coronary artery disease.

Transplantation is performed through a median sternotomy. The heart is removed from the donor by transecting the great vessels and the atria, dorsal to the atrial appendages. The recipient's heart is removed while he or she is maintained on cardiopulmonary bypass. The donor heart is anastomosed in the appropriate anatomical position.

The two major complications postoperatively are infection and rejection. Immunosuppressive therapy is used to minimize rejection; protective isolation is used to minimize the risk of infection. The first-year survival rate is 65 percent.[34]

The criteria for selection are stringent because the surgery and postoperative management are complex and the risk is high. Individuals are usually less than 50 to 60 years old; free of other chronic diseases, infection, and donor-specific antibodies; emotionally stable, and have a strong psychosocial support system.[17,34]

One of the major drawbacks to heart transplantation is the lack of available organs and the difficulties in procuring them. Currently research is ongoing in the use of the artificial heart as a mechanism to bridge the waiting period between the times when the individual's own heart fails and when a donor heart is available. Many surgeons presently feel that only temporary use of the artificial heart is appropriate because the quality of life with the artificial heart does not make its long-term use acceptable. The cost in terms of dollars, resources, and complications also weighs heavily against its use.[35]

CARDIAC REHABILITATION AND CAD

The World Health Organization defines cardiac rehabilitation as the "sum of activity required to ensure patients the best possible physical, mental and social conditions so that they may, by their own efforts, regain as normal a life as possible, a place in the community and lead an active and productive life."[39] Cardiac rehabilitation is an important adjunctive therapy in both the medical and surgical management of CAD. Medical and surgical interventions are designed to relieve the symptoms an individual experiences as a result of atherosclerosis. They do not alter the cause or the progression of the atherosclerotic process unless CAD patients concurrently recognize their risk factors and modify their lifestyles to reduce risk. With intense education and appropriate professional support, individuals are able to make and maintain specific changes in their life-styles in the general areas of diet, exercise, stress management, and compliance with medical therapy in order to reduce their own cardiac risk factors.

SUMMARY

Medical and surgical management of the individual with coronary artery disease was presented. Emphasis was placed on the following classes of drugs: nitrates, beta blockers, calcium channel blockers, cardiac glycosides, antiarrhythmics, and antihypertensives. Various combinations of these are used to control the symptoms of CAD, including pain, arrhythmias, congestive heart failure, and hypertension. Actions of the medications as well as common side effects were reviewed. The use of streptokinase as a thrombolytic agent in acute coronary artery occlusion is included.

Coronary artery bypass grafting and percutaneous transluminal angioplasty as effective means of attaining symptom relief were explained, with the emphasis that these techniques are not a cure for the progression of atherosclerosis.

Cardiac rehabilitation and risk factor reduction were briefly identified as important adjuncts to both medical and surgical management of coronary artery disease.

REFERENCES

1. Pharmacological intervention in coronary artery disease. In Vinsant, MO and Spence, MI: Commonsense Approach to Coronary Care. CV Mosby, St Louis, 1985.
2. Tannenbaum, RP, John, CA, Cantwell, R and Rogers, M: Angina Pectoris: How to Recognize; How to Manage It. Nursing 81 11:9, 1981.
3. Mathewson, MK and Umhauer, MA: Drugs affecting the cardiovascular system. In Mathewson, MK: Pharmacotherapeutics: A Nursing Process Approach. FA Davis, Philadelphia, 1986.
4. Spencer, RT: Drugs, affecting the nervous system: autonomic drugs. In Spencer, RT: Clinical Pharmacology and Nursing Management, ed. 2. JB Lippincott, Philadelphia, 1986.
5. Spencer, RT: Cardiovascular drugs: Drugs affecting the heart. In Spencer, RT: Clinical Pharmacology and Nursing Management, ed 2. JB Lippincott, Philadelphia, 1986.
6. Shepherd, JT: Circulatory response to beta adrenergic blockade at rest and during exercise. Am J Cardiol 55:810, 1985.
7. Silke B, et al: The effects on left ventricular performance of verapamil and metoprolol singly and together in exercise induced angina pectoris. Am Heart 109:1286, 1985.
8. Bigger, JT: A Primer of Calcium Ion Antagonists. Knoll Pharmaceutical, Whippany, NJ, 1980.
9. Froelicher, V, Sullivan, M, Myers, J and Jensen, O: Can patients with coronary artery disease receiving beta blockers obtain a training effect? Am J Cardiol 55:155D, 1985.
10. DeAngelis, R: Amiodarone. Crit Care Nurse 6:12, 1986.
11. Fletcher, GF: Exercise training during chronic beta blockade in cardiovascular disease. Am J Cardiol 55:1100, 1985.
12. Bruce, RA, et al: Excessive reduction in peripheral resistance during exercise and risk of orthostatic symptoms with sustained-release nitroglycerin and diltiazem treatment of angina. Am Heart J 109:1020, 1985.
13. Wenger, NK: Rehabilitation of the patient with atherosclerotic heart disease. In McIntosh, HD (ed): Cardiology Series, Vol. 3, No. 3. Parke-Davis, Morris Plains, NJ, 1980.
14. Winer, HE, Glassman, E and Spencer, FC: Mechanism of relief of angina after coronary bypass surgery. Am J Cardiol 44:202, 1979.
15. Wulff, KS and Hong, PA: Surgical intervention in coronary artery disease. In Underhill, SL, et al (eds): Cardiac Nursing. JB Lippincott, Philadelphia, 1982.
16. Kneisl, CR and Ames, SW: Adult Health Nursing. Addison-Wesley, Reading, MA, 1986.
17. Wulff, KS: Management of the cardiovascular surgery patient. In Brunner, LS and DS Suddarth: Textbook of Medical Surgical Nursing, ed 5. JB Lippincott, Philadelphia, 1984.
18. Woods, SL and Underhill, SL: Coronary heart disease: Myocardial ischemia and infarction. In Patrick, ML, et al (eds): Medical Surgical Nursing: Pathophysiological Concepts. JB Lippincott, Philadelphia, 1986.
19. Lewis, MR and Dehmer, GJ: Coronary bypass using the internal mammary artery. Am J Cardiol 56:480, 1985.
20. Barbour, DJ and Roberts, WC: Additional evidence for relative resistance to atherosclerosis of the internal mammary artery compared to the saphenous vein when used to increase myocardial blood supply. Am J Cardiol 56:488, 1985.

21. Kern, MJ, Eilen, SO and O'Rourke, R: Coronary vasomotion in angina at rest and effect of sublingual nitroglycerin on coronary blood flow. Am J Cardiol 56:488, 1985.
22. Loop FD, et al: Influence of the internal mammary artery graft on 10-year survival and other cardiac events. N Engl J Med 314:1, 1986.
23. Fowler, NO: Cardiac Diagnosis and Treatment, ed 3. Harper & Row Publishers, Hagerstown, MD, 1980.
24. Johnson, WD, Kayser, KL and Pedrazal, PM: Angina pectoris and coronary artery bypass surgery: Patterns of prevalence in occurrence in 3105 consecutive patients followed up to eleven years. Am Heart J 108:1190, 1984.
25. Kominski, K and Preston, T: Rehabilitation of the patient with coronary artery disease: Medical versus surgical. In Underhill, SL, et al (eds): Cardiac Nursing. JB Lippincott, Philadelphia, 1982.
26. Loop, LD: Atherosclerosis of the left main coronary artery: 5 year results of surgical treatment. Am J Cardiol 44:1979.
27. McGoon, DC: Cardiac surgery. In Brest, AN (ed): Cardiovascular Clinic. FA Davis, Philadelphia, 1982.
28. Behrendt, DM and Austen, WG: Patient Care in Cardiac Surgery, ed 3. Little, Brown & Co, Boston, 1980.
29. Warren, SC and Warren, SG: Coronary angioplasty: Current concepts. Am Fam Physician 32:145, 1985.
30. Hall, DP and Gruentzig, AR: Techniques of PTA of the coronary, renal, mesenteric and peripheral arteries. In Hurst, JW (ed): The Heart, Arteries and Veins, ed 5. McGraw-Hill, New York, 1986.
31. Raff, D, McKee, DC, Popio, KA and Haggerty, JJ: Life adaptation after PTCA and CABG. Am J Cardiol 56:395, 1985.
32. David, P, et al: Percutaneous transluminal angioplasty with variant angina. Circulation 66:695, 1982.
33. Diagnosis of coronary artery disease. In Vinsant, MO and Spence, MI: Commonsense Approach to Coronary Care. CV Mosby, St Louis, 1985.
34. Sokolow, M and McIlroy, MB: Clinical Cardiology. Lange Medical Publishers, Los Altos, CA, 1986.
35. A Critical Look at the Artificial Heart. In Hospital Ethics, American Hospital Association, Chicago, Jan/Feb 1986.
36. Oberman, A: Exercise and the primary prevention of cardiovascular disease. Am J Cardiol 55:100, 1985.
37. Wenger, NK and Fletcher, GF: Rehabilitation of the patient with atherosclerotic coronary heart disease. In Hurst, JW (ed): The Heart, Arteries and Veins, ed 5. McGraw-Hill, New York, 1986.
38. Shephard, RJ: The value of exercise in ischemic heart disease. A cumulative analysis. J Cardiac Rehabil 3:294, 1983.
39. Winslow, EBJ: Rehabilitation of the cardiac patient, program phases and rationale. Postgrad Med 71:114, 1982.
40. Dehn, MM, Blomquist, CG and Mitchell, JH: Clinical exercise performance. Clin Sports Med 3:319, 1984.
41. Sharma, CVRK, Ceila, G and Parisi, AF: Thrombolytic therapy. N Engl J Med 306:1268, 1982.
42. Lew, AS: Streptokinase in acute myocardial infarction: Guidelines for use. Hosp Therapy 11:35, 1986.
43. Lew, AS: Streptokinase in acute myocardial infarction: Post therapy management. Hosp Therapy 11:50, 1986.
44. Jennings, PB and Reimer, KA: Factors involved in salvaging ischemic myocardium: Effect of reperfusion of arterial blood. Circulation 68(Suppl I):25I, 1983.
45. Koren, G, et al: Prevention of myocardial damage in acute myocardial ischemia by early treatment with intravenous streptokinase. N Engl J Med 313:1384, 1985.
46. Anderson, JL, Marshall, HW and Askins, JC: A randomized trial of intravenous and intracoronary streptokinase in patients with acute myocardial infarction. Circulation 70:606, 1984.
47. Bond, EF and Underhill, SL: Antiarrhythmic drugs. In Underhill, SL, et al (eds): Cardiac Nursing. JB Lippincott, Philadelphia, 1982.

CHAPTER 6

The Electrocardiogram

An electrocardiogram (ECG) is a graphic representation of the electrical activity generated by the atria and ventricles. Impulse formation and conduction in the cardiac muscle generate weak electrical currents throughout the body.[7] The electrical impulses progressively depolarize the cardiac muscle and cause cardiac contraction.[1] By means of a galvanometer, the difference in potential between a positive and a negative area in the body is detected, amplified, and recorded. The electrocardiogram allows for indirect observation of the sequence of cardiac muscle excitation over any given period of time.

As electrical activity passes through the myocardium, it is detected by external skin electrodes placed at specific points on the body surface and recorded as a series of deflections on the ECG. The deflections or waves are known arbitrarily as P, Q, R, S, and T (Fig. 6–1). The upward deflections are positive, representing an electrical current moving toward the skin electrode. In both instances, the magnitude of the deflection represents the thickness of the muscle mass through which the current is being conducted (see section on waves, complexes, and intervals).

Each deflection or wave represents an aspect of the depolarization or repolarization of the cardiac muscle cells. Although this progressive wave of electrical current is infinitesimal, it can be detected by the skin electrodes as it passes through the heart. The wave of depolarization flows from the base of the heart to the apex. Depolarization, the change of the internal electrical potential of the cell from negative to positive, causes almost immediate myocardial contraction. Depolarization is followed by repolarization. During repolarization, the cells regain their electronegative state, and the heart is in a physically "quiet" state. Although the change in electrical potential during repolarization is seen on ECG, no physical activity accompanies this electrical activity.

It is important to note that the ECG is a recording of the electrical activity of the heart (depolarization and repolarization of the muscle cells) and not a recording of the actual contraction and relaxation of the myocardium that should occur a split second after the deflections are observed. The ECG is a composite of the total electrical activity of the heart at any given moment; therefore, every aspect of electrical activity is not discernible. Most notably, atrial repolarization, occurring in conjunction with ventricular depolarization, is "lost" in the QRS complex because of the greater voltage of the latter.

THE CARDIAC CYCLE AND IMPULSE CONDUCTION

The cardiac cycle is one complete period of depolarization and repolarization of the cardiac muscle cells. Because of the heart cells' unique properties of automaticity, rhythmicity, and conductivity, the heart may regularly initiate and propagate an impulse along its conduction pathway without nervous system influence (see Chapter 2). Every myocardial cell can initiate and propagate an impulse, but the sinoatrial node (SA node) is the "natural pacemaker" of the heart. It serves this function because the SA node cells maintain the lowest resting membrane potential in the heart's conduction system. They depolarize first, initiating the impulse [at a rate of 60 to 100 beats per minute (bpm)] that is propagated throughout the conduction system by the heart's "all or nothing" conduction property. If the SA node does not initiate an impulse at appropriate intervals (60 to 100 bpm) another ectopic focus in the atria may initiate the heart beat. An ectopic focus is a site outside the SA node that initiates an impulse. In the normal sequence of events, once the impulse leaves the SA node, it traverses the atria and ventricles in a progressive wave of depolarization. The atria have not been determined to have any specialized conduction pathways; therefore, the impulse is propagated from cell to cell within the muscle. Almost immediately, simultaneous contraction of the left and right atria occur. The impulse is relayed from the atria to the ventricles via a specialized conduction pathway known as the atrioventricular node (AV node).

The AV node also has the capacity to perform the pacemaker function (at a rate of 40 to 70 bpm) if it does not receive any stimulation from the SA node. In normal conduction, the impulse is slowed as it passes through the AV node. Ventricular depolarization rapidly proceeds as the impulse moves via the bundle of His to the left and right bundle branches and through the Purkinje fibers, terminating in the subendocardium. The ventricular septum is depolarized first, followed by almost simultaneous depolarization of the left and right ventricles. Despite the fact that the left ventricle is depolarized just a fraction of a second before the right, the ECG records all of the electrical activity of the ventricles as a composite, the QRS complex (see Fig. 6–1). Contraction of the ventricles normally occurs within a split second of depolarization of the myocardium and then ventricular recovery (cellular repolarization) begins immediately. The repolarization of the atrium occurs simultaneously with ventricular depolarization. After ventricular repolarization occurs, the entire myocardium is returned to its electronegative state, and one cardiac cycle is completed.

WAVES, COMPLEXES, AND INTERVALS

The ECG is composed of a series of waves, complexes, and intervals, including the P wave, QRS complex, T wave, ST segment, and PR interval (Fig. 6–1).

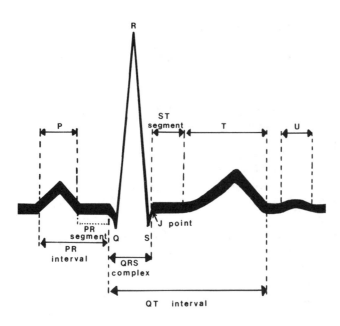

FIGURE 6–1. Normal PQRST wave configuration. ECG waves, complexes, and intervals. (From Underhill, et al: Cardiac Nursing. JB Lippincott, Philadelphia, 1983, p. 204, with permission.)

P Wave

The P wave is the first positive deflection on the ECG. It represents the depolarization of the atrial muscle cells following the release of an impulse from the SA node or some other focus in the atrium. The wave is symmetrical in appearance, usually 2.5 millimeters (mm) or less in height, and of 0.08 to 0.11 second duration (Fig. 6–2).

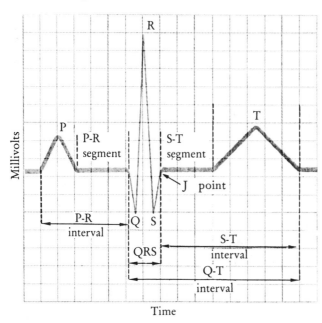

FIGURE 6–2. Normal electrocardiography and timing. Graphic representation of the normal electrocardiogram. Vertical lines represent time, each square represents 0.04 second, and every five squares (set off by heavy black lines) represents 0.02 second. The normal P-R interval is less than 0.02 second; the average is 0.16 second. The average duration of the P wave is 0.08 second; the QRS complex is 0.08 second; the S-T segment is 0.12 second; the T wave is 0.16 second; and the Q-T interval is 1.36 seconds. Each horizontal line represents voltage; every five squares equals 0.5 millivolt (mV). (From Hahn, et al: Mosby's Pharmacology in Nursing, ed. 16. CV Mosby, St. Louis, 1986, p. 432, with permission.)

P-R Interval

The PR interval is measured from the beginning of the P wave to the beginning of the QRS complex. It represents the time required for the impulse to travel from the atrium through the conduction system to the Purkinje fibers. The pause of the impulse at the AV node is within the PR interval. The entire atrial–AV node activity is 0.12 to 0.20 second in duration (see Fig. 6–2).

QRS Complex

The first negative deflection of the QRS complex is known as the Q wave and it is followed by the upward R wave. Small Q waves seen in leads I, II, V_4, and V_5 are usually insignificant. A large Q wave is not often present and may indicate a recent infarction. A diagnostically significant Q wave is usually 0.04 second in duration and one third the size of the QRS complex. The R wave is the first upward deflection followed by a downward deflection, the S wave. There are several variations of the QRS complex, but despite the variations all represent ventricular depolarization (Figure 6–3) and are collectively known as the QRS complex.[12] The QRS complex has an amplitude of 20 to 30 mm and a duration of 0.06 to 0.10 second. An increase in duration is a sign of delayed conduction through the ventricle. An amplitude of greater than 35 mm indicates ventricular hypertrophy. An amplitude of less than 5 mm may indicate coronary artery disease, emphysema, marked obesity, generalized edema, or pericardial effusion.

ST Segment

The ST segment begins at the end of the QRS complex and represents the beginning of ventricular muscle repolarization. It is generally isoelectric (returns to the baseline) but may rise above the isoelectric line 1 mm in normal individuals. (In healthy black males, the

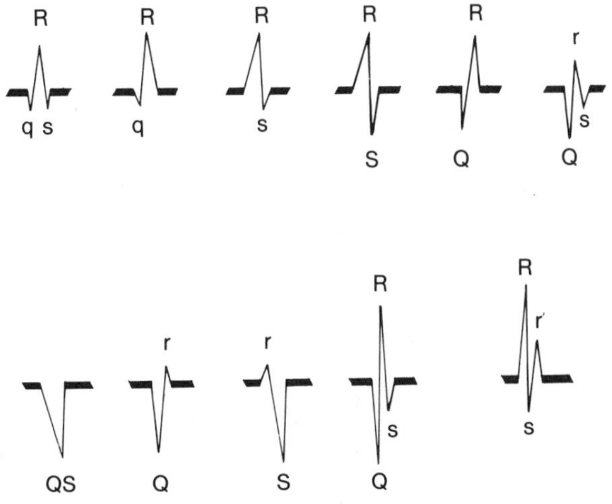

FIGURE 6–3. Variations in the QRS complexes. (From Bernreiter, M.: Electrocardiography. JB Lippincott, Philadelphia, 1963, p. 15, with permission.) Note that capital letters are assigned to large waves and lowercase letters to small waves.

ST segment may be elevated as much as 2 mm.) The point at which the ST segment begins is known as the J (junction) point (Fig. 6–4). In evaluation of the cardiac patient, the J point is significant, as ST-segment depression of greater than 1 mm occurring 0.08 second after the J point is indicative of ischemia and diagnostic of CAD (see Fig. 6–4).[21,22]

In an acute infarction, the ST segment is elevated, suggesting myocardial injury. Over time, weeks to months, the ST segment returns to the baseline. Prolonged ST-segment elevation suggests ventricular aneurysm. Generally the ST segment is an average of 0.12 second in duration and slopes gently upward to the isoelectric line and beginning of the T wave.

T Wave

Representing ventricular repolarization, the T wave is slightly rounded and slightly asymmetric. The deflection is in the same direction as the QRS, and the duration is about 0.16 second.

The time elapsed during the ST segment through the first half of the T wave is known as the absolute refractory period of the cardiac cycle. During this time, no impulse, no matter how strong, will be propagated through the ventricles. The second half of the T wave is referred to as the relative refractory period. During the relative refractory period, the vulnerable period and the cardiac cycle, a "stronger than normal" stimulus may initiate depolarization of the heart earlier than would normally be expected. A contraction resulting from this early impulse is known as a premature contraction. When premature ventricular depolarization occurs on the second half of the T wave, a lethal arrhythmia could be precipitated. This phenomenon is known as the R-on-T phenomenon.

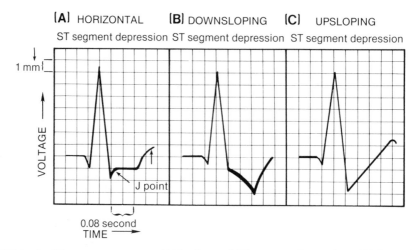

FIGURE 6–4. ST segment patterns: *(A)* horizontal ST segment depression, *(B)* downsloping ST segment depression, *(C)* upsloping ST segment depression. (From Vinsant, MO and Spence, MI: Common Sense Approach to Coronary Care. CV Mosby, St. Louis, 1985, p. 171, with permission.)

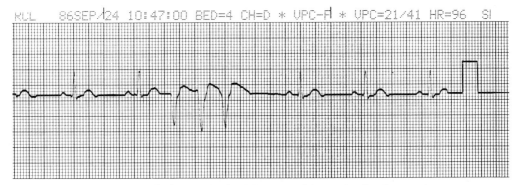

FIGURE 6-5. Standard ECG paper with standardization mark.

QT Interval

The QT interval represents electrical systole and extends from the beginning of the QRS complex to the end of the T wave.

Standard ECG Paper

ECG paper is standardized. It usually progresses through the cardiograph at a rate of 25 mm/second. Time is measured horizontally, with each small block equal to 0.04 second and each bold block 0.2 second (Fig. 6-5). Amplitude is measured vertically. Each small block equals 0.1 mV and is equivalent to 1 mm.

Standardization

Each electrocardiograph machine contains a 1 mV standard for calibration purposes which should appear on every ECG recording. The standard mark provides a manual check on the instrument's calibration. One mV of cardiac impulse should deflect the stylus exactly 1 centimeter (10 mm). The standard mark that appears on the ECG should be precisely 10 mm (1 cm) high, with a sharp upper left-hand corner. A slight sloping downward toward the right is normal. The shape and size of the standardization mark are significant, as lack of calibration may distort the ECG recording.

ECG Leads

Measurement of the normal ECG requires the use of 12 leads or reference points from which the electrical activity of the heart can be detected and subsequently viewed. Six leads are known as the limb leads (I, II, III, aVR, aVL, aVF) and six are known as the precordial or chest leads (V_1 through V_6). Leads I, II, and III are formed by three sides of a triangle connecting the right arm, left arm, and left foot. The heart is located approximately at the center of the triangle (Einthoven's triangle) formed by these three points (Fig. 6–6). An 80 to 90 percent accuracy in diagnosis can be ensured by correct interpretation of these three leads alone.

The limbs leads I, II, and III are bipolar. They represent the difference in electrical potential between two specific points in the body. Lead I is the difference of potential between the left arm (LA) and the right (RA). Lead II is the difference in potential between the left leg (LL) and the right arm. Lead III is the difference in potential between the left leg and the left arm. The unipolar leads, aVF, aVL, and aVR, represent a difference in electrical potential between one positive lead and the average of the potential between the other two leads. Lead aVR (augmented voltage right) is the difference in potential between the right arm and the average of the potential of the left arm and the left leg (Fig. 6–7). Lead aVL (augmented voltage left) is the difference in potential between the left arm and the average of the potential between the left leg and the right arm. Lead aVF (augmented voltage foot) is the difference in potential between the left leg and the average of the potential between the left arm and right arm (see Fig. 6–7).[2] The wave forms of the aV leads are augmented (increased in size) in order to get wave forms of ample magnitude for evaluation.

The six limb leads intersect at 30° angles to form six intersecting reference lines in the frontal plane of the heart (Fig. 6–8). The six chest or precordial leads (V_1, V_2, V_3, V_4, V_5, and V_6) reflect the limb leads and are marked at six different positions, right to left, across the chest (Fig. 6–9); these leads are all positive. Normally on an ECG, the QRS will become progressively more positive from V_1 to V_6 (right to left across the chest) because the chest leads follow the same vectors as the electrical activity of the heart (Fig. 6–10). The chest leads record the electrical potential under each electrode compared to the central terminal connection, or "V," which is made by connecting wires from the right arm, left arm, and left leg. The electrical potential of the V does not vary significantly throughout the cardiac cycle. Therefore, the recordings made with the V-connections show the electrical activity that is occurring under each precordial electrode. In all 12 leads, the right leg serves as the ground or indifferent lead. Extraneous electrical activity is minimized by utilizing a ground lead.

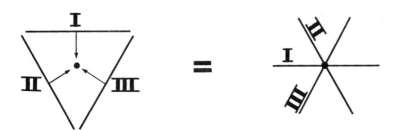

FIGURE 6–6. Vectors of Leads I, II, and III. By pushing these three leads to the center of the triangle, there are three intersecting lines of reference. (From Dubin, D.: Rapid Interpretation of EKG. Cover Publishing Co., Tampa, FL, p. 29, 1970, with permission.)

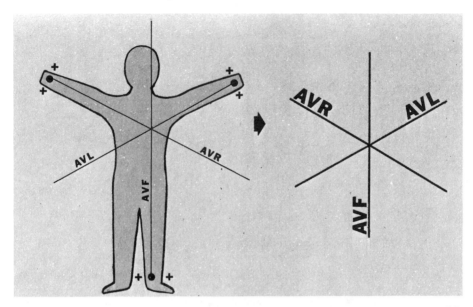

FIGURE 6–7. The unipolar limb leads. The aVR, aVL, and aVF leads intersect at different angles and produce three other intersecting lines of reference. (From Dublin, D.: Rapid Interpretation of EKG. Cover Publishing Co., 1970, p. 32, Tampa, FL, with permission.)

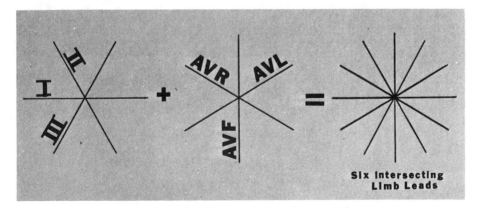

FIGURE 6–8. The limb leads. All six leads, I, II, III, aVR, aVL, and aVF, meet to form six neatly intersecting reference lines which lie in a flat plane on the patient's chest. (From Dublin, D.: Rapid Interpretation of EKG. Cover Publishing Co., 1970, p. 33, Tampa, FL, with permission.)

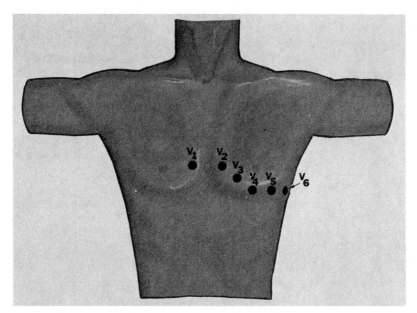

FIGURE 6–9. Chest lead reference sites. To obtain the six chest leads, a positive electrode is placed at six different positions around the chest. (From Dubin, D.: Rapid Interpretation of EKG. Cover Publishing Co., 1970, p. 37, Tampa, FL, with permission.)

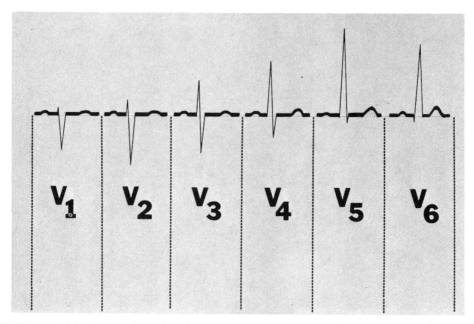

FIGURE 6–10. Progression of positive amplitude V_1–V_6. The ECG tracing will thus show progressive changes from V_1 to V_6. (From Dubin, D.: Rapid Interpretation of ECG. Cover Publishing Co., 1970, p. 39, Tampa, FL, with permission.)

Lead Placement

ECGs of the highest quality are necessary for meaningful interpretation. The quality of an ECG depends on both equipment and proper technique in recording the electrical events. Proper skin preparation (cleansing the skin with acetone or alcohol to reduce skin resistance and shaving the electrode site to ensure secure lead placement), as well as the selection of appropriate lead sites, ensures a definitive tracing. The limb leads are placed on the extremities. To ensure maintenance of good contact, they may be placed proximally when doing ECGs or monitoring during exercise testing and therapy (Fig. 6–11).

Although the 12-lead ECG gives the most complete view of the heart, it may be inappropriate during exercise therapy. Modified lead placement for exercise is effective. It

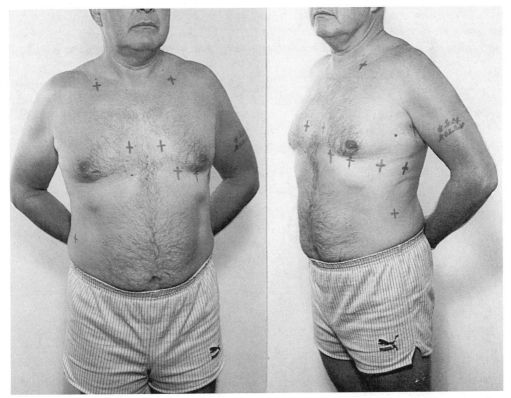

FIGURE 6–11. Electrode placement for a 12-lead exercise ECG recording. Electrode location and identification is as follows: (1) RL (Right leg): Just above the right iliac crest on the mid-axillary line. (2) LL (Left leg): Just above the left iliac crest on the mid-axillary line. (3) RA (Right arm): Just below the right clavicle medial to the deltoid muscle. (4) LA (Left arm): Just below the left clavicle medial to the deltoid muscle. (5) V_1: Fourth interspace at the right sternal margin. (6) V_2: Fourth interspace at the left sternal margin. (7) V_3: Midway between V_2 and V_4. (8) V_4: Fifth interspace at the mid-clavicular line just below the nipple. (9) V_5: Midway between V_4 and V_6 on the anterior axillary line. (10) V_6: Same traverse line as V_4 at the mid-axillary line. (From Brannon, F.J.: Experiments and Instrumentation in Exercise Physiology. Kendall-Hunt, Dubuque, 1978, p. 101, with permission.)

is not cumbersome to the individual and will not impede activity. In most cases, one lead alone will be sufficient to observe for arrhythmias.

A modified chest lead V_5 (CMV$_5$) may be recommended for exercise monitoring. It minimizes interference and permits ease of defibrillation should an emergency arise (Fig. 6–12). Ninety-eight percent of arrhythmia disturbances are thought to be detected by CMV$_5$ during exercise testing and therapy.[10,14]

The 12-Lead ECG

The interpreter of the ECG can gain a great deal of information from the 12-lead composite. Particular alterations in the depolarization and repolarization patterns reflect myocardial pathology. By carefully reviewing the 12 different views of the heart, the pathologic problem may be localized. Of course, the ECG must always be interpreted in conjunction with other clinical data, including lab results and the individual's activity tolerance and state of well-being.

Table 6–1 describes the characteristics of wave configuration for each lead of a

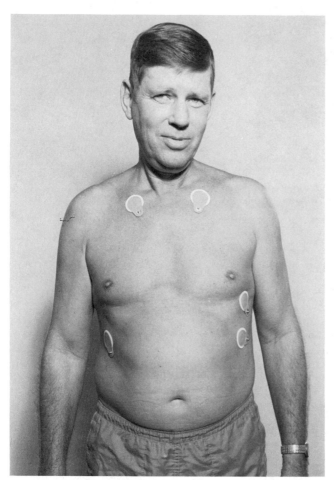

FIGURE 6–12. A modified chest lead V_5 (CMV$_5$). RL: Right leg. LL: Left leg. RA: Right arm. LA: Left arm. V_5: Left fifth intercostal space on the anterior axillary line.

TABLE 6–1. Normal Ranges & Variations in the Adult Twelve-Lead Electrocardiogram
A true understanding of the normal range and the normal variation of the ECG depends upon a basic understanding of both normal and abnormal cardiac electrophysiology. It must be remembered that many of the configurations tabulated below may represent cardiac abnormalities when interpreted in the context of the entire tracing and in the light of the clinical history and physical examination. Therefore, the information contained in the following table is intended to be used only as a rough preliminary guide to the interpretation of ambiguous and borderline tracings.

Lead	P	Q	R	S	T	ST
I	Upright deflection	Small. <0.04 s and <25% of R.	Dominant. Largest deflection of the QRS complex.	< R, or none	Upright deflection	Usually isoelectric; may vary from +1 to −0.5 mm.
II	Upright deflection	Small or none	Dominant	< R, or none	Upright deflection	Usually isoelectric; may vary from +1 to −0.5 mm.
III	Upright, flat, diphasic, or inverted, depending on frontal plane axis.	Small or none, depending on frontal plane axis; or large (0.04–0.05 s or >25% of R).	None to dominant, depending on frontal plane axis.	None to dominant, depending on frontal plane axis.	Upright, flat, diphasic, or inverted, depending on frontal plane axis.	Usually isoelectric; may vary from +1 to −0.5 mm.
aVR	Inverted deflection	Small, none, or large	Small or none, depending on frontal plane axis.	Dominant (may be QS)	Inverted deflection	Usually isoelectric; may vary from +1 to −0.5 mm.
aVL	Upright, flat, diphasic, or inverted, depending on frontal plane axis.	Small, none, or large, depending on frontal plane axis.	Small, none, or dominant, depending on frontal plane axis.	None to dominant, depending on frontal plane axis.	Upright, flat, diphasic, or inverted, depending on frontal plane axis.	Usually isoelectric; may vary from +1 to −0.5 mm.
aVF	Upright deflection	Small or none	Small, none, or dominant, depending on frontal plane axis.	None to dominant, depending on frontal plane axis.	Upright, flat, diphasic, or inverted, depending on frontal plane axis.	Usually isoelectric; may vary from +1 to −0.5 mm.
V_1	Inverted, flat, upright, or diphasic	None (may be QS)	<S, or none (QS); small r′ may be present.	Dominant (may be QS)	Upright, flat, diphasic, or inverted*	0 to +3 mm

(continued)

TABLE 6–1. *Continued*

Lead	P	Q	R	S	T	ST
V_2	Upright; less commonly, diphasic or inverted.	None (may be QS)	<S, or none (QS); small r' may be present.	Dominant (may be QS)	Upright; less commonly, flat, diphasic, or inverted.*	0 to +3 mm
V_3	Upright	Small or none	R <, >, or = S	S >, <, or = R	Upright*	0 to +3 mm
V_4	Upright	Small or none	R > S	S < R	Upright*	Usually isoelectric; may vary from +1 to −0.5 mm.
V_5	Upright	Small	Dominant (<26 mm)	S<SV$_4$	Upright	
V_6	Upright	Small	Dominant (<26 mm)	S<SV$_5$	Upright	

*Inverted in infants, children, and occasionally in young adults.
(From Goldman, MJ: Principles of Clinical Electrocardiography, 12th ed. Lange Medical Publications, Los Altos, California, 1986, with permission.)

normal 12-lead ECG, and Figure 6 – 13 represents a normal ECG. The reader is referred to any of the many excellent ECG interpretation texts for more in-depth interpretation of the ECG.[5-7] In this text, information will be reviewed regarding the basic interpretation of the most commonly occurring cardiac arrhythmias.

A standard 12-lead ECG tracing is normally used for diagnostic purposes. Arrhythmia detection in the hospital setting and in the outpatient cardiac rehabilitation setting may be accomplished easily and accurately by monitoring a single lead (lead I, II, or CMV$_5$ may be used). In cardiac rehabilitation settings, telemetry systems, in which the individual's ECG is transmitted via radio waves to a remote observer, are most often used to free the patient from the hardwire connection of the oscilloscope and to allow for unencumbered exercise.

INTERPRETING THE ECG

Learning to interpret the 12-lead ECG takes a great deal of time and practice. In this text the primary focus is the basic interpretation of single-lead ECGs or rhythm strips. Evaluation of the rate, rhythm, individual wave form, and their relationships to each other will prepare the reader for basic interpretation. This skill is necessary for safely monitoring patients during exercise testing and exercise therapy. Individuals involved in cardiac rehabilitation programs most frequently have atherosclerosis of the coronary arteries. This condition interferes with the heart's normal response to exercise and increased myocardial oxygen demand. Such an individual most likely has a lower ischemic threshold and a more limited activity tolerance than individuals with healthy coronary arteries. Therefore, the clinician must be alert to the possibility of rate-dependent blocks and rhythm disturbances at low levels of activity.

In order to properly interpret an ECG strip, the clinician must answer five questions:

1.   What is the rate?
2.   What is the rhythm? Is it regular or irregular?
3.   Are there P waves?
4.   What is the QRS duration?
5.   By evaluating the PR interval, what is the relationship between the P waves and the QRS complexes?

The following text describes how to answer these five questions and will enable the reader to identify common cardiac arrhythmias.

Calculating the Rate

The sinoatrial (SA) node is the natural pacemaker of the heart. It has an intrinsic rate of 60 to 100 bpm. When, for some reason, the SA node does not fire, there are many other pacemakers in the atria, ectopic foci, that can take over the pacemaker function. An ectopic focus is a potential pacemaker site somewhere outside the SA node that can take over as the pacemaker if the SA node is not effective.[2] Ectopic atrial pacemakers discharge at a rate of approximately 75 bpm, but this rate may increase to 150 to 250 bpm in pathologic situations. The intrinsic rate of the AV node is approximately 60 bpm, and it may assume pacemaker activity when no impulse is received from the atria. Pathologic conditions may cause an ectopic focus in the ventricle to fire at a rate of 150 to 250 bpm although the intrinsic rate of the ventricle is 20 to 40 bpm.

The heart rate is the first determination to be made in interpreting an ECG. One of the simplest methods utilized is to count the number of QRS complexes in a 6-second strip and multiply by 10 (chart speed = 25 mm/sec). (Standard ECG paper has three second marks across the top of the paper; see Fig. 6 – 15). A second method is looking at consecutive R waves. Find an R wave that falls on a heavy black vertical line on the ECG paper. Count off 300, 150, 100 on each of the heavy black lines that follow in succession. (Do not count the initial R wave that was selected.) Continue to count off 75, 60, 50 on the next three successive dark lines. (These numbers must be memorized.) Now, look for the next R wave by scanning to the right of the initial R wave identified. Where the next R wave falls will estimate the rate. If the second R wave falls between 2 heavy black lines, the location of its position between the two lines will affect the estimation of the rate (Fig. 6 – 14). This method allows the reader to quickly look at an ECG strip and roughly estimate the heart rate.[2,10] These two methods may be utilized for calculating the rate of regular rhythms, a rhythm where there is a constant interval between similar waves. Irregularly occurring rhythms are best estimated by counting the R waves that occur in a minute. Rates greater than 100 bpm are, by definition, tachycardias, and rates below 60 bpm are bradycardias.

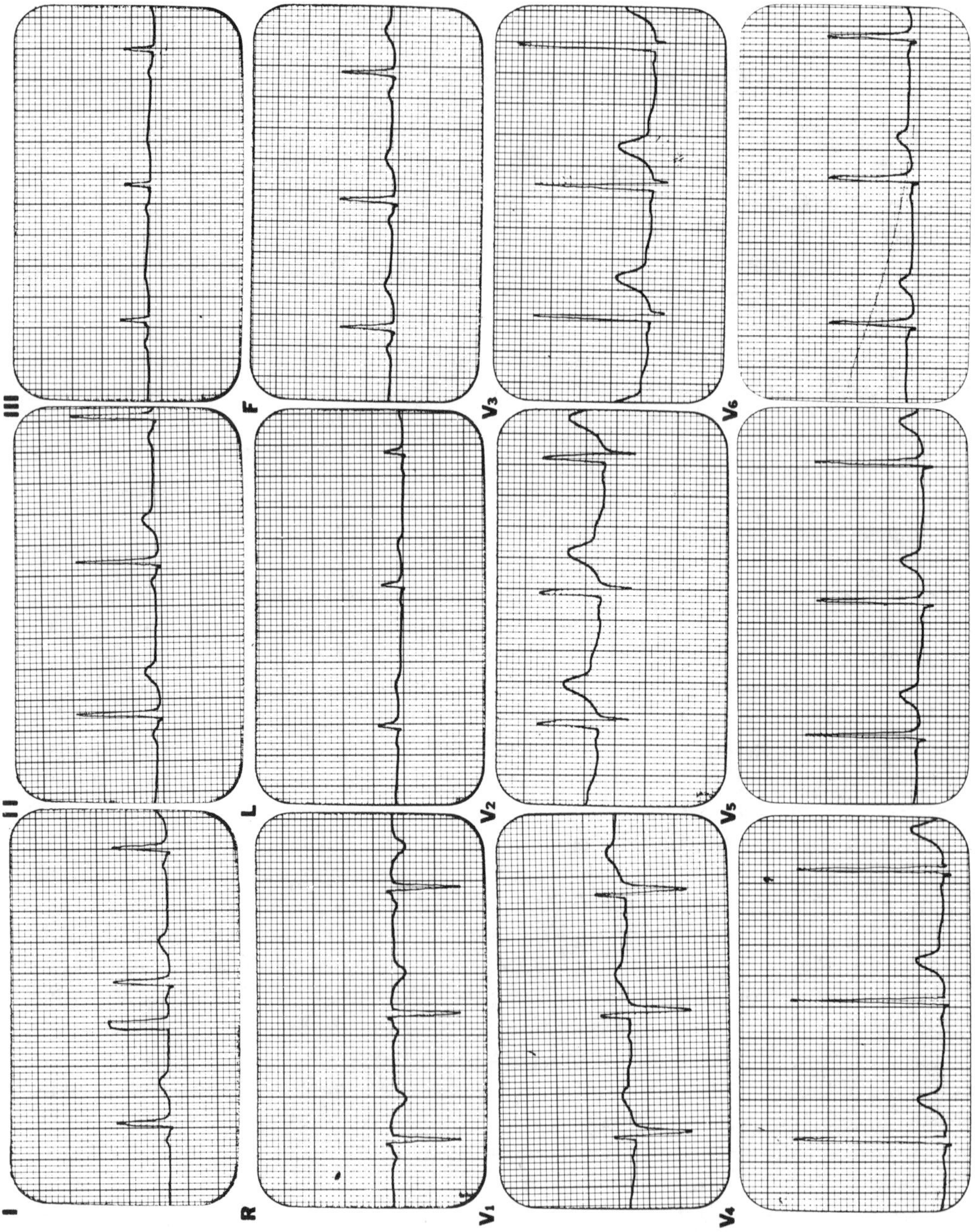

FIGURE 6–13. Normal 12-lead ECG.

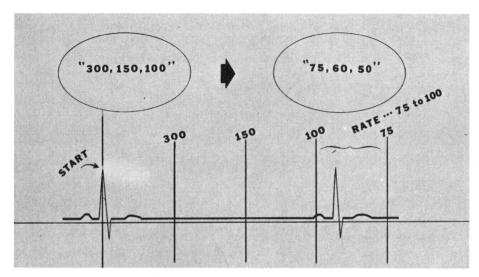

FIGURE 6–14. Calculating the heart rate. Note that the series of numbers assigned to the successive heavy black lines must be memorized: 300, 150, 100, 75, 60, 50. This figure represents an approximate rate of 90 bpm. (From Dubin, D.: Rapid Interpretation of EKG. Cover Publishing Co., Tampa, FL, 1970, p. 58, with permission.)

Determining the Rhythm

In a regular rhythm, there is a consistent distance between similar waves. The normal sinus rhythm (NSR) of the heart is a regular rhythm occurring at a rate of 60 to 100 bpm. Irregular rhythms may be regularly irregular, in which patterns of irregularity are identified and repeated, or they may be completely chaotic and termed irregularly irregular (Fig. 6–15). Disturbances in rhythm, cardiac arrhythmias, are caused by an abnormality in automaticity (initiation of the impulse), an abnormality in conduction (propagation of the impulse), or both. Disturbances in automaticity may be either decreased automaticity of the SA node, which may force an ectopic focus to take over or "escape," or enhanced

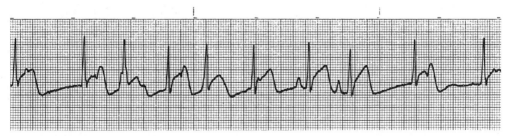

FIGURE 6–15. Ventricular response is irregularly irregular. There is no pattern to the occurrence of the R waves. Note the 3-second marks across the ECG paper.

automaticity of an ectopic focus, in which the ectopic focus may actively "usurp" or override the sinus pacemaker. The ectopic focus may be a point anywhere in the atria, AV node, or ventricles. Disturbances in conduction are the result of a block at some point in the conduction system that may be a result of ischemia to that area. Identification of arrhythmias is based on the location of their origination in the conduction system and by the characteristics of the particular rhythm.

Characteristics of Rhythms

NORMAL SINUS RHYTHM (NSR)

Definition and Cause. NSR is the conventional rhythm of the healthy heart (Fig. 6–16, Table 6–2). Arising from the SA node, the impulse follows normal conduction pathways. It is a regular rhythm, although there may be some phasic variation with respiration, increasing with inspiration and decreasing with expiration. This is frequently seen in young adults. The rate may also be influenced by exercise, emotions, environmental and body temperature, drugs, and various disease states.

Hemodynamic Implications. None.

Treatment. No treatment necessary.

SINUS BRADYCARDIA

Definition and Cause. A sinus bradycardia is a slow rhythm of less than 60 bpm originating from a supraventricular source. It occurs normally during sleep and is commonly seen in individuals who are physically fit. It also occurs in response to increased vagal tone owing to gastrointestinal (GI) distress, pain, carotid sinus pressure, ocular pressure, increased intracranial pressure, and acute myocardial infarction. Administration of digoxin, beta-adrenergic blocking agents, and calcium ion antagonists may also cause bradycardia.

ECG Appearance. All waves (Fig. 6–17) are of normal configuration with a rate of less than 60 bpm.

Hemodynamic Implications. Unless bradycardia is profound (less than 40 bpm), it is well tolerated. However, if cardiac output is not adequate, the individual is compromised hemodynamically and exhibits signs of decreased cardiac output (cold, clammy skin, low blood pressure, syncope).

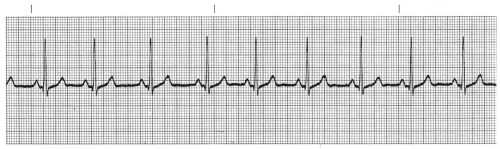

FIGURE 6–16. Normal sinus rhythm.

TABLE 6-2. Normal Configuration of ECG Waves

	Duration	Amplitude
P wave	0.8-1.2 sec	1-3 mm
PR interval	0.12-0.20 sec	Isoelectric after the P-wave deflection
QRS	0.06-0.10 sec	25-30 mm (maximum)
ST segment	0.12 sec	$-\frac{1}{2}$ to $+1$ mm
T wave	0.16 sec	5-10 mm

Treatment. Uncomplicated bradycardia requires no treatment. If the individual is compromised by the slow rate, atropine administered intravenously rapidly and dramatically increases the heart rate. Temporary or permanent pacing may be necessary if there is profound, poorly tolerated bradycardia.

SINUS TACHYCARDIA

Definition and Cause. Tachycardia is a rapid sinus rhythm of greater than 100 bpm. A sinus rhythm originates in the sinoatrial node. Anything that increases sympathetic activity, such as excitement, pain, fever, hypovolemia, hypoxia, strenuous exercise, and the consumption of caffeine and nicotine, are frequent causes of tachycardia. Cardiac failure, myocardial infarction, and many other diseases of the heart are accompanied by sinus tachycardia. It may also be induced by administration of drugs, including Isuprel, atropine, epinephrine, and alcohol.

ECG Appearance. Wave forms are normal (Fig. 6-18). The rate is greater than 100 bpm.

Hemodynamic Implications. Unless associated with a pathological state, sinus tachycardia is usually inconsequential and of brief duration. The rapid heart rate, however, increases myocardial oxygen demand and may decrease coronary artery perfusion, resulting in angina in the individual with CAD. Symptoms of low cardiac output might also be exhibited in those cases in which the decreased diastolic time prevents adequate ventricular filling.

Treatment. Intervention should include rest and treatment of the underlying pathological state. Oxygen and sublingual nitroglycerin may be necessary if the individual experiences angina. Digoxin may be administered to increase contractility, slow AV conduction, and decrease the heart rate, particularly if the patient is symptomatic.

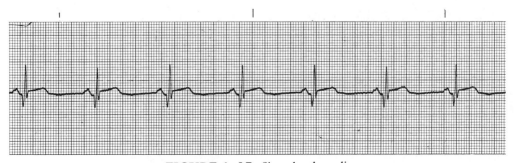

FIGURE 6-17. Sinus bradycardia.

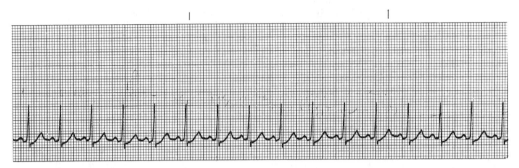

FIGURE 6–18. Sinus tachycardia.

SINUS ARRHYTHMIA

Definition and Cause. A sinus arrhythmia is a varying irregular rhythm with all impulses originating in the SA node. It may occur in the young and the elderly, in response to enhanced vagal tone, digitalis, or morphine.[3] The arrhythmia may be related to respiration, with the rate increasing with inspiration and decreasing with expiration.

ECG Appearance. All waves are normal in size and shape (Fig. 6–19), but the timing of the cycles is irregular. The rate is usually between 60 and 100 bpm.

Hemodynamic Implications. There are usually no hemodynamic consequences of sinus arrhythmia.

Treatment. No treatment necessary.

Atrial Arrhythmias

Atrial arrhythmias are caused by the rapid and repetitive firing of one or more foci in the atria outside the sinus node. They override the slower SA node pacemaker and take control of the rhythm of the heart. In atrial arrhythmias with rates of less than 200, every impulse may be conducted through the AV node to the ventricles (1 : 1 conduction). At rates greater than 200, the physiologic refractory period of the AV node introduces a block to conduction and therefore the conduction ratio (atrial : ventricular impulses) may be 2 : 1, 3 : 1, or greater. On the ECG, the P waves are variable in shape and rhythm, depending on

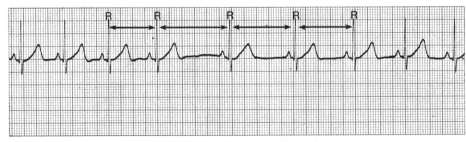

FIGURE 6–19. Sinus arrhythmia.

the location of the ectopic focus. The configuration of the QRS may be normal because the conduction pathways below the AV node are normal. However, the rhythm may be very irregular because the atrial impulses are often conducted in an irregular pattern.

WANDERING ATRIAL PACEMAKERS

Definition and Cause. The wandering atrial pacemaker is a varying rhythm caused by the changing focus of the pacemaker. It occurs when there is a change in vagal tone or changes in sympathetic stimulation to the heart.

ECG Appearance. The atrial rate is very irregular. There is no consistent pattern to the rhythm (Fig. 6–20). The shape of the P waves and the length of the PR intervals vary, depending on the pacemaker firing and the proximity of the ectopic pacemaker to the AV node. When the pacemaker site is closer to the AV node, the PR interval is shorter and the P wave becomes flatter. The ventricular rate is equal in rate and rhythm to the atrial rate, as all atrial impulses are conducted to the ventricle. The QRS is normal in appearance, as ventricular conduction is normal.

Hemodynamic Implications. There are no hemodynamic consequences because the rate is usually 60 to 100 bpm and cardiac output is maintained.

Treatment. No treatment is necessary unless the rate is too slow and then a sympathomimetic drug (Isuprel) may be administered. (Sympathomimetic drugs are synthetic substances of similar chemical structure and have many effects similar to adrenergic neurohormones. They act upon the alpha and beta receptors, increase heart rate and contractility, and accelerate conduction.) If the rate is over 100 bpm, treatment is directed toward eliminating the cause and decreasing the heart rate with a beta blocker such as propranolol.

PREMATURE ATRIAL CONTRACTIONS (PACs)

Definition and Cause. A PAC is an earlier than expected depolarization from an ectopic focus. The impulse travels through the atria by an unusual pathway and creates a P wave of a different configuration. If the ventricle is not in absolute refractory at the time the impulse reaches the AV node, the impulse will be conducted normally through the

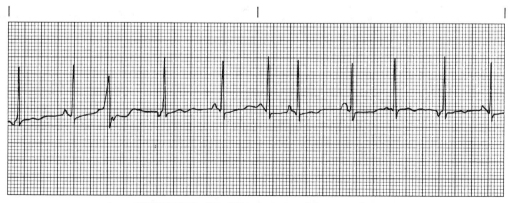

FIGURE 6–20. Wandering atrial pacemaker.

ventricles and produce a normal QRS complex. PACs are seen in the healthy heart as well as in those with CAD. Many other pathologic conditions may cause the development of PACs, including rheumatic heart disease, myocardial infarction, hypertension, and hyperthyroidism. Stress, fatigue, and anxiety may cause PACs, as will the administration of epinephrine and digoxin and the ingestion of stimulants (caffeine, nicotine).

ECG Appearance. NSR is present except for the PAC, which occurs earlier than expected (Fig. 6–21). The P wave of the PAC is abnormal, but all other waves are normal in configuration.

Hemodynamic Implications. PACs are usually well tolerated, as cardiac output is not altered.

Treatment. The only treatment is to omit the stimulus that may be precipitating the PACs (i.e., digoxin, caffeine, nicotine).

PAROXYSMAL ATRIAL TACHYCARDIA (PAT)

Definition and Cause. PAT is a rapid atrial rhythm characterized by abrupt onset and abrupt cessation. It is triggered by emotions, tobacco, fatigue, caffeine, alcohol, or sympathomimetic drugs (Isuprel). It is not usually related to organic heart disease. The rhythm may be sustained for seconds, minutes, or hours, and the patient's tolerance for this arrhythmia may depend upon the underlying pathology. The rate is usually 150 to 250 bpm, and there is a 1:1 atrial to ventricular conduction.

ECG Appearance. The P wave is slightly to grossly abnormal and may often be found in the preceding T wave (Fig. 6–22). The PR interval may be shortened (less than 0.12 second). QRS-complex and T-wave configurations are normal. In rapid rhythms, the T wave may not be discernible.

Hemodynamic Implications. PAT of short duration is of little consequence to the healthy heart. However, in the presence of an impaired left ventricle, sustained PAT may precipitate left ventricular failure. Angina may also occur as a result of decreased coronary artery blood flow.

Treatment. Treatment is directed at both eliminating the cause of the tachycardia and decreasing the heart rate. Carotid sinus massage or valsalva maneuvers are usually the

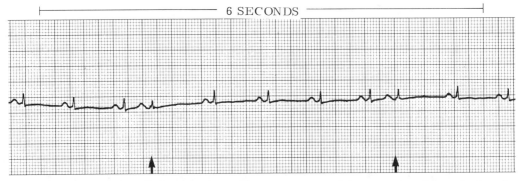

FIGURE 6–21. Normal sinus rhythm with a premature atrial contraction. Note the fourth complex from the left and the third complex from the right occur early in the cycle; the P waves are of a slightly different configuration from the other P waves.

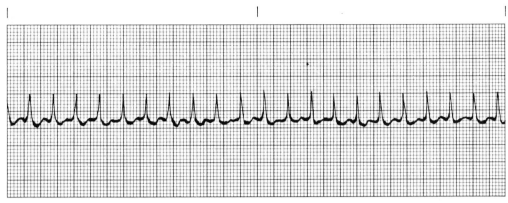

FIGURE 6–22. Paroxysmal atrial tachycardia.

first measures instituted. Pharmacologically, PAT is treated with digoxin, propranolol, quinidine, or verapamil. If drug therapy is not successful in converting PAT to normal sinus rhythm, cardioversion may be used to terminate the rapid rhythm and restore NSR. Cardioversion may be used when the individual is not tolerating the rhythm and develops symptoms of congestive heart failure or myocardial ischemia. (Cardioversion is the delivery of an electrical charge to the heart, synchronized with the R wave, that results in complete depolarization of the myocardium. The charge has the potential to interrupt certain arrhythmias, which allows the SA node, the normal pacemaker of the heart, to resume control of the rhythm.)

ATRIAL FLUTTER

Definition and Cause. Atrial flutter is a rapid, regular, atrial arrhythmia arising from one atrial focus with a rate of 250 to 350 bpm but most commonly 300 bpm. It is easily recognizable because of the regular "saw-toothed" baseline (called "F" or flutter waves). The refractory time of the AV nodal tissue prevents conduction of more than 200 impulses/minute through the AV node. The rate of impulses conducted to the ventricles is normally an *even*-numbered ratio to the atrial impulses initiated (2 : 1 and 4 : 1). Seen less frequently than atrial fibrillation, atrial flutter may convert to atrial fibrillation spontaneously or during treatment. Individuals with normal hearts experience occasional atrial flutter precipitated by anxiety, caffeine, alcohol, or nicotine. Persistent atrial flutter is usually associated with rheumatic heart disease, valvular disease, CAD, or pulmonary emboli.

ECG Appearance. The rhythm is recognizable by the regular saw-toothed baseline (Fig. 6–23). The configuration of the QRS complex is normal. Ventricular conduction follows the normal pathways. T waves are usually not identifiable because of the overriding F waves. When calculating the atrial rate, the F wave that falls within the QRS complex is also counted.

Hemodynamic Implications. The individual may experience a fluttering sensation in the chest or throat. If it is short-lived, there is probably minimal or no hemodynamic consequence. If the cardiac output is compromised by a rapid ventricular response, the individual will experience symptoms of decreased cardiac output.

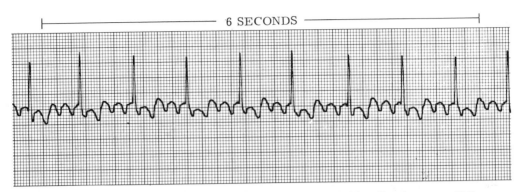

FIGURE 6-23. Atrial flutter (4:1 ratio). Note the "saw-tooth" baseline, known as "F" waves.

Treatment. The goals of therapy are to terminate the rhythm or control ventricular response, as well as to identify and treat the cause. Verapamil or vagal stimulation may be used to slow the ventricular response temporarily and to permit clear identification of flutter waves. Drugs that block AV node conduction (i.e., digitalis, verapamil, and propranolol) may be used to control the ventricular response. Long-term management may include the use of quinidine, procainamide, and disopyramide in conjunction with digitalis. Cardioversion is also effective in converting this rhythm.

ATRIAL FIBRILLATION

Definition and Cause. Atrial fibrillation is a rapid, chaotic atrial arrhythmia caused by the firing of multiple ectopic foci in the atria. The atrial rate may be 350 to 600 bpm. The ventricular response may be very rapid or controlled, but is usually irregularly irregular (Fig. 6-24) owing to the refractory period of AV nodal cells.[9] The atrial activity does not support complete atrial contraction and is out of sequence with ventricular activity. This causes a loss of the atrial "kick" (atrial contribution to left ventricular end-diastolic volume) that may result in decreased cardiac output and CHF. The etiology of atrial fibrillation is not known. It may occur paroxysmally (occurring and recurring suddenly) in the healthy heart. Chronic atrial fibrillation usually indicates heart disease and is seen in

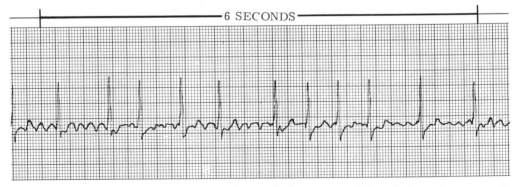

FIGURE 6-24. Atrial fibrillation with rapid ventricular response. (Note the irregular pattern of the ventricular response. There is no pattern to the irregularity, and therefore it is referred to as irregularly irregular.)

patients with CHF, CAD, and pulmonary embolism, and following coronary artery by-pass graft surgery. Atrial fibrillation occurs frequently in the elderly, with or without underlying cardiac disease. It is considered to be an "arrhythmia of old age."

ECG Appearance. P waves are not identifiable. There is an undulating baseline, or fine fibrillatory waves, representing the erratic atrial activity (Figs. 6–24 and 6–25). The ventricular response is irregularly irregular and occurs at a rate of 100 to 150 bpm in the untreated patient. The configuration of the QRS is normal. In atrial fibrillation with a controlled ventricular response, the ventricular rate is less than 100 bpm and, because of the irregular baseline, the T waves are usually unrecognizable.

Hemodynamic Implications. In atrial fibrillation with a controlled ventricular response (less than 100 bpm), the cardiac output is often adequate. However, at higher rates of ventricular response, there may be a decrease in cardiac output because ventricular fill time is decreased and coordination of atrial and ventricular systole is lost. There is a loss of the atrial "kick" that normally contributes as much as 30 to 35 percent to the left ventricular volume. Chaotic motion of the atria may also predispose the individual to the development of mural thrombi. This is frequently a concern when attempting to convert atrial fibrillation to NSR, particularly when the atrial fibrillation has been present for longer than 6 months. The more vigorous motion of the myocardia in NSR may dislodge a thrombus and pulmonary or cerebral emboli may result.

Treatment. Atrial fibrillation may be chronic or occur paroxysmally. Drugs that block AV node conduction (i.e., digitalis, verapamil, and propranolol) are the treatment of choice to convert the rhythm to NSR. No treatment is indicated when the ventricular response is controlled and the individual is asymptomatic. Cardioversion may also be successfully utilized.

SUPRAVENTRICULAR TACHYCARDIA (SVT)

Definition and Cause. Supraventricular tachycardia is any tachycardia in which the impulse initiating the rhythm arises from a location above the ventricles. These include sinus, atrial, and junctional tachycardias. The extremely rapid rates often make it difficult to identify the origin of the rhythm. Differentiating it from ventricular tachycardia may be difficult, especially if the impulse is aberrantly conducted (other than normal pathways), resulting in a QRS complex of greater than 0.12 second. In SVT, the ventricular rate is

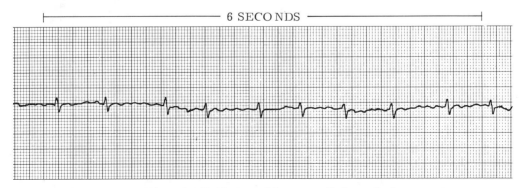

FIGURE 6–25. Atrial fibrillation with a controlled ventricular response.

regular and usually 150 to 200 bpm. SVT may be a sustained rhythm or may last only a few seconds. SVT is most often observed in an individual with ischemic heart disease or as a complication of myocardial infarction.

ECG Appearance. The origin of the arrhythmia determines the ECG appearance. If it is a sinus or atrial tachycardia, a P wave and PR interval should precede each QRS complex (Fig. 6–26). If it is a junctional tachycardia, P waves may appear before, after, or buried within the QRS complex. The QRS complex is either of normal configuration or widened and bizarre. A T wave is usually not observed.

Hemodynamic Implications. Usually the rapid rate is poorly tolerated. There is inadequate ventricular fill time, decreased cardiac output, and inadequate myocardial perfusion time.

Treatment. Treatment is aimed at controlling the ventricular rate and preventing CHF. The physician may apply carotid sinus massage or supraorbital pressure to stimulate a vagal response. Asking the patient to bear down (creating a valsalva maneuver) may have the same response. The drugs of choice are verapamil, propranolol, and digoxin. Cardioversion may also prove effective in terminating SVT.

A-V Nodal Rhythms/Junctional Rhythms

A-V nodal or junctional rhythms originate in the AV node when the SA node fails to initiate an impulse. The AV node fires intrinsically at a rate of 35 to 60 bpm. On ECG (Fig. 6–27), the P wave may be absent or inverted, appearing before, after, or buried within the QRS, as conduction in the atria occurs in a retrograde fashion. If the conduction pathways are healthy below the AV node, the QRS will be normal in configuration. With the loss of the synchronized cardiac contraction, the atrial contribution to the ventricular systolic volume (atrial kick) is lost and cardiac output may be decreased 30 to 35 percent.

PREMATURE NODAL/JUNCTIONAL CONTRACTIONS (PNC/PJC)

Definition and Cause. PNCs or PJCs are premature beats originating in the AV node. They occur in conditions that cause sinus bradycardia or in digitalis toxicity, in which there is increased automaticity of the AV node. The drugs Isuprel and atropine may also cause PNCs.

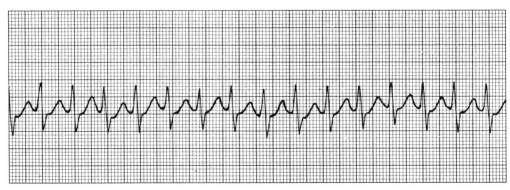

FIGURE 6–26. Supraventricular tachycardia (SVT).

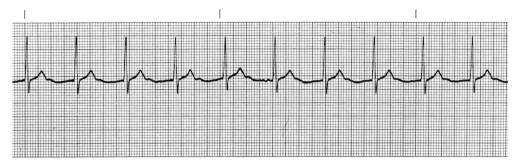

FIGURE 6-27. Junctional rhythm. Note the absence of P waves.

ECG Appearance. There is NSR or sinus bradycardia except for premature beats (Fig. 6-28). The P wave of the premature beat may precede, be buried in, or come after the QRS complex. If the PNC stimulates retrograde conduction through the atria, it will interrupt the sinus mechanism and produce a noncompensatory pause as the sinus mechanism is reset. If there is no retrograde conduction, the sinus mechanism is not interrupted and a compensatory pause will appear. (See section on premature ventricular contractions for definition of compensatory pause.)

Hemodynamic Implications. The PNC may cause decreased stroke volume because the ventricle does not have sufficient time to fill prior to the premature contraction. The radial pulse palpated following the PNC may be much fuller owing to the extra ventricular volume because the compensatory pause allows for extra fill time.

Treatment. No treatment is necessary unless the PNCs are related to digotoxin toxicity. In this case, digoxin is withheld until the digoxin level is again within the therapeutic range.

Ventricular Arrhythmias

Ventricular arrhythmias originate from foci located somewhere in the ventricles. Ventricular pacemakers are erratic, slow, and undependable. An effective cardiac output is rarely

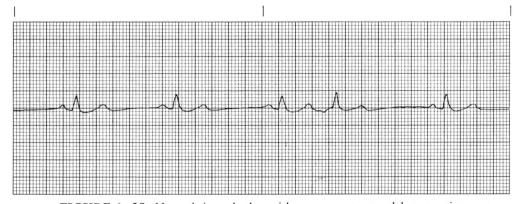

FIGURE 6-28. Normal sinus rhythm with one premature nodal contraction.

maintained, and a life-threatening situation is created for an individual experiencing a ventricular arrhythmia. Ventricular arrhythmias constitute an emergency. Immediate intervention and conversion of the arrhythmia to a rhythm that produces effective circulation is essential.

PREMATURE VENTRICULAR CONTRACTIONS (PVCs)

Definition and Cause. The most common of all arrhythmias, the PVC is a premature beat arising from the ventricle.[14] Occurring occasionally in the majority of the normal population, PVCs may be precipitated by anxiety, tobacco use, alcohol, or caffeine consumption.

Any condition resulting in ischemia of the myocardium (myocardial infarction, CAD, CHF) may cause PVCs. Hypokalemia (decreased serum potassium) may also precipitate PVCs.

ECG Appearance. The ECG may appear normal except for the premature beats (Fig. 6–29). Depolarization begins in the ventricle and follows an abnormal pathway that results in a tall and wide QRS complex (greater than 0.12 second). These complexes are said to be "bizarre." A compensatory pause follows the PVC. (A compensatory pause is longer than the regular pause between beats and is a result of the PVC coming early in the cardiac cycle.) Most often, the sinus mechanism has not been interrupted, and the next impulse is initiated, from the SA node, at the regular interval in the existing sinus rhythm. The R-R interval containing the PVC is between the sinus beats [see Fig. 6–31]. If the PVC is conducted backward and interrupts the sinus mechanism, the sinus mechanism resets and a compensatory pause does not appear.[14] The T wave is opposite in deflection to the R wave of the PVC. PVCs that occur close to the vulnerable period of the preceding T wave are of concern because they may fall on the T wave and precipitate ventricular fibrillation (the R-on-T phenomenon).

Hemodynamic Implications. Occasional PVCs have minimal consequences. Increasingly frequent or multifocal PVCs suggest an increasingly irritable ventricle with potential for the development of life-threatening ventricular arrhythmias.

Patterns of PVCs. PVCs often occur in ratios to normal sinus beats. Bigeminy (Fig. 6–30) is a PVC coupled with each sinus beat. Trigeminy is a PVC every third beat. Quadrigeminy is a PVC every fourth beat, and a couplet (Fig. 6–31) is two PVCs occurring together.

Treatment. The goal of treatment is elimination of the PVCs and their cause. The

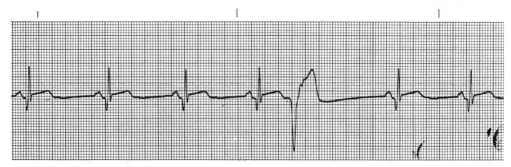

FIGURE 6–29. Normal sinus rhythm with unifocal premature ventricular contractions.

6 SECONDS

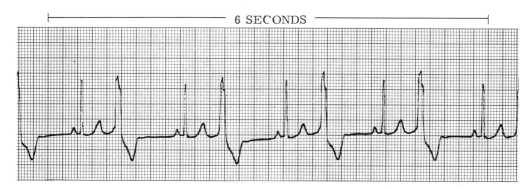

FIGURE 6–30. Ventricular bigeminy.

individual should rest and oxygen should be administered if the PVCs continue. A symptomatic individual will complain of feeling "skipped beats" or fluttering sensations in the chest or throat. In the acute care setting, intravenous lidocaine may be administered when PVCs, couplets, or multifocal PVCs occur at rates of greater than 6 per minute (a standard point for intervention). In the cardiac rehabilitation setting, some individuals may have chronic PVCs that do or do not change with exercise and do not require treatment even at rates greater than 6 PVCs per minute. Others may experience an expected increase in PVCs during some phase of their exercise or recovery period. In these individuals, the exercise prescription should include specific parameters delineating the circumstances under which the individual's exercise should be terminated and appropriate treatment initiated. Treatment of chronic PVCs is typically accomplished with procainamide or other antiarrhythmic medications such as quinidine, propranolol, and phenytoin (Dilantin). Treatment of any underlying cause is continued concomitantly.

VENTRICULAR TACHYCARDIA (VT)

Definition and Cause. Three or more PVCs, occurring sequentially at a rate of 150 to 200 bpm, constitute a run of ventricular tachycardia (VT). VT is usually the result of an

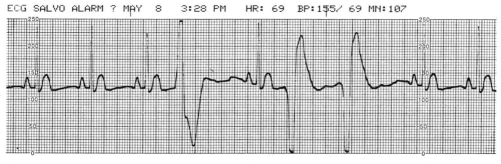

FIGURE 6–31. Premature ventricular contractions: single PVC, then a couplet. Note the compensatory pause. The R-R interval containing the PVC is two times the R-R interval between sinus beats.

irritable, ischemic ventricle. In the healthy heart, VT may occur paroxysmally, produce no symptoms, and convert spontaneously to an effective cardiac rhythm. Sustained VT is life-threatening because a sufficient cardiac output is not maintained. As the ventricle becomes increasingly ischemic, VT degenerates to ventricular fibrillation. This progression of arrhythmias is believed to be responsible for sudden cardiac death following myocardial infarction.

ECG Appearance. The QRS is wide, bizarre, and usually of high amplitude (Fig. 6–32). There is no P wave, and the R-R intervals are usually regular.

Hemodynamic Implications. Coronary artery flow is estimated to decrease 60 percent in VT owing to ineffective cardiac output from a rapidly contracting ventricle. Syncopal episodes occur. (If the patient remains alert with no signs of decreased cardiac output, the arrhythmias may actually be supraventricular, a rhythm that may also begin paroxysmally and have large, regular QRS complexes.)

Treatment. Once the rhythm has been identified, treatment should begin immediately and without hesitation. In the acute care setting, oxygen, intravenous lidocaine, and defibrillation are the immediate treatment of choice. If lidocaine is ineffective, bretylium may be used. The Food and Drug Administration (FDA) recently approved an automatic implantable defibrillator for use in patients who have intractable VT or fibrillation that cannot be controlled by drug therapy. When tachycardia or fibrillation is sensed by the implanted pulse generator, it sends an electrical shock to the heart. This shock depolarizes the entire myocardium and allows the sinus node to regain control of the rhythm.

VENTRICULAR FIBRILLATION (VF)

Definition and Cause. VF is chaotic activity of the ventricle originating when multiple foci in the ischemic ventricle fire simultaneously. Because of electrical disorganization, the ventricles do not contract as a unit. There is absolutely no effective cardiac output or coronary perfusion. VF is associated with severe myocardial ischemia. VF may also be precipitated by drug overdose (digitalis, procainamide, potassium chloride, and others), anesthesia, electrical shock, or cardiac surgery. This is a life-threatening arrhythmia that usually results in death if not treated within 4 minutes.

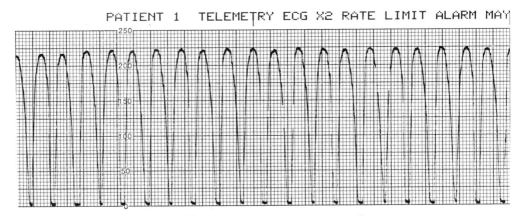

FIGURE 6–32. Ventricular tachycardia.

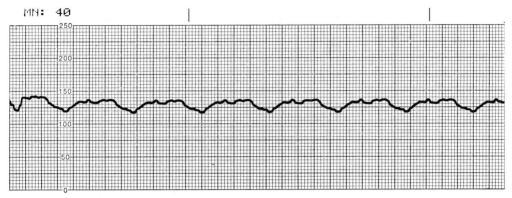

FIGURE 6–33. Ventricular fibrillation.

ECG Appearance. There are no recognizable P waves, QRS complexes, or T waves. The erratic wave forms vary in size and may initially be unrecognizable waves of large amplitude (coarse VF) that quickly decrease in amplitude (fine VF) as myocardial death occurs. A flat baseline (asystole) indicates absolute electrical silence and death (Figs. 6–33 and 6–34).

Hemodynamic Implications. There is no systemic or coronary circulation. Clinical death occurs within 4 minutes.

Treatment. Immediate defibrillation with 200 to 400 watt-seconds. If unavailable or ineffective, cardiopulmonary resuscitation must be initiated immediately.

Heart Blocks

Heart blocks are anatomic or functional interruptions to the normal conduction of an impulse through the heart's conductive pathways. This text briefly describes some of the more common blocks.

SINOATRIAL BLOCK (SA BLOCK)

Definition and Cause. In SA node block, the impulse is discharged from the SA node, but for some reason the impulse is unable to reach the surrounding atrial tissue.

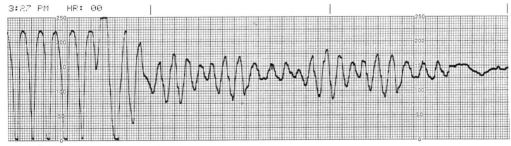

FIGURE 6–34. Progression of ventricular arrhythmias. Note the rhythm rapidly changes from VT to course VF and then to fine VF.

Although SA block is most frequently the result of drug therapy (digoxin or quinidine), it may occur in CAD.

ECG Appearance. The appearance of all waves is normal. There is an occasional or frequent interruption in the rhythm, in which one or more cardiac cycles are missed. The rhythm is the same before and after the pause. If the pause is prolonged, an ectopic focus may fire. The sinus node usually continues to function as the pacemaker.

Hemodynamic Implications. There are hemodynamic implications only if the pause is prolonged. Prolonged pauses may be associated with signs of decreased cardiac output.

Treatment. Treatment is not necessary unless bradycardia is profound and the individual becomes symptomatic. Atropine, epinephrine, or isoproterenol may be administered to increase the heart rate if this occurs. Medications should be withdrawn if the block is the result of drug therapy.

Atrioventricular Blocks (AV Blocks)

AV conduction blocks are abnormal delays or failure of conduction through the AV node or bundle of His. The electrical impulse arises normally from the SA node and depolarizes the atria but, upon reaching the AV node or bundle of His, the conduction is slowed to greater than 0.20 second or completely blocked. The block may be a result of CAD, rheumatic heart disease, or myocardial infarction. Therapy with quinidine, digitalis, and/or procainamide may also delay AV conduction. Treatment is based on the symptomatology the patient demonstrates and the etiology of the block.

FIRST DEGREE AV BLOCK

Definition and Cause. In first-degree AV block, all impulses arise normally from the SA node. The impulse is, however, slowed for greater than 0.20 second at the AV node or bundle of His and is then conducted to the ventricle. The delay may be as great as 0.8 second and usually remains constant. The most common causes of first-degree AV block include congenital heart disease, digitalis therapy or toxicity, myocardial infarction, and complications of coronary artery bypass surgery.

ECG Appearance. The configuration of all waves is normal. The P-R interval is, however, prolonged (Fig. 6–35).

Hemodynamic Implications. There are no hemodynamic implications. First-degree AV block must be observed for progression to further block, especially in acute onset.

Treatment. Correction of first-degree block requires treatment of the underlying cause. If it is pharmacologic, the benefits of treatment are weighed against the complication of heart block.

SECOND-DEGREE AV BLOCK MOBITZ TYPE I (WENCKEBACH)

Definition and Cause. In the Wenckebach phenomenon, there is a repeated pattern of progressively lengthening P-R intervals until finally an atrial impulse is completely blocked at the AV node. Myocardial infarction, electrolyte imbalance, or digoxin, quini-

6 SECONDS

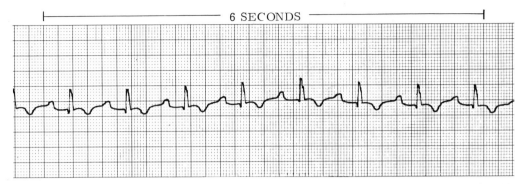

FIGURE 6–35. Normal sinus rhythm with first degree AV block. (Note the P-R interval, 0.28 second.)

dine, or procainamide therapy may bring on this unusual transient arrhythmia. Wenckebach phenomenon rarely progresses to complete heart block.

ECG Appearance. The rate is usually slow because of AV conduction block. The P-R interval is progressively lengthened until the P wave is completely blocked and there is no ventricular complex (Fig. 6–36). It is a cyclical phenomenon.

Hemodynamic Implications. The Wenckebach rhythm is fairly well tolerated unless profound bradycardia, a rate less than 40 bpm, results. If bradycardia is profound and the cardiac output is inadequate, the individual will exhibit signs of decreased cardiac output (cold, clammy skin, syncope, low blood pressure).

Treatment. Treatment is necessary only if the heart rate is slow and the individual exhibits symptoms of low cardiac output. Atropine may be utilized to increase the heart rate. Medications that slow AV conduction (digoxin, quinidine, calcium channel blockers, and procainamide) may be withheld. In rare instances, an artificial pacemaker may be necessary to establish a rate consistent with an adequate cardiac output.

SECOND DEGREE AV BLOCK MOBITZ TYPE II

Definition and Cause. Mobitz type II block is rare. It is clinically very significant. In Mobitz type II block, atrial impulses occur at a regular rate but are irregularly conducted to

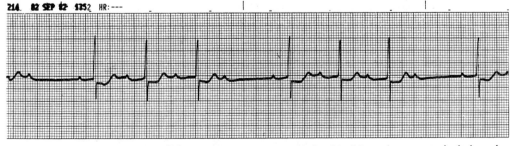

FIGURE 6–36. Second degree AV block type I (Wenckebach). (Note the progressively lengthening P-R interval and then the absence of the QRS complex.)

the ventricle. The P waves occur in a regular ratio to the QRS (i.e., 2 : 1 or 3 : 1). However, a progressive lengthening of the P-R interval before the blocked P wave is absent. The site of the block is usually below the bundle of His and is a form of bilateral bundle branch block. This block usually progresses to complete heart block and, therefore, requires immediate therapeutic intervention. Mobitz type II block may occur as a result of a large anterior myocardial infarction.

ECG Appearance. The atrial rate is regular. P waves are normal in appearance. The ventricular rate is slow and irregular. Conduction of the atrial impulse to the ventricle is intermittent. The P-R interval is consistent (Fig. 6–37). The QRS complex may either be normal in appearance or have a bundle branch pattern, depending on the level of the block.

Hemodynamic Implications. Symptoms experienced depend on the ventricular rate. When impulses are conducted from the atria to the ventricle, the normal atrioventricular sequence remains intact. If the ventricular rate is adequate, the individual will not experience symptoms of low cardiac output. Symptoms of low cardiac output appear as the ventricular rate slows.

Treatment. The insertion of a permanent pacemaker and the withdrawal of medications that may increase AV conduction time are the treatment of choice. Atropine may be administered initially in an attempt to increase the conduction of impulses across the AV node. However, this is usually not effective because of the level of the block.

COMPLETE HEART BLOCK

Definition and Cause. In complete heart block, the atrial and ventricular rhythms are independent of one another, and therefore the rhythm is termed AV dissociation. There is a failure of conduction of impulses from the atria to the ventricle. Any apparent sequence of these independent rhythms is coincidental. Impulses originating in the SA node are completely blocked at the AV node. An escape rhythm from the junctional or ventricular area must take over as the pacemaker of the ventricle. The ventricular rate is 20 to 40 bpm. Complete heart block is usually seen as a complication of acute myocardial infarction or severe angina in which sustained ischemia of the AV node has occurred.

ECG Appearance. The atrial and ventricular rhythm appear as independent regular

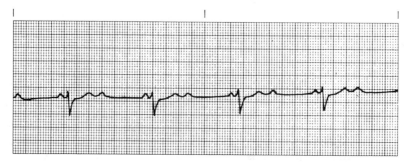

FIGURE 6–37. Second degree AV block Mobitz type II. The AV node selectively conducts some beats while blocking others. Those that are not blocked are conducted through to the ventricles, although they may encounter a slight delay in the node. Once in the ventricles, conduction proceeds normally.

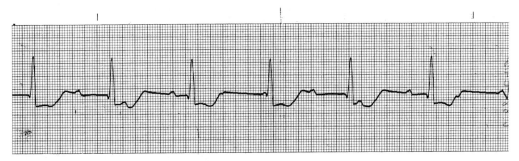

FIGURE 6–38. Complete heart block. (Note that the atrial and ventricular rates are independendently occurring rhythms.)

rhythms. The P wave is of normal configuration. The appearance of the QRS depends on the location of the ventricular pacemaker. P-P and R-R intervals are regular. There is no relationship between the P and R waves. Ventricular irritability may be seen, as a result of the slow heart rate and the resulting myocardial ischemia (Fig. 6–38).

Hemodynamic Implications. A slow heart rate, low cardiac output, and compromised coronary perfusion may result in acute congestive heart failure. Individuals may also experience syncope. Syncope as a result of complete heart block is known as the Stokes-Adams syndrome.

Treatment. Complete heart block is a life-threatening emergency because the ventricle is an unreliable pacemaker. Emergency treatment with intravenous atropine or isoproterenol may be used until an artificial pacemaker can be implanted.

Bundle Branch Blocks

Bundle branch blocks (BBB) are blocks in conduction along either the right or left bundle branch or both. (The bundle branches refer to the major branches of the intraventricular conduction system.) A block in the bundle of His or bundle branches slows the depolarization of that ventricle because the impulse must travel to the "blocked" ventricle from the ventricle with the "normal" conduction pathway. The depolarization, now occurring at separate times, is represented on the ECG by two joined QRS complexes. The QRS is wider than 0.10 second with a notched configuration that represents two R waves, R and R prime (R'). The tracing reflects the nonsimultaneous depolarization and is diagnostic of BBB. A 12-lead ECG is necessary for diagnosis. BBB is best seen in leads V_1 and V_6.

RIGHT BUNDLE BRANCH BLOCK (RBBB)

Definition and Cause. RBBB is an anatomical or functional block in the right bundle branch that slows the depolarization and contraction of the right ventricle. Although also seen in healthy hearts, RBBB is most frequently seen in anterior myocardial infarction.

ECG Appearance. Atrial conduction is normal. The QRS is greater than 0.12 second and is notched ("rabbit ears") in V_1. The T wave is opposite in deflection to the QRS (Fig. 6–39).

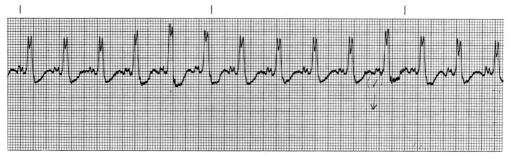

FIGURE 6–39. Right bundle branch block.

Hemodynamic Implications. There are no hemodynamic implications. Despite delayed conduction, diastolic fill time and cardiac output remain normal.

Treatment. No treatment is necessary.

LEFT BUNDLE BRANCH BLOCK (LBBB)

Definition and Cause. LBBB is caused by a block in the left bundle branch that delays conduction and contraction of the left ventricle. LBBB occurs in ischemic heart disease, myocardial infarction, valvular heart disease, and in other cases of serious heart disease. In some instances, BBB may be rate dependent (i.e., it appears only when a "critical rate" is reached). The significance of this event is yet to be determined. The LBBB will disappear immediately when the individual's heart rate falls below the critical rate and can be immediately reproduced by raising the heart rate to the critical level.

ECG Appearance. The rate and rhythm are normal, with a widened QRS greater than 0.12 second that appears notched in the left chest leads (V_5–V_6) (Fig. 6–40).

Hemodynamic Implications. There are no complications of the rhythm itself.

Treatment. No treatment is necessary for the rhythm itself.

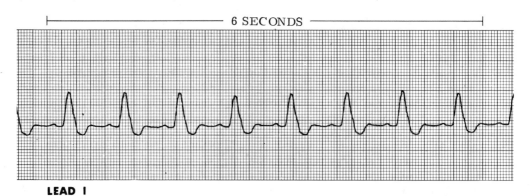

LEAD I

FIGURE 6–40. Normal sinus rhythm with complete left bundle branch block (Lead 1).

ARTIFICIAL PACEMAKERS

An artificial pacemaker is an electronic device that provides repetitive electrical stimuli to the heart muscle. These stimuli, like the heart's natural pacemaker, allow for the origination and conduction of energy through the heart. Pacemakers may be inserted on a temporary or permanent basis. They are generally used when an individual has an arrhythmia that has caused or may potentially cause a decreased cardiac output. This may occur with complete heart block, severe bradycardia, or tachycardia. Pacemakers are also used to control tachyarrhythmias. There has been only limited clinical applicability of the antitachycardic mode to date.[10,19]

Pacemaker Equipment

Pacemakers are composed of a pulse generator (a battery and electrical circuit) and a lead wire. The pulse generator initiates the electrical stimulus to the heart. It may also have a sensing mechanism with which it senses the individual's heartbeat.

Pacemaker generators have various types of power sources with varying life spans including: mercury zinc (3 to 4 years), lithium (approximately 10 years), and plutonium-nuclear (20 years to a lifetime). They are replaced according to their life spans. In addition, there are batteries that are externally rechargeable. With permanently implanted pacemakers, the pulse generator usually "fails" over a period of weeks to months. The symptoms exhibited depend on the underlying rhythm. The failure of the battery is usually detected by a change in heart rate, either bradycardia or uncontrolled tachyarrhythmias.

The lead is the conducting wire and electrode tip. It extends from the generator to the patient's heart. The lead may be placed transvenously by threading it through the subclavian into the right atrium. When properly positioned, the electrode tip lies against the atrial or ventricular endocardium. It is held in place by a tine-like tip. The lead may also be sutured directly to the epicardium. This is usually done through a transthoracic approach during open heart surgery, or it may be done via a transmediastinal approach through an incision in the subxiphoid area.

Types of Pacemakers

Pacemakers may be used either temporarily or permanently. Temporary pacing, usually via the transvenous approach, is used when the arrhythmia is believed reversible to evaluate the effects of a pacer-supported rhythm or as an emergency intervention until the permanent pacer can be inserted. In temporary pacing, the generator remains external to the patient.

A permanent pacemaker is most commonly indicated in cases of complete heart block. The lead is passed transvenously into the right atrium or directly sutured to the epicardium. The pulse generator is implanted in a subcutaneous pocket either in the pectoral area or in the abdominal wall. This procedure is usually done under local anesthesia.

Classification

Pacemakers are classified according to five parameters: chamber paced, chamber sensed, mode of response, programmable features, and special tachyarrhythmia features.

"Chamber paced" and "chamber sensed" refer to the chamber of the heart in which the electrode lies (atrial, ventricular, dual chamber, or AV sequential). Chamber sensed depends on the presence and function of the sensing mechanism. "Mode of pacing" refers to sensing function and how it relates to stimulus release. Programmable pacemakers have a variety of modes and specific functions that can be adjusted by external reprogramming. Special antitachycardia functions are available only on a few highly specialized pacemakers. With this type of pacemaker, the fixed-rate mode is activated by external application of a magnet or radio-frequency unit over the pulse generator during tachycardic episodes. Pacemaker signals are initiated and eventually interrupt the tachycardic cycle.

Modes of Pacing

There are five pacing modes: fixed rate or asynchronous, demand or inhibited, triggered or synchronous, dual, and reverse pacing.

Fixed-rate pacemakers fire continuously without regard to the patient's own rhythm. This preset firing may result in competition; that is, the ventricles may receive impulses simultaneously from both natural and artificial pacemakers, which compete for dominance. This competition may cause chaotic rhythm disturbances and is the primary disadvantage associated with fixed-rate pacemakers.

A demand or inhibited pacemaker senses the inherent rhythm of the heart and does not discharge an impulse if the heart initiates its own impulse. The pacemaker fires only when needed.

A triggered or synchronous pacemaker paces constantly when there is no intrinsic beat. When the pacemaker senses a ventricular depolarization owing to natural pacing, the pacemaker releases its impulse. Because the ventricle is already depolarized and refractory to another stimulus, the pacer impulse is ineffectual.

Dual-chamber pacemakers are capable of sensing and pacing both the atria and the ventricles. This enables each atrial contraction, whether spontaneous or paced, to be followed at a preset interval with a ventricular contraction. These are AV sequential pacemakers. Their primary advantage is that they preserve the normal sequence of cardiac events. The atrial contribution to ventricular filling is maintained. These pacemakers are more versatile than single-chamber units. AV sequential pacemakers may be reprogrammed to either single-chamber (atrial or ventricular) or dual-chamber function as needed.

Reverse pacemakers fire opposite to what is normally expected. They sense tachyarrhythmias and interrupt the rhythm disturbance.

ECG Appearance

On the ECG, the pacemaker impulse is recorded as a spike immediately preceding the depolarization of the atria and/or ventricles (Figs. 6–41 and 6–42). The spike may be of varying amplitude. It is instantaneous and has no real duration. When a pacemaker is

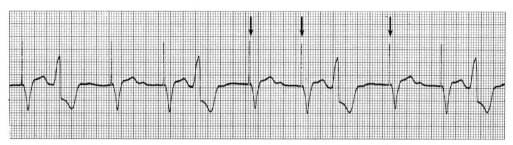

FIGURE 6–41. Ventricular pacemaker rhythm. (Note the "spike" preceding each ventricular complex. The ventricular complex is wide and bizarre because the ventricle is the site where the impulse is initiated.)

stimulating adequately, each pacing spike produces a cardiac response. If the electrode is in the atria, each spike should produce a P wave. If the electrode is in the ventricles, each spike should produce a QRS complex. When a pacing spike fails to produce a response, the pacemaker is said to be out of "capture." Frequent causes of failure to capture are a loss of contact between the electrode and the chamber wall, depletion of the power source, or a fracture in the electrode.

The appearance of the waves of the cardiac cycle differs from the appearance of the waves of the individual's natural rhythm because the pacemaker impulses arise from a different site in the myocardium. Conduction does not follow normal pathways. In a ventricularly paced rhythm, the QRS will often be wide and bizarre in appearance.

Complications

Complications associated with pacemaker function include: local infection or hematoma formation at the lead or pulse generator insertion sites, arrhythmias from irritation of the ventricle, perforation of the right ventricle from the catheter, and loss of capture. The individual is treated symptomatically for each complication, with appropriate adjustments made to the pacemaker to ensure optimal functioning.

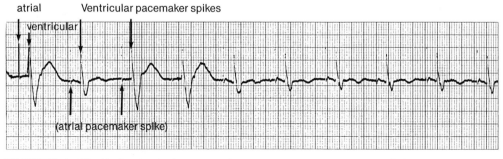

FIGURE 6–42. Atrioventricular pacemaker rhythm. (Note the "spike" before each atrial and each ventricular complex.)

ECG CHANGES SEEN WITH EXERCISE

Individuals with healthy hearts demonstrate a number of expected and insignificant ECG changes during exercise (Table 6–3). Most notable is the significant tachycardia that occurs with moderate to heavy physical exertion, accompanied by a rapid return to the pre-exercise heart rate following cessation of the exercise (during recovery). The healthy individual may experience single or rare premature atrial, junctional, or ventricular contractions during exercise. These arrhythmias are without hemodynamic consequences.[23] Beneficial ECG changes and a low heart rate (at rest and during submaximal exercise) that occur as a result of physical conditioning are demonstrated by both healthy individuals and those with CAD. Individuals with CAD also develop the ability to engage in more vigorous activity before reaching their ischemic threshold.

Abnormal ECG responses observed during exercise reflect an imbalance between myocardial oxygen supply and demand. Usually they are either exertional arrhythmias or alterations in the ST segment and T wave (see Table 6–2).[10,21] Exertional arrhythmias occur during both exercise and the recovery period. They are significant in their relationship to an individual's cardiac output. If the arrhythmia causes inadequate cardiac output, it may induce syncope, angina, or congestive heart failure. Alterations in the ST segment and T wave (see Fig. 6–4) fall into three categories: horizontal, downsloping, and upsloping. ST-segment depression or elevation of 1 mm or greater measured at 0.08 second from the J point indicates ischemia of the myocardium. It is an abnormal response to exercise. When monitoring exercise in cardiac rehabilitation, this parameter should be assessed carefully in relation to other clinical symptoms to determine intervention. There is little or no agreement concerning the significance of the varying shapes of both the ST segment and T wave that occur with exercise.[21]

Many pathophysiologic conditions, including anemia, hypoxemia, and ventricular aneurysm, as well as cardioactive drugs cause the same ST segment and T wave changes commonly induced by exercise. In determining the significance of ST-segment depression during exercise, it is important not only to observe and evaluate the associated symptoms,

TABLE 6–3. ECG Changes During Exercise

Healthy Individual*	Individual with CAD†
1. Slight increase in amplitude of P wave	1. Appearance of a BBB at a "critical heart rate"
2. Shortening of P-R interval	2. Recurrent or multifocal PVCs during exercise and/or recovery
3. Slight shift to right of QRS axis	3. VT
4. ST-segment depression of less than 1 mm	4. Appearance of bradyarrhythmias/ tachyarrhythmias — rapid rate abruptly slowing or vice versa, not related to exercise
5. Decreased amplitude of the T wave	5. ST-segment depression/elevation of greater than 1 mm, 0.08 second after the J point
6. Single or rare PVCs during exercise and recovery	6. Bradycardia in response to exercise
7. Single or rare PJCs or PACs	

Decreases in the resting heart rate and the submaximal heart rate are observed in both groups with physical conditioning.

*These ECG changes are all normal in response to exercise.

†Occurrence of any one of these changes should result in cessation of exercise and thorough evaluation of the ECG change and related symptoms.

but also to observe and evaluate how quickly the individual's ECG returns to normal upon cessation of the exercise. Table 6–3 lists other abnormal ECG changes that may be observed. For all of these abnormalities, and any other new potentially significant clinical symptom, exercise should be terminated and appropriate treatment instituted. Observation of the arrhythmia and the patient should continue in order to detect the appearance of other symptoms, should they occur. Prompt evaluation by the individual's physician should be completed, with appropriate results forwarded to the cardiac rehabilitation staff before the individual exercises again. Additionally, new arrhythmias or other new symptoms observed prior to exercise should always be evaluated before the individual is permitted to exercise. Exercise is contraindicated in any individual found to be in complete heart block or demonstrating symptoms of congestive heart failure. Such individuals should seek immediate medical attention.

DRUG EFFECTS ON ECG

Drugs that affect the heart rate may have some effect on the ECG pattern. Cardiac glycosides, antiarrhythmics, and beta blockers all have varying effects on the cardiac cycle. Beta blockers, in particular, may cause bradycardia. They may produce heart rates in the range of 40 to 50 bpm. Digitalis preparations and calcium ion antagonists increase AV conduction time, with the most prominent characteristic of digitalis toxicity, AV block. Digitalis may also produce sagging in the ST segment (Fig. 6–43) and shortening of the Q-T interval (measured from the Q wave through the T wave). In digitalis toxicity, arrhythmias of all types (atrial, junctional, and ventricular) have been documented[1] (Table 6–4).

Quinidine and procainamide may prolong the AV conduction time and result in a prolonged P-R interval. A wide QRS complex and a wide, notched T wave or even an inverted T may also be seen. In toxicity, patients will frequently demonstrate an AV block, widening of the QRS (to as much as one and a half normal duration), or ventricular arrhythmias.[12]

Drugs used in the treatment of concurrent illnesses may also cause changes in the ECG. Phenothiazines (Phenergan, Thorazine) and tricyclic antidepressants (Elavil, Sinequan) cause T-wave changes, P-R and Q-T prolongation, conduction disorders, and

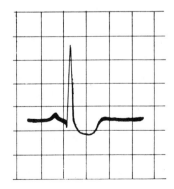

FIGURE 6–43. Digitalis effect. Notice the rounded sagging appearance of the ST segment. (From Brunner, LS and Suddarth, DS: Textbook of Medical Surgical Nursing, ed. 5. JB Lippincott, Philadelphia, 1984, p. 571, with permission.)

TABLE 6–4. Effects of Selected Drugs on the ECG[8,16]

Drug	ECG Effect
Digitalis	1. Shortens ventricular activation time 2. Increases AV conduction time 3. Shortens Q-T interval 4. Depresses ST segments and makes them sag 5. In large doses: decrease T wave amplitude prolong P-R interval sinus bradycardia PACs, PVCs, and bigeminy multiple conduction abnormalities 6. Toxicity: AV block
Quinidine and Procainamide	1. Prolonged P-R interval 2. Wide QRS complex; lengthened Q-T interval 3. Depressed, widened, or notched T wave 4. Toxicity: SA or AV block Ventricular arrhythmias Up to 50% increase in QRS duration
Phenothiazines (Phenergan, Thorazine)	1. Nonspecific T-wave changes 2. Decreased T-wave amplitude 3. Intraventricular conduction disturbances 4. Supraventricular and ventricular arrhythmias
Tricyclic antidepressants (Elavil, Sinequan)	1. T-wave changes 2. P-R interval, Q-T interval, and QRS complex prolongation 3. Conduction disturbances 4. Supraventricular and ventricular arrhythmias

supraventricular and ventricular arrhythmias.[16] It is therefore important to keep current records of patients' complete medical and pharmacologic regimens. Patients should be encouraged repeatedly to keep the cardiac rehabilitation team aware of any changes in their medications, as changes could have a dramatic effect on their exercise prescription and their response to exercise.[12]

SUMMARY

Electrocardiography is discussed in this chapter. Information regarding the significance of electrocardiograms (ECGs) in the diagnosis and treatment of cardiac pathology is presented. The individual wave forms are identified and related to the heart's corresponding electrical and muscular activity. Lead placements for proper ECG recording at rest and during exercise are identified and illustrated.

In addition, the basic concepts of rate, rhythm, and waveform configuration for the interpretation of ECGs most commonly encountered in a cardiac rehabilitation setting are presented. Arrhythmias, abnormalities in initiation and/or conduction of the heart beat, are described, with sample electrocardiographic strips for the purpose of illustration. Information outlining each arrhythmia's specific etiology, hemodynamic implications, and treatment is included for common arrhythmias and conduction blocks. Brief discussions of pacemakers and the effects of drug therapy on the ECG conclude the chapter.

Review questions and ECG rhythm strips in workbook fashion are given after the References for the purpose of providing an opportunity for evaluation of basic arrhythmia identification skills.

REFERENCES

1. Kniesl, CR and Ames, SW: Adult Health Nursing. Addison-Wesley, Reading, MA, 1986.
2. Dubin, D: Rapid Interpretation of EKGs, ed 2. Cover Publishing Co, Tampa, 1970.
3. Woods, SL and Underhill, SL: Cardiac Arrhythmias and Conduction Abnormalities. In Patrick, ML, et al (eds): Medical-Surgical Nursing: Pathophysiological Concepts. JB Lippincott, Philadelphia, 1986.
4. Littman, D: The Electrocardiogram: Examination of the Heart, Part 5. American Heart Association, Dallas, 1973.
5. Marriott, HJL: Practical Electrocardiography, ed 7. Williams & Wilkins, Baltimore, 1983.
6. Conover, M: Understanding Electrocardiography: Physiological and Interpretive Concepts, ed 4. CV Mosby, St. Louis, 1984.
7. Goldman, MJ: Principles of Electrocardiography, ed 11. Lange Medical Publications, Los Altos, CA, 1982.
8. Woods, SL: Electrocardiograms and Heart Arrhythmias. In Brunner, LS and Suddarth, DS: Textbook of Medical-Surgical Nursing, ed 5. JB Lippincott, Philadelphia, 1984.
9. Norsen, L, Telfair, M and Wagner, AL: Detecting dysrhythmias. Nursing '86 16:11, 1986.
10. Vinsant, MO and Spence, MI: Common Sense Approach to Coronary Care. CV Mosby, St. Louis, 1985.
11. Sumner, SM and Grau, PA: Guidelines for running a 12-lead EKG. Nursing '85 15:12, 1985.
12. Liss, JP (ed): Reference Guide—Preventative Rehabilitative Exercise Specialist Workshop/Certification. American College of Sports Medicine, Madison, WI, 1981.
13. Introduction to Arrhythmia Recognition. California Heart Association, San Francisco, 1968.
14. Pearl, MJ: Electrocardiography. In Amundsen, LA (ed): Cardiac Rehabilitation. Churchill Livingstone, New York.
15. Brannon, FJ: Experiments and Instrumentation in Exercise Physiology. Kendall-Hunt, Dubuque, 1978.
16. Woods, SL: Electrocardiography, Vectorcardiography and Polarcardiography. In Underhill, SL, et al (eds): Cardiac Nursing. JB Lippincott, Philadelphia, 1982.
17. Poyatos, ME, et al: Predictive value of changes in R-wave amplitude after exercise in CHD. Am J Cardiol 54:10, 1984.
18. Lipman, BS, Dunn M, Massic, E: Clinical Electrocardiology, ed 7. Year Book Medical Publishers, Chicago, 1984.
19. Braunwald, E (ed): Heart Disease: A Textbook of Cardiovascular Medicine. WB Saunders, Philadelphia, 1984.
20. Sokolow, M and McIlroy MB: Clinical Cardiology. Lange Medical Publications, Los Altos, 1986.
21. Sivarajan, ES: Exercise Testing. In Underhill, LS, et al (eds): Cardiac Nursing. JB Lippincott, Philadelphia, 1982.
22. Wenger, NK: Exercise Therapy for Patients with Coronary Artery Disease. Consultant, 1980.
23. Dehn, MM: Rehabilitation of the cardiac patient: The effects of exercise. Am J Nurs 80:5, 1980.
24. Shephard, RJ: The value of exercise in ischemic heart disease: A cumulative analysis. J Cardiac Rehabil 3:294, 1983.
25. Berkovits, BV: AV sequential demand pacemakers for treatment of cardiac arrhythmias. CVP Feb/March, 1980.
26. Cardiovascular Disorders: Nursing 84 Books. Springhouse Corporation, Springhouse, PA, 1984.
27. Feldman, MS and Helfant, RH: Cardiac Pacing. In Bellet, S (ed): Essentials of Cardiac Arrhythmias, ed 2. WB Saunders, Philadelphia, 1980.
28. Hahn, AB, Barkin, RL and Oestreich, SJK: Pharmacology in Nursing, ed 15. CV Mosby, St. Louis, 1982.
29. Mangiola, S and Ritota, MC: Cardiac Arrhythmias, ed 2. JB Lippincott, Philadelphia, 1982.
30. Phillips, RE and Feeney, MK: The Cardiac Rhythms, ed 2. WB Saunders, Philadelphia, 1980.
31. Purcell, JA and Haynes, L: Using the ECG to detect MI. Am J Nurs 84:5, 1984.
32. Stapleton, JF: Essentials of Clinical Cardiology. FA Davis, Philadelphia, 1983.

CHAPTER 6 REVIEW QUESTIONS

Instructions: Briefly answer the following questions as they apply to electrocardiography as discussed in chapter 6. (Answers follow.)

1. ECG interpretation is based upon _____ ,
_____ , _____ , and
_____ .

2. _____ is the hallmark ECG sign of myocardial ischemia.
3. Disturbances in cardiac rhythm, cardiac arrhythmias, are caused by abnormalities in either _____ or _____ or in both.
4. The _____ , the "natural pacemaker of the heart," fires intrinsically at a rate of _____ times per minute.
5. _____ _____ leads and
_____ _____ leads make up the 12 standard ECG leads. _____ is often used as a single monitoring lead during exercise.
6. Match the wave or waves of the ECG in Figure 6–44 that are described by one of the following definitions or phrases.

    a. _____ ventricular depolarization

    b. _____ the cardiac cycle

    c. _____ absolute and relative refractory period

    d. _____ ventricular repolarization

    e. _____ atrial depolarization

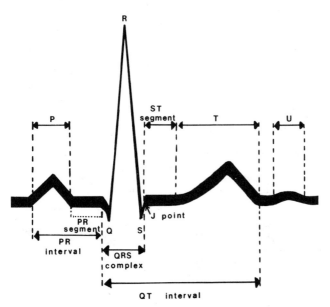

FIGURE 6–44. Illustration of ECG wave configuration. (From Underhill, SL, et al: Cardiac Nursing. JB Lippincott, Philadelphia, 1983, p. 200, with permission.)

7. Identify the most common heart blocks.
   a.
   b.
   c.
   d.
   e.
8. All are characteristics of NSR *except*:
   a. The rhythm is essentially regular.
   b. The impulse arises from the sinoatrial node at a rate of 60 to 100 bpm.
   c. The appearance of the QRS complex is variable.
   d. The rate may decrease slightly with deep inspiration and increase with expiration.
9. In individuals with coronary artery disease and angina, sinus tachycardia:
   a. increases myocardial oxygen demand.
   b. may significantly decrease coronary artery perfusion because of the decrease in the duration of diastole.
   c. may result in an anginal episode if the underlying cause is not identified and treated to decrease the heart rate.
   d. all of the above.
10. Regularly occurring premature ventricular contractions (PVCs) may be identified as
    _____ when a PVC is coupled with every normal beat and as
    _____ when the PVC occurs every third beat.
11. Briefly explain the mechanism by which the heart meets the increased oxygen demand of exercise.

    How does this differ in the individual with atherosclerosis?

12. Sinus bradycardia:
    a. may be well tolerated.
    b. is often seen in individuals who are physically fit and in many individuals during sleep.
    c. may be profound (less than 40 bpm) and lead to signs and symptoms of low cardiac output.
    d. may be seen in individuals on digoxin therapy.
    e. all of the above.

13. Identify the average duration of the:

    a. P wave _____

    b. PR interval _____

    c. QRS complex _____

    d. ST segment _____

    e. T wave _____

14. When an abnormal ECG change is detected and persists or increases in frequency with exercise, the health professional should do all of the following *except*:

    a. terminate the exercise with the appropriate monitored cool-down period.

    b. check and record the individual's vital signs and associated symptoms.

    c. allow the individual to resume exercise as soon as the abnormality disappears.

    d. notify the client's physician of the ECG change.

    e. caution the client against exercise until the ECG change is evaluated.

    f. none of the above.

15. All of the following are *normal* ECG changes seen with exercise except:

    a. depression of the ST segment of less than 1 mm.

    b. tachycardia.

    c. recurrent and/or multifocal PVCs during exercise or in the recovery phase.

    d. decreased amplitude of T wave.

16. An anatomic or functional interruption to conduction of an impulse through the normal conductive pathway is:

    a. atrial fibrillation.

    b. heart block.

    c. heart failure.

    d. ventricular muscle depolarization.

17. Identify four characteristics of PVCs.

    a.

    b.

    c.

    d.

18. Premature ventricular contractions may be precipitated by:

    a.

    b.

    c.

19. Briefly describe why arrhythmias, arising in the ventricles (other than occasional PVCs) require immediate treatment.

20. Atrial flutter is characterized by all of the following *except*:
   a. ventricular response may be irregular or regular and stated in a ratio of atrial to ventricular activity.
   b. the atrial activity has a saw-toothed configuration on ECG and is known as "F" or flutter waves.
   c. there is an abnormal configuration to the QRS waves.
21. List the categories of cardiac drugs that will most commonly affect the ECG and give their effects.

22. Atrial arrhythmias
   a. include atrial fibrillation, atrial flutter, and premature atrial contractions as the most common.
   b. arise from ectopic foci in the atria.
   c. have P waves of abnormal or various configurations, or there may be an absence of identifiable P waves.
   d. may have normal QRS configurations.
   e. all of the above.
23. Why is it essential to maintain up-to-date medication profiles on all patients in a cardiac rehabilitation program?

24. What is the biggest advantage of atrioventricular sequential pacemakers?

25. How is a pacemaker detected on ECG?

ANSWERS TO REVIEW QUESTIONS

1. Rate, rhythm, regularity, and the individual wave configurations
2. ST-segment depression/elevation of greater than 1 mm occurring 0.08 second after the J point
3. Automaticity, conduction
4. Sinoatrial node, 60 to 100
5. Six limb, six chest, modified chest lead V_5 (CMV_5)
6. a. QRS complex
   b. The entire PQRST complex
   c. ST segment and T wave
   d. T wave
   e. P wave
7. a. sinoatrial node block (SA node block)
   b. first-degree AV block (Mobitz I)
   c. second-degree AV block (Mobitz II)
   d. complete heart block
   e. bundle branch block
8. C is the correct answer.
9. D is the correct answer.
10. bigeminy, trigeminy (in that order)
11. Because the heart is extremely efficient in extracting oxygen from the blood at normal rates, the healthy heart meets increased oxygen demand brought on by exercise by increasing the heart rate (and consequently, increasing the coronary artery blood flow) and through dilation of the coronary arteries.
    In CAD there are changes in the vessel walls that inhibit dilation, and therefore the increase in heart rate is the only mechanism that increases oxygen supply to the myocardium during exercise.
12. E is the correct answer.
13. a. P wave: 0.08 to 0.12 second
    b. PR interval: less than 0.20 second
    c. QRS: 0.06 to 0.12 second
    d. ST segment: 0.12 second
    e. T wave: 0.16 second
14. C is the correct answer.
15. C is the correct answer.
16. B is the correct answer.
17. Any four of these answers:
    a. QRS is prolonged owing to the abnormal pathway of myocardial conduction and depolarization
    b. A compensatory pause follows the PVC
    c. Often occurs in the cool-down or recovery phase following exercise
    d. If untreated, may degenerate into life-threatening arrhythmias of ventricular tachycardia or ventricular fibrillation
    e. The T wave is opposite in deflection to the R wave of the PVC

18. Premature ventricular contractions may be precipitated by any three of these answers:
   a. caffeine
   b. alcohol
   c. anxiety
   d. tobacco
   e. any ischemia-producing event

19. With the exception of occasional PVCs, arrhythmias that have their origin in the ventricles are life-threatening because the ventricular pacemakers are undependable, and chaotic rhythms may result in a cardiac output that may be well below what is necessary to meet the body's metabolic demands.

20. C is the correct answer.

21. a. Cardiac glycosides. *Effect:* Increased AV conduction time; sagging ST segment; shortened Q-T interval
   b. Beta blockers. *Effect:* Bradycardia at rest; slower heart rate than may be predicted with exercise
   c. Calcium antagonists. *Effect:* Increased AV conduction time; slowing of heart rate
   d. Antiarrhythmics. *Effect:* Varies with the drug and the arrhythmia it is being used to treat

22. E is the correct answer.

23. Different medications have various effects on patients when they exercise and may cause some complications or ECG changes. Knowledge of patient's medication profile allows for more appropriate interpretation of a change in the ECG or a new symptom brought on by any exertion.

24. The atrioventricular pacemaker mimics the normal conduction system of the heart, the atria, and the ventricle pump in sequence. The atrial kick is maintained.

25. The properly functioning pacemaker is detected by the appearance of a spike (a deflection with no duration) just prior to the atrial and/or the ventricular depolarization wave.

RHYTHM STRIP REVIEW

Interpret each of the following rhythm strips by answering the following questions:

1. What is the rate?
2. What is the rhythm? Regular or irregular?
3. Are there P waves?
4. What is the QRS duration?
5. By evaluating the P-R interval, what is the relationship between the P waves and the QRS complexes?
   (Answers follow.)

RHYTHM STRIP REVIEW NOTES

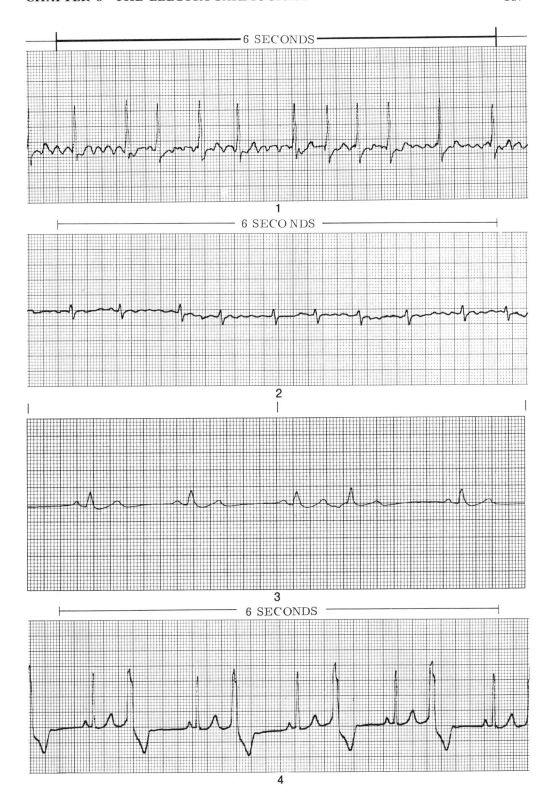

RHYTHM STRIP REVIEW NOTES

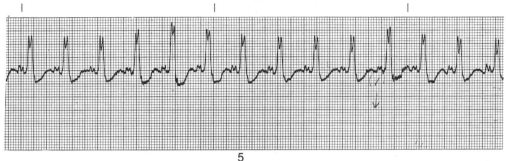

5

ECG SALVO ALARM ? MAY 8   3:28 PM   HR: 69   BP:155/ 69 MN:107

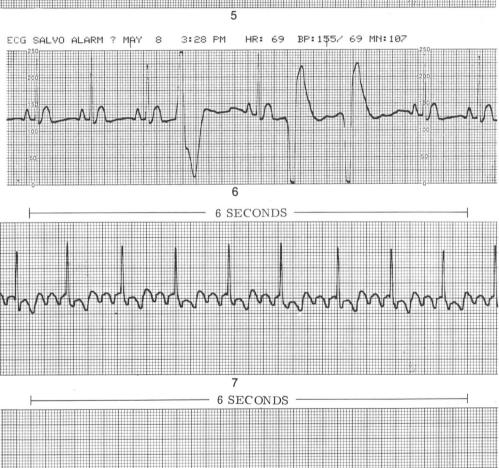

6

—————————————— 6 SECONDS ——————————————

7

—————————————— 6 SECONDS ——————————————

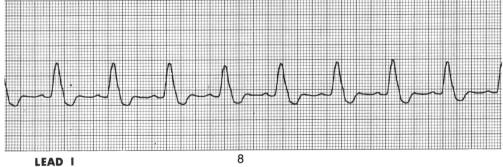

LEAD I   8

RHYTHM STRIP REVIEW NOTES

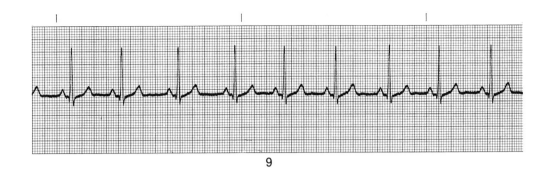

9

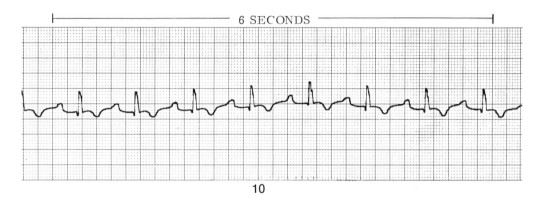

6 SECONDS

10

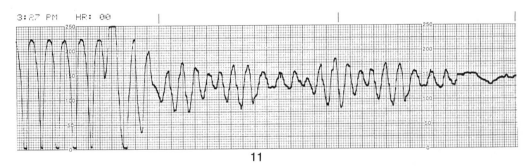

3:27 PM   HR: 00

11

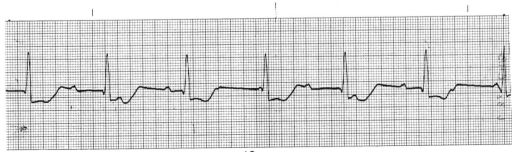

12

RHYTHM STRIP REVIEW NOTES

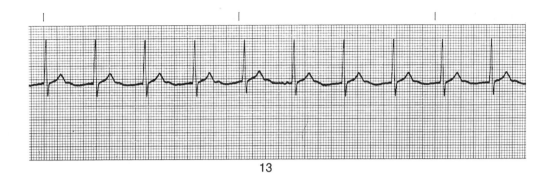

13

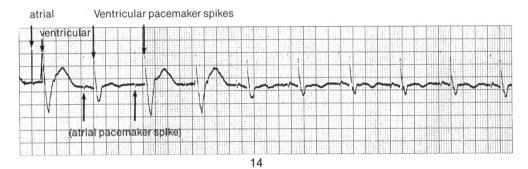

14

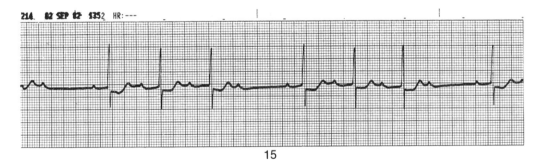

15

PATIENT 1   TELEMETRY ECG X2 RATE LIMIT ALARM MAY

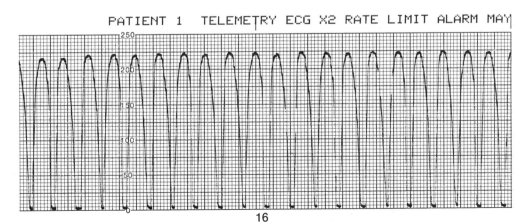

16

RHYTHM STRIP REVIEW NOTES

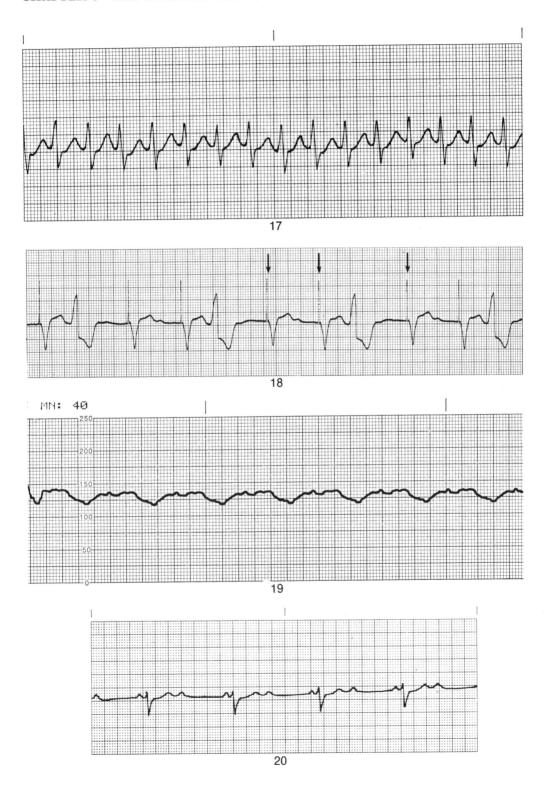

17

18

MN: 40

19

20

RHYTHM STRIPS REVIEW ANSWERS

1. Atrial fibrillation with rapid ventricular response.
2. Atrial fibrillation with controlled ventricular response.
3. Sinus bradycardia with one premature nodal contraction.
4. Ventricular bigeminy.
5. Normal sinus rhythm with right bundle branch block (RBBB).
6. Normal sinus rhythm with unifocal premature ventricular contractions.
7. Atrial flutter.
8. Normal sinus rhythm with left bundle branch block (LBBB).
9. Normal sinus rhythm.
10. Normal sinus rhythm with first-degree AV block.
11. Progression of ventricular arrhythmias. Ventricular tachycardia degenerates to course ventricular fibrillation and then fine ventricular fibrillation.
12. Complete heart block or third degree heart block.
13. Junctional rhythm.
14. Atrioventricular sequentially paced rhythm.
15. Second-degree AV block, type I (Wenckebach).
16. Ventricular tachycardia.
17. Supraventricular tachycardia (SVT).
18. Ventricular paced rhythm.
19. Ventricular fibrillation.
20. Second-degree AV block, type II.

CHAPTER 7

Laboratory Assessment and Procedures

It is not within the scope of this text to discuss the many more technical diagnostic tests that may be employed by the referring physician to determine accurately a cardiac patient's medical status. Many of these tests will have been performed prior to the referral of a patient for outpatient cardiac rehabilitation. The purpose of these more technical tests is to determine the etiology and the severity of the cardiac disease. They are, therefore, necessary for the classification of patients according to diagnosis(es), cardiac function, and risk, thereby determining whether a particular patient is a candidate for cardiac rehabilitation. Ideally, these tests should be comprehensive and, in addition to screening for cardiac disease, should evaluate the patient for concomitant vascular, pulmonary, and/or metabolic disorders.

These technical diagnostic tests, which may include echocardiography, coronary angiography, thallium stress testing, and Doppler screening for peripheral vascular disease in symptomatic patients, have been extensively described from a clinical standpoint in various texts.[1-5] Therefore, the following discussion of laboratory assessment and procedures focuses not on these more technically sophisticated tests, but rather on the basic assessment procedures most commonly employed in the outpatient cardiac rehabilitation setting. These basic tests provide the necessary information for writing and executing an accurate, effective exercise prescription. These procedures include: (1) a physical examination (if not performed by the referring physician); (2) a medical history and risk factor analysis; (3) pulmonary function testing; (4) miscellaneous physical measurements, including body composition analysis; (5) blood and urine analysis (if not performed by the referring physician); (6) electrocardiography, including a monitored graded exercise tolerance test (GXTT); and (7) functional heart classification based on the results on the GXTT. In this section, the administrative forms required to perform the laboratory assessment are also discussed and examples are provided.

INFORMATION REGARDING PATIENT MEDICAL STATUS

Prior to scheduling laboratory assessments, specific information regarding a patient's medical status must be obtained. This information is gathered from two primary sources: the patient and the referring physician. Tests performed by the referring physician do not have to be repeated if they were performed within a reasonable length of time prior to the initiation of therapy and if a full report of the results is made available to the cardiac rehabilitation staff. The "reasonable" length of time that may elapse from the test date to the initiation of therapy varies with each test but, in most cases, eight weeks is considered reasonable.[2,3,5] In some cases, however, because of recurring cardiovascular complications, medication changes, or illness, the GXTT may have to be repeated just prior to the initiation of exercise therapy.

The information required to determine medical status prior to laboratory assessment should be inclusive, as this information will assist in not only the determination of the testing procedures and techniques, for example, the exercise test modality and protocol, but also in the exercise prescription and the strategies used to modify risk factors as well.

Information Provided by the Patient

Specific forms have been developed to obtain information from, as well as to provide information for, the patient. In most cases these forms are mailed to the prospective patient after the patient makes the initial request for information. Although the packet of application forms can be expensive to mail, properly completed forms in advance of the laboratory assessment can save considerable staff time and expense. Five separate forms should be included in the patient program application packet: the patient information letter, the medical history form (including the risk factor questionnaire), an insurance information form, a medical release authorization form, and an exercise evaluation instruction sheet (see examples, Appendix A).

The patient information letter, which should be individually addressed and signed by the program director, contains general information about the purpose and goals of the cardiac rehabilitation program. The staff facilities and geographic location of the rehabilitation center may also be mentioned. The primary purpose, however, is to inform the prospective patient of the appropriate entry procedures, that is, the accurate completion of the enclosed forms, the information to be supplied by the referring physician, and the scheduling of the laboratory assessment. Information regarding the cost of the program and insurance reimbursement may also be included. To be most effective, this letter should be clear and concise.

The medical history and risk factor analysis forms are included in the packet of patient application forms and should be reviewed for accuracy in a later interview. This interview is an essential part of the laboratory assessment conducted by the cardiac rehabilitation staff. The laboratory procedures essentially begin with this interview.

There are many ways to administer a medical history. Medical histories may be patient- (self) administered, computer-administered, obtained through interview by physicians or paramedical personnel, or obtained by a combination of these methods. There are advantages and disadvantages to each method.[6] However, the self-administered history in combination with a patient interview conducted by trained paramedical staff or the physician is generally the most effective in a variety of situations.[2,6] The effectiveness of the interview is maximized by the skill of the interviewer. A well-trained interviewer familiar with the medical history form and skilled in the use of the technique of active listening is needed.[7,8] Active listening is a technique developed by Rogers that helps clarify the patient's response, thereby preventing misinterpretation of the question and faulty responses.[8]

Although the cardiovascular history (including symptoms and medications) is the most significant part of the medical history for cardiac patients, the medical history should also include information pertaining to the major systems of the body and may be divided into three categories: past history, family history, and present symptoms. In addition, information regarding allergies, medications, injuries, operations, and hospitalizations should be reviewed and documented. The self-administered history may take various forms but is most effective with clear and precise questions and a short-answer format (see example, Appendix A).

Information regarding the patient's life-style and health habits should be included as part of the comprehensive medical history. This information may be regarded as "social" history and should include a risk factor appraisal. It should include assessments of an individual's smoking and drinking habits, physical activity (occupational and leisure time), and dietary habits and a stress profile. This information is helpful in planning counseling and patient education and in enhancing modification of those habits that are detrimental to the cardiac patient.

In addition to the aforementioned information, a social history may review the following items:[2]

Job description
Job satisfaction
Family responsibilities
Family socioeconomic history
Marital status
Socioeconomic background
Sexual activity
Geographic history

However, the most useful information gleaned from the social history is data about the patient's lifestyle, health habits, and risk factors. This information may be included in the medical and personal history form or may be obtained separately (see examples, Chapter 10).

Much of the optional information may be reviewed informally with the patient after the rehabilitation program has been initiated. Patients feel more comfortable discussing personal information when they understand the relevance of the information to the rehabilitative process.[7] Also, after working with patients for a short period of time, it is easier for the health-care team to identify those patients for whom this information may be more important. All information reviewed in regard to a patient's social history should be documented and placed in the patient's permanent file. The permanent file should be available to all rehabilitation professionals working with the patient.

There are many examples of medical history and risk factor appraisal forms.[2,5,6,9-13]

However, it is best to develop the required forms in accordance with individual needs. Forms should be adapted to specific needs before being accepted for use.

Information Provided by the Referring Physician

The information that is requested on the referring physician's form influences the testing procedures performed in the physical examination. An example of a referring physician's form appears in Appendix B.

Although various suggestions have been made regarding when the physical examination should take place in relation to the initiation of cardiac exercise therapy,[1,2,6] patients with known CHD should have a physical examination immediately prior to the exercise test.[1] However, as previously mentioned, tests performed within eight weeks of the initiation of therapy in most cases need not be repeated.

Information requested of the referring physician may include the following:[2,6]

1. Specific etiology of the disease
2. Findings of cardiovascular evaluation:
   a. Coronary angiography
   b. Thallium stress test
   c. Echocardiography
   d. Chest x-ray
   e. A copy of a 12-lead electrocardiogram with interpretation (special note of rhythm and/or other abnormalities)
   f. Additional tests for peripheral vascular disease, etc. (as needed)
3. Diagnosis(es) (including those other than cardiac, for example, diabetes or musculoskeletal)
4. Medications
5. Dated results of urinalysis: albumin, glucose, micro.
6. Dated results of blood analysis: complete blood count (Hbg, Hct, WBC, differentials) and lipid profile (triglycerides, cholesterol, HDL, LDL, HDL/cholesterol)
7. Blood pressure
8. Results of graded exercise tolerance test (GXTT)

Often the referring physician does not have current data regarding the urinalysis, blood analysis, electrocardiogram, or GXTT findings. These tests may then be performed as a part of the cardiac rehabilitation center's laboratory assessment. If necessary, the center may perform the physical examination, but from a practical standpoint it is often better for the referring physician to perform the exam.

The referring physician's form must be completed by the referring physician for each patient and returned to the rehabilitation center prior to the initiation of treatment. The referring physician's form clarifies the objectives and procedures of the rehabilitation program, requests specific information regarding the physician's physical examination of the patient (see Appendix B), and requests the physician's signature on the STAT and PRN emergency orders as well as a prescription for cardiac rehabilitation.

The referring physician's form also establishes a line of communication between the cardiac rehabilitation staff and the patient's primary care physician. This initial contact should lead to the good rapport that is important in maintaining a high standard of patient care and that may also increase the likelihood of future referrals.

If, during the course of treatment, a patient experiences a medically significant cardiac episode at the rehabilitation center, the patient must again be referred to the program by the primary care physician (see physician re-referral form in Appendix B). The primary care physician must be informed of medically significant episodes directly and in the patient's monthly progress report. Such episodes may include the onset of new symptoms such as dysrhythmias, angina, or atypical blood pressure or heart rate responses to exercise; syncopal episodes; and episodes requiring transportation of the patient for in-hospital emergency care. The decision regarding which episodes require the immediate attention of and response from the referring physician should be made by the medical director.

As with all the forms previously discussed, the referring physician's forms must be adapted according to specific needs and properly evaluated before they are adopted for use.

The referring physician's form should always be accompanied by the patient's medical information release authorization form (see Appendix A). This form must be signed by the prospective patient (or other legally authorized individual), witnessed (usually by the spouse), and dated in order to request information from the patient's referring physician. This form should be retained in the referring physician's file for that patient. This form gives the rehabilitation center the legal right to request information regarding the results of the physical examination and various diagnostic tests performed on the patient.

Once the information is gathered from the patient and the referring physician, it is possible to determine the battery of tests that will comprise the patient's laboratory assessment at the rehabilitation center. Because the physical examination, blood and urine analyses, electrocardiogram (12-lead), and more technical cardiovascular screening tests have been performed prior to the rehabilitation center's laboratory assessment, the center is involved primarily in pulmonary function testing, physical measurements including body composition analysis, GXTT (if current data are unavailable or the referring physician requests that the GXTT be performed by the rehabilitation center), and functional heart classification based on the results of the GXTT. The exercise prescription is also formulated by the rehabilitation center's staff as a part of the assessment procedures. The prescription is thoroughly discussed in Chapter 8.

LABORATORY ASSESSMENT AT THE CARDIAC REHABILITATION CENTER

When a patient comes to the rehabilitation center for a scheduled laboratory assessment, the patient is interviewed and the medical history and risk factor appraisal forms are confirmed for accuracy. At this time, the patient signs informed consent and release forms prior to the conduction of any laboratory assessments.

Informed Consent

Specific policies for the protection of the legal rights and safety of patients must be developed. Obtaining informed consent assures preservation of patient's rights and documents patients' voluntary assumption of risk. All staff members must understand the document as well as the importance of obtaining the informed consent.

Informed consent forms should be developed through careful study of national and local practices relating to this area and adopted only after approval by medical and legal advisors. As all situations are not similar, following these guidelines will help to assure the best standard of reasonable and prudent care.

Rehabilitation centers that provide diagnostic services for patients who may not subsequently participate in rehabilitation therapy should have two separate informed consent forms: one for use prior to exercise testing and another for use prior to beginning the cardiac rehabilitation program (see example, Appendix C).

INFORMED CONSENT/EXERCISE TESTING FORM

Prior to administration of the exercise test, the patient must receive an explanation of the testing procedures. This explanation is contained in the written informed consent form. The form should explain the possible risks and discomforts involved with the testing, as well as the possible benefits to be expected. If the patient is unable to read the form, the form must be read to the patient. Following the explanation, the patient, other legally authorized individual, or both must be asked if there are any questions that have not been answered. The questions and the replies must be documented. The patient (or legally authorized individual) and the individual responsible for the test administration must sign and date the informed consent form[1] (see example, Appendix C).

INFORMED CONSENT/REHABILITATION PROGRAM FORM

All forms of this nature must suit the needs of the individual rehabilitation center. Again, this form should be adopted only after the approval of medical and legal advisors. However, nine concepts are standard to all forms and should be included:[1]

1. The form should explain the intent of the program, the scheduling of the exercise therapy and other counseling, the re-evaluation process, and the progress reports and other forms of communication with the referring physician.
2. The method in which the patient will be monitored should be discussed as well as the possibility of other tests that may be recommended if needed.
3. The risks and discomforts associated with exercise therapy must be fully disclosed, including the possibility of a heart attack. This information should be balanced with reassuring statements related to the screening process, professional staff, and emergency procedures.
4. The benefits resulting from exercise therapy and rehabilitation programs, which have been demonstrated by research, should be explained. A statement should be included that indicates that the rehabilitation center in no way "guarantees" that these benefits will be derived from participation.
5. The concept of patient responsibility should be fully explained and lists of behavioral objectives, including specific DOs and DO NOTs, are helpful in reinforcing proper conduct.
6. Policy regarding the use of medical records for statistical analysis or scientific purpose as well as the confidentiality of medical records should be explained.

7. Inquiries regarding any aspect of the rehabilitation program should be encouraged and an opportunity for questions and further explanation should be provided. Questions and replies should be documented.
8. A statement of freedom of consent should be included, as well as a statement indicating the patient's comprehension of the form and willingness to accept the policies described (see example in Appendix C).
9. A clause that legally releases the rehabilitation center from liability is optional but, in many cases, desirable. This clause must also include a description of the services rendered by the rehabilitation center to the patient.

The informed consent form must be signed and dated by the patient (or other legally authorized individual) and the program director. The form should also be witnessed by either another staff member or the patient's spouse (see example in Appendix C).

After all preliminary forms have been completed and the procedures described thus far have been performed, all information required to perform the cardiorespiratory exercise evaluation should be in the possession of the rehabilitation center's test administrators. In the next section, various modalities and protocols utilized in the administration of laboratory tests, including the graded exercise tolerance test (GXTT), are presented.

Pulmonary Function Testing

Pulmonary function testing is indicated for the cardiac patient primarily to determine: (1) the presence of lung disease or abnormal lung function; (2) the extent of the abnormality, should one exist; (3) the disabling effect of the abnormality; and (4) the appropriate exercise prescription for the patient with abnormal lung function. Although comprehensive testing may be desirable or indicated in many cases, this text defines and briefly discusses the significance of the major tests that are minimally required, namely: vital capacity (VC), forced expiratory volume over time (FEV_T), and midexpiratory flow rate ($FEF_{25-75\%}$).[2,6,14]

VITAL CAPACITY (VC)

Vital capacity is the volume of air exhaled following maximal inhalation. Vital capacity is usually recorded in liters or milliliters. Decreases in vital capacity can be caused by many factors:[14,15]

1. Loss of distensible lung tissue, e.g., pulmonary edema, pneumonia, pulmonary restriction, or congestion
2. Depression of the respiratory centers
3. Neuromuscular diseases
4. Reduction of available thoracic space, e.g., cardiac enlargement, hiatus hernia, or pleural effusion
5. Limitation of thoracic movement, e.g., kyphoscoliosis

The vital capacity may vary as much as 20 percent from predicted normal values in healthy individuals and may vary from time to time in the same individual, depending on medical status, body position, and other factors. Vital capacity varies directly with height and indirectly with age.

FORCED EXPIRATORY VOLUME OVER TIME (FEV_T)

FEV_T is the volume of expired gas measured over a given time period during a forced vital capacity maneuver. The FEV is normally stated in liters and the subscript "T" is expressed in seconds. Because the FEV_T maneuver measures a volume of gas expired over a unit of time, it is a measure of flow. By assessing the flow at specific intervals, the severity of airway obstruction can be determined. Decreased FEV_T values are common in patients with obstructive lung disease. The FEV_T should be related to the patient's forced vital capacity. The ratio contributes to a diagnosis of chronic obstructive and restrictive disease.[14,15]

FORCED EXPIRATORY FLOW ($FEF_{25-75\%}$)

The $FEF_{25-75\%}$ is the average rate of flow during the middle half of a forced expiratory maneuver (FEV_T). It is recorded in liters per second or liters per minute. This test is also recognized as maximum midexpiratory flow rate (MMFR). This test is a good indicator of the status of medium-sized airways. Decreased flow rates are common in the early stages of obstructive disease. The values for $FEF_{25-75\%}$ decrease with age.[14,15]

Pulmonary function tests evaluate (1) the response of the airway to specific stimuli such as allergens; (2) ventilatory regulation, for example, the effect of hypoxic (reduction in blood oxygen) and hypercapneic (increase in blood carbon dioxide) stimulation on the rate and depth of breathing; and (3) ventilatory mechanics, which include lung volumes and flow rates.[16] The assessment of ventilatory mechanics provides the rehabilitation staff with information regarding the effectiveness of therapy, the general progression of the disease process, and an estimation of the extent of permanent impairment. In addition to enabling the staff to discriminate between cardiac and pulmonary dyspnea, this information assists the staff in making appropriate adjustments in the exercise prescription to accommodate the physiologic restrictions imposed by pulmonary impairment (see chapter 9).

Physical Measurements

Physical measurements are also important in assessing the patient. They may be performed on a separate visit to the rehabilitation center either prior to or after the scheduling of the GXTT or on the same day the GXTT is performed. These measurements can be obtained quickly and do not require extensive equipment. The information provided by these measurements is useful in the planning, evaluation, and motivational aspects of the program. Usually, the physical measurements are obtained at the rehabilitation center by any of the trained staff, that is, a nurse, laboratory technician, or exercise specialist. Although most of the procedures are simple, adequate time and training must be provided to ensure that they are properly performed. The physical measurements generally include height, body weight, body girth measurements, and percentage body fat (estimation determined by skinfolds and anthropometric measurements), and may include various measurements for strength and range of joint motion as needed. Instructions for obtaining physical measurements follow.

HEIGHT

Accurate height is desirable for utilizing height-weight charts[17] and for use in various formulas for the prediction of percentage body fat[18] or metabolic equivalents. Use of a stadiometer is recommended for measurement (see Fig. 7–1). The patient should remove both socks and shoes prior to measurement. The patient should stand with his or her back to the measuring device, with feet together and arms relaxed at the sides of the body. Eyes should be directed straight ahead. The measuring square should be adjusted to rest lightly on the scalp and the measurement should be recorded to the nearest quarter inch or centimeter.

BODY WEIGHT

A standard balance scale is preferred to a spring-balance or digital scale because it is more easily calibrated. All weighings should be performed using the same scale. The scale

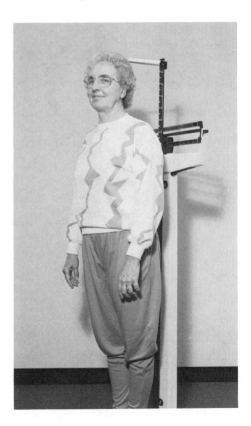

FIGURE 7–1. Use of stadiometer for measurement of height.

should be checked in the zero position before each weighing and the balance returned to zero after each weighing. The scale should be recalibrated periodically. Patients may be weighed at the same time height measurement is obtained. Weight recorded during the patient's participation in the rehabilitation program may be measured with or without socks and shoes as long as the measurement technique is consistent.

BODY GIRTH MEASUREMENTS

Various girth measurements are valuable in assessing obesity and evaluating changes in body composition.[18] For example, diet and exercise may cause a decrease in abdominal, hip, or thigh measurements with no appreciable change in body weight. The selection of body girths for measurement depends on the evaluator's intent. Some evaluation techniques require that many sites be measured; in other cases, only one or two sites are measured to give a gross indication of obesity. In either case, the measurements should be obtained with a steel or heavy plastic measuring tape. The tape should wrap smoothly and snugly around the body part being measured without kinking or indenting the skin. The measurement should be read to the nearest ⅛ inch or 0.5 centimeter. Instructions for the Wilmore and Behnke method of measuring body girth are as follows (see Fig. 7−2):[18]

1. Upper arm circumference — measure the maximum girth of the dominant limb, midpoint between the head of the humerus and the elbow with the arm extended shoulder height in the sagittal plane, hand supinated.

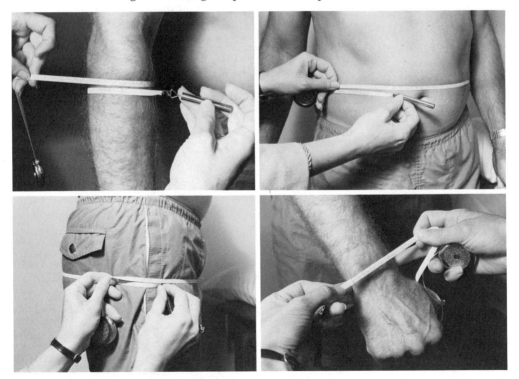

FIGURE 7−2. Measurement of three body circumferences and one body diameter for use in estimation of percent body fat.

2. Forearm circumference—measure the maximum girth of the dominant arm just below the elbow with the elbow extended and hand supinated.
3. Maximum abdominal circumference—measure the maximum abdominal protrusion at the level of the navel following a normal exhalation.
4. Hip circumference—measure around the fullest part of the hips with the patient's heels together.
5. Wrist diameter—measure the dominant limb between the styloid processes using a small sliding caliper or small metric ruler.

PERCENTAGE BODY FAT

Body composition can be divided into two components: lean body mass and body fat. The lean body mass encompasses all the body's nonfat tissues including the skeleton, water, muscle, connective tissue, organ tissues, and teeth. The body fat component includes both the essential and the nonessential lipid stores. Essential fat includes fat that is a part of organs and tissues such as nerves, brain, heart, lungs, liver, and mammary glands.[19] The storage of nonessential fat is primarily within the adipose tissue. Average values for nonessential body fat have been established for men and women (see chapter 8).

Various methods can provide precise estimations of body composition. However, these laboratory methods (hydrostatic or underwater weighing) are not practical for use in most cardiac rehabilitation centers. Therefore, the indirect methods of anthropometry and skinfold measurement are commonly used.

Wilmore and Behnke Method. The Wilmore and Behnke method of estimating percentage body fat from lean body weight is a technique that utilizes anthropometric data and requires only a measuring tape.[18]

Equation for Men:
    Maximum Abdominal Circumference (MAC) _____ inches
    Body weight (BW) _____ lb (subtract 2–3 lb for clothing)
    LBW = 98.42 + [(1.082 × BW) − (4.15 × MAC)] = _____

To calculate percent fat:

$$\% \ FAT = \frac{BW - LBW}{BW} \times 100 = \underline{\hspace{1cm}}$$

Equation for Women:
    Body weight (BW) _____ kg (weight in pounds ÷ 2.2)
    Wrist diameter (WD) _____ cm
    Maximum Abdominal Circumference (MAC) _____ cm
    Hip Circumference (HC) _____ cm
    Forearm Circumference (FC) _____ cm
    LBW = 8.987 + [(0.732 × BW) + (3.786 × WD) − (0.157 × AC) − (0.249 ×
        HC) + (0.434 × FC)] = _____ kg
    LBW (kg) × 2.2 = LBW _____ lb

To calculate percentage fat:

$$\% \ FAT = \frac{BW \ (lb) - LBW \ (lb)}{BW \ (lb)} \times 100 = \underline{\hspace{1cm}}$$

Skinfold Method. Skinfold measurements are probably the most common method of assessing body composition. The skinfold equations are derived using multiple regressions that predict the result of hydrostatic weighing (the most accurate indirect means of measuring body composition) from the measurement of various skinfold sites.[20] Hydrostatic weighing equations have been developed from the direct chemical analysis of human cadavers; the two most widely used equations are derived by Brozek and associates[21] and by Siri.[22]

Several models of skinfold calipers are available. The ideal caliper should have parallel jaw surfaces and a constant spring tension, regardless of the degree of opening (see example of Lange caliper, Fig. 7–3).

The skinfold method of assessing body composition has the potential for considerable error, even when employed by skilled evaluators. Dehydration can decrease a skinfold thickness by as much as 15 percent; therefore, an attempt must be made to schedule re-evaluations at the same time of day. The accuracy of the method can be increased by the use of multiple measurements performed by the same experienced evaluator.

In obtaining the skinfold measurement, a fold of skin and subcutaneous tissue is pinched between the thumb and forefinger and lifted firmly away from the underlying muscle. (Active contraction of the muscle in the skinfold site prior to measurement helps the test administrator to discriminate between the muscle and the subcutaneous tissue.)

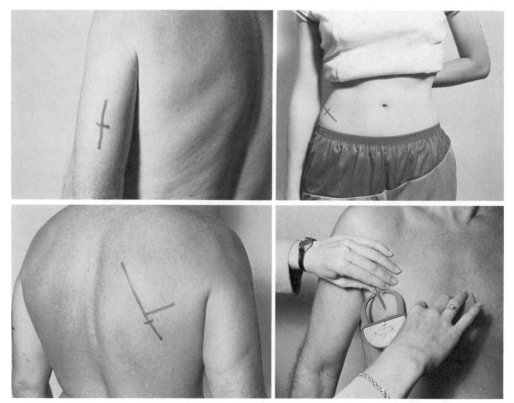

FIGURE 7–3. Lange skinfold calipers and location of three skinfold measurement sites.

The fold should be held between the finger and thumb when the measurement is being made, and the calipers should be applied to the fold at a point approximately 1 cm below the finger. The measurement should be recorded to the nearest millimeter. Most skinfolds are measured in the vertical plane except where the natural skinfold lines distort the skinfold, for example, the suprailiac skinfold, in which case the skinfold is taken along the natural line. Skinfolds should be measured on the dominant side of the body (see Table 7–1).

Table 7–2 provides an equation for the prediction of percentage body fat from three skinfold measurements as developed by Durnin.[23] The three skinfold sites and instructions for measurement are:

1. Triceps skinfold—locate the midpoint between the tip of the acromial process and the olecranon process on the posterior aspect of the upper arm with the elbow flexed at a 90° angle. Measure the skinfold by pinching in the vertical plane with the arm relaxed and extended.
2. Suprailiac skinfold—locate the site immediately above the iliac crest at the midaxillary line. Measure the skinfold by pinching along the diagonal natural body lines.
3. Subscapular skinfold—locate the site just below the inferior angle of the scapula. The skinfold should be angled upward medially and down laterally to follow the body's natural lines.

Graded Exercise Tolerance Test

THE EXERCISE ELECTROCARDIOGRAM

Equipment basic to the gathering of ECG data during exercise include a cardiograph with multilead capabilities and a monitor to continuously view the ECG. Although individual preferences vary, most practitioners require a 12-lead cardiogram at rest (either supine, sitting, standing, or hyperventilating), during, and after the stress test has been completed. Some experts feel that the standard 12-lead system is impractical in emergency situations, as the electrodes covering the chest impede defibrillation procedures. As a result, a lead system referred to as CMV_5 (see Chapter 6) is frequently used; this system has been reported to be 98 percent accurate in detecting cardiac problems during exercise testing.[18]

Some practitioners prefer to record a variety of ECG leads during the stress testing process. Assuming the electrocardiograph has this capability, an example of one format might be:

TABLE 7–1. Summary of Instructions for Skinfold Measurement

1. Pinch the fold of skin and subcutaneous tissue between thumb and forefinger.
2. Lift the fold of tissue away from underlying muscle and hold while measurement is taken.
3. Apply calipers approximately 1 cm below the finger.
4. Measure:
   In the vertical plane (except where natural skinfolds distort the line).
   The dominant side.
   To the nearest millimeter.

TABLE 7-2. Estimation of Percentage Body Fat From Three Skinfold Measurements*

	Fat (% body weight)	
Total Skinfold (mm)	Males	Females
10.0	2.8	7.8
15.0	7.3	13.3
20.0	10.5	17.2
25.0	13.0	20.3
30.0	15.1	22.8
35.0	16.9	25.0
40.0	18.5	26.9
45.0	19.8	28.6
50.0	21.1	30.2
55.0	22.2	31.6
60.0	23.2	32.8
65.0	24.2	34.0
70.0	25.1	35.1
75.0	25.9	36.2
80.0	26.7	37.1
85.0	27.4	38.0
90.0	28.1	38.9
95.0	28.7	39.7
100.0	29.4	40.5
105.0	30.0	41.2
110.0	30.5	41.9
115.0	31.1	42.6
120.0	31.6	43.3
125.0	32.1	43.9
130.0	32.6	44.5
135.0	33.0	45.1
140.0	33.5	45.7
145.0	33.9	46.2
150.0	34.4	46.7

*Regression equation for the prediction of body density (Y) from the log of the sum of skinfold thicknesses at three sites in millimeters (X):

Y = Density
X = Log of sum of 3 skinfolds
Density = $1.1536 - 0.0605 \, (X)$
% Fat = $\left(\dfrac{4.95}{Y} - 4.5\right) (100)$

Desired weight = lean body mass + 15% fat (males), 25% fat (females).
(From Durnin and Rahaman,[23] p. 681, with permission.)

Pre-Exercise: 12-lead sitting
                12-lead standing
                12-lead hyperventilating
Exercise: 3-lead (II, aVF, V_5) during last 10 seconds of each minute
Post Exercise: 12-lead cool-down each minute
                12-lead recovery each minute

When necessary, 12-leads and/or rhythm strips are obtained, or individual leads can be selected for recording.

The ECG Recording

Good ECG recordings during exercise are more difficult to obtain than ECGs at rest, even when the practitioner has followed proper procedures for patient preparation in applying the electrodes. ECG tracings can be poor owing to electromagnetic interference such as AC interference and static electricity created by the patient wearing nylon or other synthetic clothing (cotton clothing should be recommended prior to testing). Other reasons for poor ECG tracings include loose electrodes, movement artifact, and large amounts of fatty tissue present at electrode sites. Methods for checking poor tracings in any lead recording are outlined in Table 7–3.

COMPARISON OF MODALITIES

Modalities for stress testing generally include a treadmill, a bicycle ergometer, or a bench for stepping. Each modality has advantages and disadvantages, and personnel responsible for making decisions as to choice of modality must do so with their specific needs and situations in mind. Some patients may be too deconditioned or too uncoordinated to perform quantitative testing on either the treadmill or bicycle ergometer. Although a variety of tests and modalities exist for stress testing populations with specific needs (e.g., arm ergometric testing of orthopedically impaired patients), this text will describe the most commonly used modalities and tests.

   The treadmill has become the first choice among these three testing modalities. Walking on a treadmill requires little skill, is a more accurate predictor of VO_2max, and uses more leg muscles, thus reducing leg fatigue, one of the most common reasons for premature test termination. The main disadvantages of the treadmill are its expense, inability to test persons with balance problems, difficulty in obtaining good ECG tracings, and difficulty in determining accurate blood pressure measurements because of treadmill noise and patient movement. Equipment manufacturers have attempted to solve these problems by minimizing the noise on newer model treadmills and increasing the accuracy of electronic sphygmomanometers.

   Use of the bicycle ergometer for testing is particularly attractive because of its relatively low cost and ease in calibration. It is also the modality to utilize when testing patients

TABLE 7–3. Troubleshooting Poor ECG Tracings

Troublesome ECG Lead	Electrode and Leadwire Check
II and III	LL
I and II	RA
I and III	LA
I, II, and III	RL
aVR, aVL, aVF	I, II, III (as above)
V_1, V_2, V_3, etc.	V_1, V_2, V_3, etc.

with poor balance, poor vision (such as diabetics), or limited range of motion in the joints of the lower extremities (such as arthritic patients). Blood pressure measurements are more accurate during bicycle tests, and ECG recordings are usually good because upper body movement is minimal in comparison with other modalities. It should be noted that some patients find the bicycle seat uncomfortable and have difficulty in keeping their feet on the pedals or maintaining a regular pace. In addition, localized muscle fatigue (quadricep) may prevent maximal testing of the cardiovascular system.

Bench stepping is the least expensive of the three modalities utilized for stress testing. The major disadvantages of bench stepping include leg fatigue, lack of allowance for different stepping heights when considering differences in individual body heights, and the coordination required to step properly. Blood pressure measurements utilizing standard equipment are almost impossible to obtain. Bench stepping, however, may be modified successfully for use when testing individuals with low physical and functional capacities (see section on bench stepping tests).

ESTIMATION OF $\dot{V}O_2$max

Data gathered from stress tests are usually reported in terms of metabolic equivalent (MET). A MET is the amount of oxygen consumed at rest (sitting) and is equal to approximately 3.5 ml/kg/min.[1,24] Thus, MET levels (multiples of resting $\dot{V}O_2$) attained during maximal stress testing are determined by dividing the estimated $\dot{V}O_2$max achieved during the test by the resting $\dot{V}O_2$. Fortunately, various experiments of actual $\dot{V}O_2$max measurements have been conducted, and tables of MET equivalents have been devised to save time and error in mathematically computing actual METs achieved.

In using a standardized GXTT to predict $\dot{V}O_2$max, one must remember that MET equivalents for specific protocols have been based upon the exercise responses of specific populations; for example, the Bruce treadmill protocol utilized data from apparently healthy young men to formulate the MET values. Therefore, using these values to predict $\dot{V}O_2$max for a cardiac patient may result in a considerable error (overestimate).[25] Some population-specific equations are available for patients with cardiac disease and for other populations.[25] The use of such equations results in estimated $\dot{V}O_2$max values that are more accurate and reliable than values calculated without the equations. For practical purposes, however, the estimated $\dot{V}O_2$max values calculated in METs for specific workloads on the treadmill, bicycle ergometer, or bench step may be used as guidelines for the purpose of exercise prescription.

A maximal stress test is generally defined in terms of a specific endpoint target heart rate (since heart rate and $\dot{V}O_2$max are linearly related; see Chapter 3) based on the patient's age. This is usually referred to as the "age-adjusted maximum heart rate" (AAMHR) and may be estimated by subtracting the individual's age from 220. In most cases tests that do not elicit a heart rate equal to 100 percent of the AAMHR are considered submaximal. However, use of the AAMHR method to predict maximal heart rate is inherently inaccurate because of the wide variation in actual maximal heart rates. Shephard[26] indicates that the heart-rate formula (220 − age in years) underpredicts maximum heart rates for most older adults by 10 to 15 beats per minute. In addition, some cardiovascular medications lower the heart rate, thereby rendering inaccurate the AAMHR as a predictor of maximal effort. Therefore, the clinician must remember that the heart-rate formula should be used as a guideline only when predicting maximal responses to a GXTT.

For the cardiac patient or otherwise physically impaired individual, the GXTT endpoint may not be based on AAMHR but rather on symptoms such as the onset of angina, ECG changes, and dysrhythmias. Therefore, the classification of the GXTT as "maximal" or "submaximal" is not determined by heart rate but by the onset of symptoms. This type of GXTT is described as "symptom-limited." The heart rate achieved at the endpoint of the GXTT is generally expressed as a percentage of the predicted maximal heart rate (AAMHR). If a GXTT is terminated because of localized muscle fatigue or at the patient's request, the test is described as a "maximal volitional" test, and the endpoint heart rate is also expressed as a percentage of AAMHR. Although studies indicate that estimates of VO_2max derived from submaximal performance on a GXTT may vary by ± 10 to 15 percent from actual VO_2max,[27] the estimated VO_2max in METs achieved at the endpoint of the symptom-limited or maximal volitional test is considered the "maximal" capacity for that individual for the purpose of exercise prescription.

At this point, it should be apparent that the use of METs in prescribing exercise must be done carefully. For patients with cardiovascular disease, heart rate is a much better indicator of the myocardial oxygen status than is estimated MET level. Therefore, the GXTT endpoint heart rate is more practical for determining the exercise prescription than the MET level attained. Patients also relate more easily to the concept of heart rate than to METs.

BLOOD PRESSURE RESPONSE TO GXTT

During the stress test, ECGs as well as blood pressure measurements must be frequently recorded. It is recommended that blood pressure measurements be recorded at rest and at least every 3 minutes during exercise (more if conditions warrant) (Fig. 7–4) and during recovery from the test. During the exercise test, systolic blood pressure should rise with increasing workloads and the diastolic pressure should remain about the same. The highest systolic blood pressure should be achieved at the maximal workload. Blood pressure should be taken in the supine, sitting, and standing position prior to exercise.[1,28] After exercise, systolic blood pressure is elevated in the supine position, gradually returns to normal during recovery, and may drop below normal for several hours after the test. In response to exercise testing, a decline in diastolic pressure is encouraging, particularly if it has been over 86 mmHg at rest or during the test.[28] Also, if the test administrator hears an extension of sounds toward or to zero with no cuff or stethoscope pressure on the artery, this response indicates both cardiodynamic and peripheral adaptive competence.[28]

RATE-PRESSURE PRODUCT (DOUBLE PRODUCT)

The rate-pressure product (RPP) is the product of the heart rate times the systolic blood pressure.[28,29] It is usually a five-digit number, of which the last two digits are dropped.[28,29] This product is an excellent indicator of aerobic conditioning, as the RPP decreases for a given workload as the patient becomes more conditioned. Cardiac and deconditioned subjects generally have higher RPPs for a given workload than physically trained individuals. The RPP relates well to measured myocardial oxygen consumption,[30,31] and it is

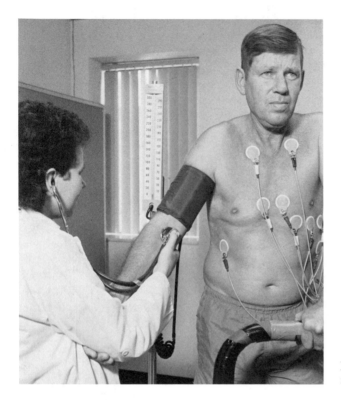

FIGURE 7 – 4. Blood pressure measurement technique.

possible to precipitate a patient's angina pectoris repeatedly at the same RPP when a standardized workload or exercise test is performed.[32] The RPP illustrates the importance of considering both heart rate and blood pressure responses when writing an appropriate exercise prescription.

Test Protocols

Regardless of the modality selected for the stress test, there is a variety of standard protocols available for the practitioner's use. This text presents only the most common protocols, and stress test administrators should keep in mind that standard protocols may have to be adapted for individuals with low functional capacity or orthopedic limitations, such as arthritis.

Adequate warm-up periods as well as provisions for a cool-down should be included as standard procedure in any test protocol. A major criticism of some stress testing situations is that there is no allowance for warm-up and cool-down because of the extra time required. Proper warm-up allows the heart to adjust gradually to increased demands and reduces the incidence of ST-segment depression during exercise.[32] Although this may not be the goal of some test administrators who are interested in detecting clinical abnormalities, when the test administrator is primarily interested in determining functional work capacity, the warm-up not only decreases the incidence of muscular injuries but also decreases patient anxiety.[34] The decision to include proper warm-up and cool-down must be made by the test administrator, although some test protocols (see Tables 7–5 and 7–11) begin at such a low level that adequate warm-up is an inherent part of the test. Most protocols do not specifically state what the cool-down should be, but the minimal length of time directed to cool-down should be 3 minutes. The cool-down helps to prevent pooling of the peripheral circulation (see Chapter 3). When exercise is stopped, a number of patients (approximately 10 percent)[28] will demonstrate significant decreases in systolic pressure due to peripheral pooling. To avoid fainting, allow the patient to be seated after cool-down.

TREADMILL TESTS

The Bruce Protocol (see Table 7–4) is the test of choice for most physicians because of its ease of administration and economy of time. In many cases, however, the Bruce Protocol may be too strenuous to use for the initial evaluation of a deconditioned cardiac patient. In such cases, protocols with more gradually increasing intensities may be used, for example, the Adapted Bruce.

The Adapted Bruce Protocol is a graded exercise tolerance test (GXTT) in which the speed or the grade of the treadmill are increased every 3 minutes (see Table 7–5). The Adapted Bruce is particularly good to use with cardiac patients because it begins at a very low level and the initial stage allows an adequate warm-up for most persons.

BICYCLE ERGOMETER TESTS

The bicycle tests are also graded (GXTT). The rate of pedaling is usually 50 to 60 revolutions/min but the resistance to pedaling usually increases every 3 or 6 minutes. Because treadmill tests are utilized more frequently than bicycle tests, analyses of data in terms of MET levels achieved are lacking. The bicycle test utilized by the YMCA[35] and the Astrand-Rhyming bicycle test[27,36] base their norms on predictions of maximal oxygen uptake in liters per minute and, VO_2max predictions along with age determine an individual's score. In order to convert the liters per minute to METs, the appropriate mathematical calculations have to be made.

TABLE 7–4. Bruce Treadmill Protocol

Stage No.	Speed (mph)	Grade (%)	Time (min)	METs
1	1.7	10	3	5
2	2.5	12	3	7
3	3.4	14	3	10
4	4.2	16	3	13
5	5.0	18	3	16
6	5.5	20	3	19
7	6.0	22	3	22

(From Computer Assisted Exercise System. Marquette Electronics, Milwaukee, 1980, with permission.)

TABLE 7-5. Adapted Bruce Treadmill Protocol

Stage No.	Speed (mph)	Grade (%)	Time (min)	METs
1	1.7	0	3	2
2	1.7	5	3	3
3	1.7	10	3	5
4	2.5	12	3	7
5	3.4	14	3	10
6	4.2	16	3	13
7	5.0	18	3	16
8	5.5	20	3	19
9	6.0	22	3	22

(From Computer Assisted Exercise System. Marquette Electronics, Milwaukee, 1980, with permission.)

An example of a bicycle ergometer protocol for multistage stress testing is given in Table 7-6.

There are a number of ergometers currently utilized for conducting stress tests. Some workloads are set in terms of KP (kiloponds), others in kilograms per minute, while others are in watts. These variances create some difficulty in standardizing tests. Although interpolations will most probably have to be made, Tables 7-7 and 7-8 should help in converting the stress test data into MET levels achieved.

BENCH STEPPING TESTS

The Master's step-test, or some variation thereof,[36] has been utilized most frequently in the past by the physician as a feasible test to administer in the office to assess cardiovascular function. Currently, the Master's step-test is being replaced by the treadmill or bicycle and therefore is not included in this text. However, in situations where older individuals are unable to utilize the treadmill or bicycle as a means for assessing cardiorespiratory function, it may be advisable to utilize a sitting-chair step test.[37] During this test, the patient sits in a straight-backed chair facing a step (which may be a bench or a pile of books). The step is placed a distance from the patient that is equal to the length of his or her leg when it is extended. Prior to the beginning of the test, the patient is sitting with both

TABLE 7-6. A Protocol for Multistage Stress Testing With the Bicycle Ergometer

Stage	Speed (RPM)	Workload	Time (min)
Warm-Up	50	0	2-3
1	50	.5 KP	3
2	50	1.0 KP	3
3	50	1.5 KP	3
4	50	2.0 KP	3
5	50	2.5 KP	3
6	50	3.0 KP	3
7	50	3.5 KP	3
8	50	4.0 KP	3
Cool-Down	50	0	3

(Adapted from American College of Sports Medicine,[1] p. 17.)

TABLE 7-7. Conversion of Workload in Kiloponds (KP) to METs for Bicycle Ergometry

Body Weight (lb)	Workloads (KP*)								
	.5	1	1.5	2	2.5	3	3.5	4	5
110	3.6	5.1	6.9	8.6	10.3	12.0	13.7	15.4	16.3
132	3.3	4.3	5.7	7.1	8.6	10.0	11.4	12.9	14.0
154	3.1	3.7	4.9	6.1	7.3	8.6	9.8	11.0	13.5
176	3.0	3.2	4.3	5.4	6.4	7.5	8.6	9.6	11.0
198	2.9	2.9	3.8	4.8	5.7	6.7	7.6	8.6	10.0
220	2.8	2.6	3.4	4.3	5.1	6.0	6.9	7.7	9.2

*0.5 KP = 150 kgm/min = 25 watts
1.0 KP = 300 kgm/min = 50 watts
1.5 KP = 450 kgm/min = 75 watts, etc.
(Adapted from American College of Sports Medicine,[1] p. 171.)

TABLE 7-8. Oxygen Requirements of Bicycle Ergometric Workloads

	Workload									
Watts	25	50	75	100	125	150	175	200	250	300
Kgm/min	150	300	450	600	750	900	1050	1200	1500	1800
Total Oxygen Used	600	900	1200	1500	1800	2100	2400	2700	3300	3900
Kcal/min	3.0	4.5	6.0	7.5	9.0	10.5	12.0	13.5	16.5	19.5
Body Weight					Oxygen Used (ml/kg/min of body weight)					
(lb) (kg)										
88 40	15.0	22.5	30.0	37.5	45.0	52.5	60.0	67.5	82.5	97.5
110 50	12.0	18.0	24.0	30.0	36.0	42.0	48.0	54.0	66.0	78.9
132 60	10.0	15.0	20.0	25.0	30.0	35.0	40.0	45.0	55.0	65.0
154 70	8.5	13.0	17.0	21.5	25.5	30.0	34.5	38.5	47.0	55.5
176 80	7.5	11.0	15.0	19.0	22.5	26.0	30.0	34.0	41.0	49.0
198 90	6.7	10.0	13.3	16.7	20.0	23.3	26.7	30.0	36.7	43.3
220 100	6.0	9.0	12.0	15.0	18.0	21.0	24.0	27.0	33.0	39.0
242 110	5.5	8.0	11.0	13.5	16.5	19.0	22.0	24.5	30.0	35.5
264 120	5.0	7.5	10.0	12.5	15.0	17.5	20.0	22.5	27.5	32.5

(From Ellestad, MH: Stress Testing: Principles and Practice, ed 2. FA Davis, Philadelphia, 1980, with permission.)

feet flat on the floor. A metronome should be set at 120, and at the count of 1, the arch of one foot comes up to touch the edge of the step and on the count of 2, the foot returns to the floor. On the next count of 1, the other foot touches the step edge and on 2, returns to the floor. This process is continued, alternating right and left feet, so that 60 ''steps'' per minute are completed. The performance of stages 1, 2, and 3 are the same.

The heart rate is monitored continuously and recorded after 2 minutes. If the patient is able to complete the 2 minutes without symptoms, the test is repeated at the same level for 5 minutes. The heart rate should be recorded after both the 2- and 5-minute intervals. If the heart rate at the 5-minute endpoint is less than 75 percent of AAMHR, the patient should be advanced to the next stage of the test.

The first stage uses a 6-inch-high step, the second a 12-inch-high step, and the third stage an 18-inch-high step, with the same testing procedure (see Fig. 7–5). The fourth stage also uses an 18-inch-high step and if a patient can continue the test to stage 4, the touching of the step with the foot remains as in stages 1 to 3. In addition the patient should be instructed to raise the arm (on the same side as the leg with which he or she is touching the step) and extend it over the leg. As the touching foot returns to the floor, the arm should be lowered so that the hand rests on the knee (Table 7–9).

TEST AND EXERCISE TERMINATION

In most cases, the guidelines utilized for terminating the stress test are also employed during the exercise therapy sessions. These guidelines for test and exercise therapy termination should be established according to the particular situation and must be developed by the personnel in charge of the rehabilitation program. Some indications for exercise and test termination are given in Table 7–10 (and later in Tables 7–15 to 7–23 in the section on case histories).

INTERPRETATION OF GXTT TEST RESULTS

Interpretation of test results and their application to exercise therapy require knowledge of physiology, pathophysiology, and exercise and should always be supervised by the medi-

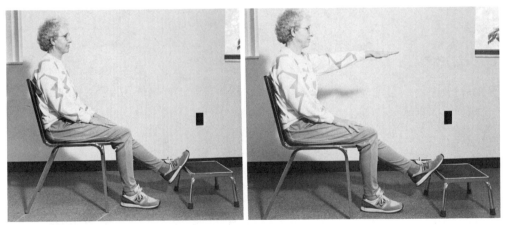

FIGURE 7–5. Proper technique for step-touching: Stages 1–3 *(left)* and Stage 4 *(right)*.

TABLE 7-9. Chair Step Test Protocol

Stage	Time (min)	Step Height (in)	METs
1	5	6	2.3
2	5	12	2.9
3	5	18	3.5
4	5	18	3.9

(From Smith and Gilligan,[37] p. 94, with permission.)

cal director. Exercise prescription (according to heart rate) begins at a percentage (see Chapter 8) of the maximum heart rate attained during the stress test. The endpoint for test termination may be related to the subject's age but may also be related to the point at which such symptoms as angina, dysrhythmias, adverse blood pressure responses, and the like occur. Occasionally, patients may be too unstable to participate in exercise therapy. Such decisions must be made on an individual basis and with the medical and legal consequences in mind.

After completion of the GXTT, it is possible to classify a patient according to functional capacity (see Tables 7-11 and 7-12).

This functional classification is helpful in predicting subsequent cardiac events and determining prognosis for survival,[38,39] and assists in the determination of maintenance levels for cardiac exercise therapy. Classification also aids in advising patients about recreational and occupational activities. If a patient achieves a maximal aerobic capacity of 8 METs as measured by performance on a GXTT, this does not represent the level at which the patient can safely exercise (see calculation of target zone in Chapter 8). A patient must achieve a maximal aerobic capacity in the area of 12 METs in order to perform cardiorespiratory exercise for an extended period of time (see steady state in Chapter 3) at the 8-MET

TABLE 7-10. Indications for Test and Exercise Therapy Termination

1. Subject requests to stop.
2. Failure of the monitoring system.
3. Progressive angina (stop at 3+ level or earlier on a scale of 1+ to 4+).
4. Two millimeters horizontal or downsloping ST depression or elevation.
5. Sustained supraventricular tachycardia.
6. Ventricular tachycardia.
7. Exercise-induced left or right bundle branch block.
8. Any significant drop (10 mmHg) of systolic blood pressure, or failure of the systolic blood pressure to rise with an increase in exercise load after the initial adjustment period.
9. Lightheadedness, confusion, ataxia, pallor, cyanosis, nausea, or signs of severe peripheral circulatory insufficiency.
10. Excessive blood pressure rise: Systolic greater than 250 mmHg; diastolic greater than 120 mmHg.
11. R on T premature ventricular complexes.
12. Unexplained inappropriate bradycardia—pulse rise slower than two standard deviations below age-adjusted normals.
13. Onset of second- or third-degree heart block.
14. Multifocal PVCs.
15. Increasing ventricular ectopy (>30%).

(Adapted from American College of Sports Medicine,[1] p. 21, with permission.)

TABLE 7–11. Establishing Functional Classification Based on GXTT Results in METS

FUNCTIONAL CLASS	CLINICAL STATUS	O₂ REQUIREMENTS ml O₂/kg/min	STEP TEST	TREADMILL TESTS				BICYCLE ERGOMETER**
			NAGLE, BALKE, NAUGHTON*	BRUCE†	KATTUS†	BALKE**	BALKE**	
			2 min stages 30 steps/min	3-min stages	3-min stages	% grade at 3.4 mph	% grade at 3 mph	
NORMAL AND I	PHYSICALLY ACTIVE SUBJECTS	56.0	(Step height increased 4 cm q 2 min)			26		For 70 kg body weight
		52.5			mph %gr	24		kgm/min
		49.0		mph %gr	4 | 22	22		
		45.5	Height (cm)	4.2 | 16		20		1500
		42.0	40		4 | 18	18	22.5	1350
		38.5	36			16	20.0	1200
	SEDENTARY HEALTHY	35.0	32	3.4 | 14	4 | 14	14	17.5	1050
		31.5	28			12	15.0	900
		28.0	24		4 | 10	10	12.5	750
	DISEASED, RECOVERED	24.5	20	2.5 | 12	3 | 10	8	10.0	
II		21.0	16			6	7.5	600
	SYMPTOMATIC PATIENTS	17.5	12	1.7 | 10	2 | 10	4	5.0	450
		14.0	8			2	2.5	300
III		10.5	4				0.0	
		7.0						150
IV		3.5						

(From Wells et al,[29] p. 104, with permission.)

level. This distinction in the interpretation of functional classification must be made clear to patients in order to avoid misinterpretation of test results.

In order to interpret correctly the results of a GXTT, one must also be aware of the specificity and sensitivity of the test. An exercise test that is interpreted as abnormal in a person who is not found to have disease is called a false-positive test and, conversely, a test interpreted as normal in a person who is found to have disease is called a false-negative test.[1] The probability of a false-positive test is related to the specificity of a test; in this case, if 100 normal persons (free of disease) are tested and 90 percent of those tested are normal and 10 percent are abnormal (false-positive), the test *specificity* is 90 percent for prediction of CAD. The specificity of the GXTT is reported to be in the range of 80 to 90 percent for men and 70 percent for women.[1,40,41] On the other hand, false-negative test results are related to the sensitivity of the test; in this instance, if 100 diseased persons are tested and

TABLE 7–12. Metabolic Measurements During GXTT for Functional Classification of the Cardiac Patient

Functional Class A (corresponds to I and II, Table 7–11)
   max. $VO_2 >$ ml/min/kg
   (>5.7 METs)
   little or no impairment in aerobic capacity
Functional Class B (corresponds to II, Table 7–11)
   max. VO_2 16–20 ml/min/kg
   (4.6–5.7 METs)
   mild to moderate impairment in aerobic capacity
Functional Class C (corresponds to III, Table 7–11)
   max. VO_2 10–15 ml/min/kg
   (2.9–4.3 METs)
   moderate to severe impairment in aerobic capacity
Functional Class D (corresponds to III and IV, Table 7–11)
   max. $VO_2 <$ 10 ml/min/kg
   (<2.9 METS)
   severe impairment in aerobic capacity

(From Weber, KT and Janick, JS: Cardiopulmonary Exercise Testing for Evaluation of Chronic Cardiac Failure. American Journal of Cardiology 55:22A, 1985, with permission.)

90 percent of those tested are found to be diseased and 10 percent are not identified as having disease (false-negatives), the *sensitivity* of the test is 90 percent for prediction of CAD. Sensitivity for exercise testing is reported to be in the range of 60 to 80 percent. However, many of the studies that reported low sensitivity for exercise testing were not conducted under standardized conditions and thus the true sensitivity of this type of testing may be higher than previously reported. Conditions that contribute to increased incidence of false-positive and false-negative tests are listed in Tables 7–13 and 7–14.

Interpretation of GXTT results is strongly influenced by an individual's age, sex, risk factors, and symptoms. An abnormal response must be interpreted in light of these factors.

TABLE 7–13. Conditions Contributing to Increased Incidence of False-Positive Tests

1. A pre-existing abnormal resting ECG (e.g., ST-T abnormalities)
2. Cardiac hypertrophy
3. Wolff-Parkinson-White syndrome and other conduction defects
4. Hypertension
5. Drugs (e.g., digitalis)
6. Cardiomyopathy
7. Hypokalemia
8. Vasoregulatory abnormalities
9. Sudden intense exercise
10. Mitral valve prolapse syndrome
11. Pericardial disorders
12. Pectus excavatum
13. Technical or observer error

(Adapted from American College of Sports Medicine,[1] p. 28.)

TABLE 7–14. Conditions Contributing to Increased Incidence of False-Negative Tests

1. Failure to reach an adequate exercise workload
2. Insufficient number of leads to detect ECG changes
3. Failure to use other information, such as systolic blood pressure drop, symptoms, dysrhythmias, heart rate response, etc., in test interpretation
4. Single vessel disease
5. Good collateral circulation
6. Musculoskeletal limitations before cardiac abnormalities occur
7. Technical or observer error

(Adapted from American College of Sports Medicine,[1] p. 28.)

EMERGENCY PROCEDURES, MEDICATIONS, AND BASIC EQUIPMENT

Written emergency procedures should be established and signed by the appropriate medical authorities. Equipment and medications for emergencies must be available during all testing and exercise sessions. An example of emergency procedures and a list of standard emergency medications and equipment[42–44] may be found in Appendix D. Emergency procedures must be updated to keep pace with changes in technology and research in emergency medicine. Because situations and the laws that govern them are different, personnel in charge of such programs would be prudent to have a carefully documented plan for dealing with emergency situations. This plan should include specific instructions for the administration of basic and advanced life support, the periodic review of emergency procedures, and the plans for emergency drills for all members of the staff. These plans should be approved by the appropriate medical and legal advisors. The safety of patients involved in rehabilitation programs is the highest priority.

STRESS TESTING CASE HISTORIES

One of the most difficult decisions an inexperienced practitioner may have is that of determining precisely when the stress test is of adequate duration for diagnostic and/or exercise prescription purposes to warrant test termination. The case histories presented in this section may provide some insight into this decision-making process, as they illustrate that test termination most often is a result of factors other than those attributed to age-related maximum heart rates.

Case Study 1. The patient is a 57-year-old woman with a history of CAD and CABG. Her medications are Persantine and Synthroid, her body fat is 32 percent, and her AAMHR is 163 bpm. Table 7–15 gives a summary of the results of her GXTT.

TABLE 7–15. Raw Data—Case History 1

AGE: 57	SEX: F	AAMHR: 163 bpm	80% AAMHR: 130 bpm

BRIEF HISTORY: CAD, CABG, Angina

MEDICATIONS: Persantine, Synthroid

RESTING EKG: Slight ST-T flattening, No PVCs or other dysrhythmias

RESTING HR:	65 bpm	RESTING BP: 128/84

PROTOCOL: Adapted Bruce (Treadmill)

STAGE:	HR (bpm)	BP (3-min)	METs	COMMENTS AND REASON FOR TEST TERMINATION:
1	80			
	82			
	80	. . . . 146/84	2	
2	84			
	84			
	86	. . . . 150/86	3	
3	96			
	92			
	96	. . . . 158/86	5	
4	112			
	118			
	118	. . . . 168/86	7	Dyspnea, fatigue; ECG showed ST-T sagging increasing to −2 mm. RPP = 198.

ENDPOINT HR: 118 bpm	ENDPOINT BP: 168/86

CONCLUSION: A mildly positive treadmill test with no dysrhythmias: heart rate and blood pressure responses were good. The test was terminated at the end of stage 4, which was considered adequate for prescription purposes.

Case Study 2. The patient is a 60-year-old woman with a history of CAD, angina, and post-MI. Her medications are Inderal, Lanoxin, Lasix, and Isordil, her body fat is 28 percent, and her AAMHR is 160 bpm. Table 7–16 gives a summary of her GXTT.

TABLE 7–16. Raw Data—Case History 2

AGE: 60	SEX: F	AAMHR: 160 bpm	80% AAMHR: 128 bpm

BRIEF HISTORY: CAD, Angina, Post-MI

MEDICATIONS: Inderal, Lanoxin, Lasix, Isordil

RESTING EKG: ST-T depression of −1 mm, No dysrhythmias

RESTING HR:	52 bpm	RESTING BP: 140/80

PROTOCOL: Adapted Bruce (Treadmill)

STAGE:	HR (bpm)	BP (3-min)	METs	COMMENTS AND REASON FOR TEST TERMINATION:
1	63			
	68			
	68	. . . . .140/88	2	
2	72			
	74			
	75	. . . . .168/88	3	
3	80			
	82	. . . . .176/90 (2-min)	~4	Throat dryness, chest pain and burning. RPP = 144.

ENDPOINT HR: 82 bpm	ENDPOINT BP: 176/90

CONCLUSION: The test was terminated after 2 minutes into Stage 3 owing to chest pain and chest burning and is positive for angina. The ST-T changes are mild and difficult to interpret because the patient is taking Lanoxin. The blood pressure responses were fairly normal, although somewhat hypertensive in view of the mild workload the patient was able to achieve.

Case Study 3. The patient is an 81-year-old man with ASHD, post-MI, hypertension, arthritis, and a pacemaker implant. His body fat is 28 percent, his AAMHR is 139, and his medications are Pronestyl, Lanoxin, Cardizem, Dyazide, Clinoril, and Transderm-Nitro 10. Table 7–17 summarizes the results of his GXTT.

TABLE 7–17. Raw Data—Case History 3

AGE: 81	SEX: M	AAMHR: 139 bpm	80% AAMHR: 112 bpm

BRIEF HISTORY: ASHD, Post-MI, Arthritis (knees), Pacemaker implant

MEDICATIONS: Pronestyl, Lanoxin, Cardizem, Dyazide, Transderm-Nitro 10, Clinoril

RESTING EKG: Frequent pacer beats, ST-T sagging, 1½ mm

RESTING HR: 74 bpm   RESTING BP: 110/70

PROTOCOL: Adapted Bruce

STAGE:	HR (bpm)	BP (3-min)	METs	COMMENTS AND REASON FOR TEST TERMINATION:
1	84			
	84			
	82	112/70	2	
2	86			
	86			
	88	120/70	3	
3	88			
	86			
	88	124/72	5	
4	90			
	92			
	92	132/78	7	Patient exhibits dyspnea, is fatigued. T-wave inversion noted. RPP = 121.

ENDPOINT HR: 92 bpm   ENDPOINT BP: 132/78

CONCLUSION: Pacer beats were not apparent during last stage of GXTT, but T waves were inverted. Inverted T waves indicate possible ischemia, but as the patient was asymptomatic, the inversion was most likely due to an old MI or post-pacemaker activity—difficult to interpret due to medications.

Case Study 4. The patient is a 52-year-old man whose body fat is estimated to be 38 percent. He is a smoker with a history of hypertension and a pacemaker implant. His medications are Quinidine, Minipress, and HydroDIURIL. Table 7–18 summarizes the results of his GXTT.

TABLE 7–18. Raw Data—Case History 4

AGE: 52	SEX: M	AAMHR: 168 bpm	80% AAMHR: 134 bpm

BRIEF HISTORY: Hypertension, Pacemaker, Obesity

MEDICATIONS: Quinidine, Minipress, HydroDIURIL

RESTING EKG: Pacer spikes evident with occasional PVCs (<10 min) and 1 episode of coupling noted.

RESTING HR:	72 bpm	RESTING BP: 120/80

PROTOCOL: Adapted Bruce

STAGE:	HR (bpm)	BP (3-min)	METs	COMMENTS AND REASON FOR TEST TERMINATION:
1	82			2 episodes of coupling,
	85			frequent (>10 min) PVCs
	82	140/82	2	with some bigeminy, asymptomatic
2	85			
	86			1 episode of coupling,
	86	140/90	3	occasional PVCs, asymptomatic.
3	86			
	90			1 episode of coupling,
	96	140/92	5	occasional PVCs, asymptomatic
4	102			
	102			
	102	142/92	7	Dyspnea, Leg fatigue. RPP = 144.

ENDPOINT HR: 102 bpm	ENDPOINT BP: 142/92

CONCLUSION: Fairly frequent ventricular coupling and episodes of bigeminy that decreased in frequency during Stages 3 and 4. Pacer firings were intermittent with no ST-T changes noted. Treadmill test was negative for angina and positive for ventricular dysrhythmia.

Case Study 5. The patient is a 70-year-old woman with an estimated body fat of 44 percent. She is hypertensive, obese, and arthritic, and her medications are HydroDIURIL and Aldomet. Owing to the limitations imposed by her arthritis, she is being tested on a bicycle ergometer. A summary of the test results is shown in Table 7–19.

TABLE 7–19. Raw Data—Case History 5

AGE: 70	SEX: F	AAMHR: 150 bpm	80% AAMHR: 120 bpm

BRIEF HISTORY: Hypertension, Obesity, Arthritis (knees, wrists, spine)

MEDICATION: HydroDIURIL, Aldomet

RESTING EKG: Normal

RESTING HR: 62 bpm   RESTING BP: 146/92

PROTOCOL: Adapted Astrand-Rhyming Bicycle Test

STAGE:	HR (bpm)	BP (3-min)	METs	COMMENTS AND REASON FOR TEST TERMINATION:
1 (at one-half workload)	88			Headache with pounding sensation. Test terminated owing to severe hypertensive response to exercise. RPP = 248.
	95			
	113	. . . . 220/136	<2	

ENDPOINT HR: 113 bpm   ENDPOINT BP: 220/136

CONCLUSION: Severe hypertensive response to exercise; severely deconditioned. No dysrhythmias or chest pain noted. Negative test for ischemia to level tested.

Case Study 6. The patient is a 73-year-old man with a history of hypertension, chronic obstructive pulmonary disease, arthritis, and cancer of the colon. His body fat estimation is 30 percent, and his medications are Procainamide, Ativan, Antivert, Ecotrin, and Tylenol. He is a smoker and the results of his GXTT are shown in Table 7–20.

TABLE 7–20. Raw Data—Case History 6

AGE: 73	SEX: M	AAMHR: 147 bpm	80% AAMHR: 118 bpm

BRIEF HISTORY: Hypertension, COPD, Arthritis (generalized), CA (colon), Colostomy, Rectal Sensitivity, Hyperlipidemia

MEDICATIONS: Procainamide, Antivert, Ativan, Ecotrin, Tylenol

RESTING EKG: Normal

RESTING HR: 76 bpm   RESTING BP: 148/92

PROTOCOL: Adapted Bruce

STAGE:	HR (bpm)	BP (3-min)	METs	COMMENTS AND REASON FOR TEST TERMINATION:
1	98			
	98			
	98	194/98	2	
2	102			
	106			
	112	206/104	3	Slight Dyspnea
3	114			
	116			Moderate Hypertensive Response,
	122	220/106	5	Dyspnea, Fatigue, Achieved >83% AAMHR. RPP = 268.

ENDPOINT HR: 122 bpm   ENDPOINT BP: 220/106

CONCLUSION: No dysrhythmias noted during test but PACs were observed during recovery. ST-T depression of 1 mm in leads II, III and aVF indicate a mildly positive treadmill test suggesting possible right coronary artery disease. A moderate hypertensive response to exercise was noted.

Case Study 7. The patient is a 51-year-old man with a history of CAD, post-MI, and hypertension. His body fat is estimated to be 25 percent, and his medications are Corgard and Procainamide. Because the patient had been involved in a cardiac rehabilitation program, the Bruce protocol seemed appropriate for his GXTT. The results of his treadmill test are shown in Table 7–21.

TABLE 7–21. Raw Data—Case History 7

AGE: 51	SEX: M	AAMHR: 169 bpm	80% AAMHR: 135 bpm

BRIEF HISTORY: CAD, Post-MI, Hypertension

MEDICATIONS: Corgard, Procainamide

RESTING EKG: Normal

RESTING HR: 56 bpm   RESTING BP: 126/86

PROTOCOL: Bruce

STAGE:	HR (bpm)	BP (3-min)	METs	COMMENTS AND REASON FOR TEST TERMINATION:
1	76			
	76			
	80	148/90	5	
2	92			Frequent PVCs, bigeminy,
	110			and 1 episode of coupling.
	110	168/94	7	Test terminated. RPP = 184.

ENDPOINT HR: 110 bpm   ENDPOINT BP: 168/94

CONCLUSION: At peak exercise, PVCs became more frequent with bigeminy and 1 episode of coupling, when test was terminated. No ST-T changes were noted, but the treadmill test is considered positive for ischemia due to dysrhythmias.

Case Study 8. The patient is a 50-year-old man with a history of an MI, CAD, coronary artery bypass graft (X3), peripheral vascular disease, and hyperlipidemia. His body fat is estimated to be 20 percent, and his medications are Cardizem, Isordil, and Transderm-Nitro 5. Table 7–22 shows the results of his GXTT.

TABLE 7–22. Raw Data—Case History 8

AGE: 50	SEX: M	AAMHR: 170 bpm	80% AAMHR: 136 bpm

BRIEF HISTORY: CAD, Post-MI, CABG, PVD, Hyperlipidemia

MEDICATIONS: Cardizem, Isordil, Transderm-Nitro 5

RESTING EKG: Baseline ST abnormalities noted with ST-T flattening in II, III, and aVF

RESTING HR:	48 bpm	RESTING BP: 138/84

PROTOCOL: Adapted Bruce

STAGE:	HR (bpm)	BP (3-min)	METs	COMMENTS AND REASON FOR TEST TERMINATION:
1	68			
	78			
	82	138/84	2	
2	84			Patient complained of
	82			bilateral leg tightness,
	84	146/90	3	pain level 1.
3	94			Patient complained of
	94			bilateral leg pain. Some ST-T
	94	150/94	5	depression in V_5 noted.
4	98	156/98		Bilateral leg pain intense (pain level 2) and test was terminated after 1 min into Stage 4. ST-T depression apparent (−3 mm). RPP = 152.

ENDPOINT HR: 98 bpm	ENDPOINT BP: 156/98

CONCLUSION: Mild hypertensive response to exercise. Positive treadmill test for ischemia with 3 mm of depression noted in V_5 at maximal exercise. No angina occurred, but the test was positive for claudication. PVCs and occasional episodes of bigeminy were noted during cool-down and recovery.

Case Study 9. The patient is a 55-year-old woman with a history of mitral valve prolapse, atypical angina, possible coronary artery spasms, hypertension, and hyperlipidemia. Her body fat is estimated to be 18 percent, and her medications are Inderal and HydroDIURIL. The results of her GXTT are shown in Table 7–23.

TABLE 7–23. Raw Data—Case History 9

AGE: 55	SEX: F	AAMHR: 165 bpm	80% AAMHR: 132 bpm

BRIEF HISTORY: MVP, Atypical angina, Possible coronary artery spasms, Hypertension, Hyperlipidemia

MEDICATIONS: Inderal, HydroDIURIL

RESTING EKG: Resting ST flattening, T-wave inversion in V_4 during hyperventilation

RESTING HR: 62 bpm   RESTING BP: 150/86

PROTOCOL: Adapted Bruce

STAGE:	HR (bpm)	BP (3-min)	METs	COMMENTS AND REASON FOR TEST TERMINATION:
1	110			
	110			
	110	140/88	2	Some ST depression apparent.
2	112			ST depression continuing,
	114			patient complained of
	114	142/90	3	slight chest pain.
3	114			
	116			
	116	158/92	5	Same as for Stage 2.
4	130			Chest pain severe, radiating
	136			into neck and both arms.
	142	164/94	7	Test terminated. RPP = 232.

ENDPOINT HR: 142 bpm   ENDPOINT BP: 164/94

CONCLUSION: Positive treadmill test for angina and for ischemia, although it may be a false-positive for CAD due to MVP. Recommend thallium stress test for further evaluation.

These case histories provide examples of responses to graded exercise tolerance testing. In each case, the reason for test termination should be clear to the reader. Test termination guidelines have been provided in Table 7–10 and Chapters 5 and 6.

SUMMARY

The procedures commonly utilized to evaluate patients with cardiovascular disease have been reviewed. The prudent clinician should be initially concerned with evaluating the medical status of a prospective patient through the comprehensive medical history. The information should include personal, medical, family health histories, life-style health habits, and results from the most recent physical examination by the patient's physician.

Results from laboratory evaluations give valuable information about the medical status of a patient. Those of particular significance include blood test results, pulmonary function testing, and electrocardiograms. Information gathered through assessments, such as body weight and percent body fat, is also valuable to the understanding of the medical status of a patient.

Prior to the administration of the exercise evaluation or stress test, several forms need to be read, completed, and in some cases signed by the patient. A primary concern for the clinician is the informed consent form, which should be devised with the aid of legal counsel and signed by each patient before any stress test or exercise program is undertaken.

The evaluation of cardiorespiratory capacity through stress testing has value not only for diagnosis of ischemic heart disease and similar disorders, but also for formulating exercise prescriptions. Although the clinician may administer a stress test utilizing a treadmill, a bicycle ergometer, or a bench step, the mode of choice in most cases is the treadmill. Rather than the single level test, a graded test such as the Adapted Bruce or the Bruce Protocol is preferred.

The clinician administering the stress test should be alert for patient symptoms such as angina, dyspnea, and ECG changes that indicate the test should be terminated. Equipment and medications to be used in case of an emergency situation must be available during all testing and exercise sessions. Case studies illustrating criteria for test termination have been included.

REFERENCES

1. American College of Sports Medicine: Guidelines for Graded Exercise Testing and Prescription. Lea & Febiger, Philadelphia, 1986.
2. Wilson, PK, Fardy, S and Froelicher, VF: Cardiac Rehabilitation, Adult Fitness, and Exercise Testing. Lea & Febiger, Philadelphia, 1981.
3. Hellerstein, HK and Wenger NK: Rehabilitation of the Coronary Patient, ed 2. John Wiley & Sons, New York, 1984.
4. Wenger, NK: Management of the Patient with Myocardial Infarction. Primary Care. WB Saunders, Philadelphia, 1981, pp. 353–541.
5. Fardy, S, et al: Cardiac Rehabilitation: Implications for the Nurse and Other Health Professionals. CV Mosby, St. Louis, 1980.
6. Wilson, PK et al: Policies and Procedures of a Cardiac Rehabilitation Program: Immediate to Long-Term Care. Lea & Febiger, Philadelphia, 1978.

7. Rogers, C: Client Centered Therapy. Houghton-Mifflin, Boston, 1951.
8. Riffenburgh, RS: Active listening in the medical interview. Postgrad Med J 55:91, 1974.
9. Rose, GA, et al: Cardiovascular Survey Methods, ed 2. World Health Organization, Geneva, 1982.
10. Diethrich, EB: The Heart Test. Cornerstone Library, Simon & Schuster, New York, 1981.
11. Friedman, M and Ulmer, D: Treating Type A Behavior and Your Heart. Knopf, New York, 1984.
12. Gunderson, EK, Rahe, E and Rahe, RH: Life Stress and Illness. Charles C Thomas, Springfield, IL, 1974.
13. Guss, SB: Heart Attack Risk Score. Cardiac Alert, Nov. 1982.
14. Ruppel, G: Manual of Pulmonary Function Testing, ed 2. CV Mosby, St. Louis, 1979.
15. Chusid, LE: The Selective and Comprehensive Testing of Adult Pulmonary Function. Futura, Mount Kisco, NY, 1983.
16. Humberstone, N: Cardiopulmonary Physical Therapy. Irwin, S and Tecklin, JS (eds): CV Mosby, St. Louis, 1985, p. 223.
17. Metropolitan Life Insurance Co: Four Steps to Weight Control. Metropolitan Life Insurance Co, New York, 1969.
18. Brannon, FJ: Experiments and Instrumentation in Exercise Physiology. Kendall-Hunt, Dubuque, 1978.
19. McArdle, WD, Katch, FI and Katch, VL: Exercise Physiology: Energy, Nutrition and Human Performance. Lea & Febiger, Philadelphia, 1981.
20. Brooks, GA and Fahey, TD: Exercise Physiology: Human Bioenergetics and Its Applications. John Wiley & Sons, New York, 1984.
21. Brozek, J, et al: Densitometric analysis of body composition: Revision of some quantitative assumptions. Ann NY Acad Sci 110:113–140, 1963.
22. Siri, WE: The Gross composition of the body. Biological and Medical Physics IV:239–280, 1956.
23. Durnin, JV and Rahaman, MM: The assessment of the amount of fat in the human body from measurements of skinfold thickness. Br J Nutr 21:681, 1967.
24. Wenger, NK: Exercise and the Heart. FA Davis, Philadelphia, 1978.
25. Bruce, RA, Kusumi, F and Hosmer, D: Maximal oxygen intake and nomographic assessment of functional aerobic impairment in cardiovascular disease. Am Heart J 85:546–562, 1973.
26. Shephard, RJ: Physical Activity and Aging. Year Book Medical Publishers, Chicago, 1978.
27. Astrand, PO and Rodahl, K: Textbook of Work Physiology, ed 2. McGraw-Hill, New York, 1977.
28. Koppes, G et al: Treadmill testing: Part I. In Harvey, WP (ed): Curr Prob Cardiol VII (8): 1977.
29. Wells, SJ, et al (ed), New York Heart Association: Manual of Cardiovascular Assessment. Reston Publishing Co, Reston, VA, 1983, pp. 101–105.
30. Jorgenson, CR, et al: Effect of propranolol on myocardial oxygen consumption and its hemodynamic correlates during upright exercise. Circulation 50:1173, 1973.
31. Nelson, RR, et al: Hemodynamic predictors of myocardial oxygen consumption during static and dynamic exercise. Circulation 50:1179, 1974.
32. Redwood, DR et al: Importance of design in an exercise protocol in evaluation of patients with angina pectoris. Circulation 43:618, 1971.
33. Barnard, RJ, et al: Ischemic responses to sudden strenuous exercise in healthy men. Circulation 48:936–942, 1973.
34. Brannon, FJ and Geyer, MJ: A study of electrocardiographic responses to various multi-stage treadmill tests in an adult cardiac population. Unpublished Study, Bio-Energetiks Rehabilitation, Prospect, PA, 1984.
35. Myers, C, Golding, L and Sinning, W: The Y's Way to Physical Fitness: A Guide Book for Instructors. Rodale Press and National Council YMCA, Emmaus, PA, 1973.
36. Bruce, RA, et al: Cardiovascular function tests. Heart Bulletin 14:9, 1965.
37. Smith, EL and Gilligan C: Physical activity prescription for the older adult. The Physician and Sportsmedicine 11:91–101, 1983.
38. Hamm, LF, et al: Short- and long-term prognostic value of graded exercise testing soon after myocardial infarction. J Am Phys Therapy Assoc 66 (No 3): 334–338, 1986.
39. American Heart Association Committee on Exercise: Exercise Testing and Training of Individuals With Heart Disease or at High Risk. American Heart Association, Dallas, 1975.
40. Ellestad, MH: Stress Testing: Principles and Practice, ed 2. FA Davis, Philadelphia, 1980.
41. Ellestad, MH: Stress Testing: Principles and Practice, ed 3. FA Davis, Philadelphia, 1985.
42. Campbell, JE: Basic Trauma Life Support: Advanced Prehospital Care. Brady Communications, Bowie, MD, 1985.
43. Ellis, DP and Billings, DM: Cardiopulmonary Resuscitation: Procedures for Basic and Advanced Life Support. CV Mosby, St. Louis, 1980, pp. 183–200.
44. McIntyre, K and Lewis, JA (eds): Textbook of Advanced Cardiac Life Support. American Heart Association, Dallas, 1983, pp. 297–305.
45. Bruce, RA and McDonough, JR: Coronary disease and exercise. Tex Med, 5:73–7, 1969.
46. Blomquist, G: The Frank Lead Exercise Electrocardiogram. Acta Med Scand [Suppl] 440:178, 1965.

47. Astrand, I: A Method for prediction of aerobic work capacity for 49 females and males of different ages. Acta Med Scand, [Suppl] 169:45–60, 1960.
48. Master, AM and Rosenfeld, L: Two step exercise test current status after twenty-five years. Mod Concepts Cardiov Dis 36:19, 1967.
49. Shephard, RJ: The prediction of maximal oxygen consumption: A new progressive step test. Ergonomics 10:1–15, 1967.
50. Bruce, RA and Hornsten, TR: Exercise stress testing in evaluation of patients with ischemic heart disease. Prog Cardiovasc Dis 11:371–390, 1979.
51. Bruce, RA: Multistage treadmill test of submaximal and maximal exercise. In The Exercise Standards Book. American Heart Association, Dallas.
52. Wenger, NK: Rehabilitation of the Patient With Symptomatic Atherosclerotic Coronary Heart Disease. In Hurst JW, et al (eds): The Heart, ed 5. McGraw-Hill, New York, 1982.
53. Kasser, IS and Bruce RA: Comparative effects of aging and coronary heart disease on submaximal and maximal exercise. Circulation 39:759–74, 1969.
54. Wong, HO and Bruce, RA: Impaired maximal exercise performance with hypertensive cardiovascular disease. Circulation 39:633–38, 1969.
55. Niemel, K: Role of a progressive bicycle exercise test in evaluating the functional capacity in healthy subjects and patients with valvular heart disease. Acta Universitatis Ouluensis, Series D, Medica, 99, 1983.
56. Leff, AR: Cardiopulmonary Exercise Testing. Grune & Stratton, Orlando, 1986.
57. Hall, LK, Meyer, CG and Hellerstein, HK (eds): Cardiac Rehabilitation: Exercise Testing and Prescription. SP Medical and Scientific Books, New York, 1984.
58. Froelicher, VF: Exercise Testing and Training. LeJacq, New York, 1983.
59. Mellerowicz, VN, et al: Ergometry: Basics of Medical Exercise Testing. Urban and Schwarzenberg, Baltimore, 1981.
60. Koppes, GM: Treadmill exercise testing. Curr Prob Cardiol 2:8–9, 1977.
61. Jones, NL, et al: Clinical Exercise Testing. WB Saunders, Philadelphia, 1975.
62. Fox, SM: Coronary Heart Disease: Coronary Disease Learning System. International Medical Corporation, Denver, 1974.
63. Weber, KT and Janicki, JS: Cardiopulmonary exercise testing for evaluation of chronic failure. Am J Cardiol 55:22A–31A, 1985.
64. Karvonen, MJ, Kentala E, and Mustala, O: The effects of training on heart rate. Annales Medicinae Experimentalis et Biologiae Fenniae 35:307–315, 1957.
65. Rahe, RH: Life change measurement as a predictor of illness. Proc R Soc Med, 61:1124–1126, 1968.
66. Phillips, RE and Zohman, LR: Medical Aspects of Exercise Testing and Training for the Prevention and Treatment of Coronary Heart Disease. In Progress in Cardiac Rehabilitation. Intercontinental Medical Book, New York, 1972.
67. Hellerstein, HK, Mohler, IC and Naughton, J: Exercise Testing and Exercise Training in Coronary Heart Disease. Academic Press, New York, 1973.
68. Detry, JMR: Exercise Testing and Training in Coronary Heart Disease. Williams & Wilkins, Baltimore, 1973.
69. Ameil, M, et al: Coronary Disease: Diagnostic and Therapeutic Imaging, 1984.
70. Jaffe, CC: Clinics in Diagnostic Ultrasound, Vol 10. Churchill Livingstone, New York, 1984.
71. Boucek, RJ: Coronary Artery Disease: Pathologic and Clinical Assessment. Williams & Wilkins, Baltimore, 1984.
72. Cohn, PF: Diagnosis and Therapy of Coronary Artery Disease, ed 2. Nijhoff, Boston, 1985.
73. American Heart Association: Exercise Testing and Training of Apparently Healthy Individuals. A Handbook for Physicians. AHA, New York, 1972.

CHAPTER 8

The Exercise Prescription

To write a comprehensive exercise prescription for an individual patient, the clinician must: (1) demonstrate an understanding of the physiologic factors that are essential to the attainment of normalized function and physical fitness, (2) identify through evaluative procedures the status of an individual with regard to these factors, and (3) recognize and skillfully apply the training principles associated with physiologic adaptation to improve the functional status of impaired patients and to assist patients in maintaining normalized function once it has been attained. The following discussion will identify and define the factors that contribute to physical fitness. The principles governing physiologic adaptation and how these principles are applied to rehabilitate the patient with cardiovascular disease effectively and safely are also discussed. Examples of exercise prescriptions using the case histories from the preceding chapter have been included in this section. In this way, knowledge of training principles may be integrated with the information attained from the evaluation procedures (Chapter 7) and applied to the formulation of initial exercise prescriptions that establish scientifically based, personalized goals for some of the patients whose case histories have been presented (Chapter 7). This method of presentation will illustrate the process of writing an exercise prescription in a clear, practical manner.

In recent years, the major factors essential to the attainment and maintenance of physical fitness have been identified. These factors have been found to improve through regular exercise (training): cardiorespiratory endurance, body composition (percentage body fat), muscular strength and endurance, and flexibility (range of joint motion). The development of each of these factors requires a different training technique. To be effective, training methods designed to improve muscular strength must differ from those employed to improve flexibility. This requirement of variance in training methods illustrates the principle of "specificity of training."[1-3] Although training is specific and training programs differ, inherent in each well-designed program are principles relating to the type, intensity, duration, and frequency of the exercise performed. All these factors are essential to general physical fitness; however, the highest priority must be placed on the development of cardiorespiratory endurance, as this factor appears to be most beneficial in the maintenance of health. It is the primary concern of the cardiac rehabilitation specialist. This is not to say that cardiac exercise therapy should exclude training to enhance the other factors, but certainly the majority of training time should be spent in cardiorespiratory activities. The discussion of fitness factors that follows is included to illustrate the role each plays in cardiac exercise therapy. A comprehensive exercise prescription includes recommendations for the enhancement of all fitness factors, with emphasis on cardiorespiratory endurance training.

CARDIORESPIRATORY ENDURANCE

No single exercise can promote improvement in all factors identified as major contributors to physical fitness. A complete exercise prescription for the cardiac patient, therefore, includes exercises to effect changes in all parameters. However, throughout this discussion the importance of one factor, cardiorespiratory endurance, is emphasized, for the maintenance of health and the rehabilitation of individuals with cardiorespiratory disease. In writing an exercise prescription, no other component demands more specialized knowledge than that of cardiorespiratory endurance.

Although health-care providers are among those who strongly advocate exercise for health maintenance as well as to augment their patients' rehabilitation or treatment, not all receive formal training in exercise physiology. Many are unfamiliar with cardiorespiratory training principles and methodologies. Therefore, when exercise is prescribed, it tends to be rather vague. "Walk as far as you feel you can each day" or "Do what you feel comfortable doing." As with all types of training, to be most effective, the cardiovascular exercise prescription must be specific in terms of the type, intensity, duration, and frequency of the exercise performed.

Type of Exercise

The rules of specificity of training apply to cardiorespiratory (CR) and cardiovascular (CV) endurance, and therefore not all types of exercise are equally useful for promoting CR fitness. To achieve the desired degree of CR adaptation, the exercise must produce prolonged increases in metabolic, cardiovascular, and respiratory functions. As aerobic exercise (see Chapter 3) requires the CR system to supply oxygen continuously to the exercising muscles, it is generally considered to be the type of exercise that can best promote and maintain CR fitness.[4] In aerobic exercise, a balance is achieved between the amount of oxygen utilized by the working muscles and the amount delivered to the working muscles. Any physical activity that is rhythmical and sustained and dynamically uses large muscle groups may be classified as aerobic exercise. Various activities and their abilities to promote CR fitness are listed in Table 8–1.[5,6]

In addition to the involvement of large-muscle groups, CR exercises should be easy to perform—not requiring any special skills (such as walking, stationary cycling, bench stepping)—and amenable to fine gradations in intensity that are easily measured.

Some thought should also be given to the various factors that are important in

TABLE 8–1. Cardiorespiratory-Endurance-Promoting
Potential of Various Activities

Intensity (70-kg Person)	Endurance Promoting	Occupational	Recreational
1½–2 METs 4–7 ml/kg/min 2–2½ kcal/min	Too low in energy level	Desk work, driving auto, electric calculating machine operation, light housework, polishing furniture, washing clothes	Standing, strolling (1 mph), flying, motorcycling, playing cards, sewing, knitting
2–3 METs 7–11 ml/kg/min 2½–4 kcal/min	Too low in energy level unless capacity is very low	Auto repair, radio and television repair, janitorial work, bartending, riding lawn mower, light woodworking	Level walking (2 mph), level bicycling (5 mph), billiards, bowling, skeet shooting, shuffleboard, powerboat driving, golfing with power cart, canoeing, horseback riding at a walk
3–4 METs 11–14 ml/kg/min 4–5 kcal/min	Yes, if continuous and if target heart rate is reached	Brick laying, plastering, wheelbarrow (100-lb load), machine assembly, welding (moderate load), cleaning windows, mopping floors, vacuuming, pushing light power mower	Walking (3 mph), bicycling (6 mph), horseshoe pitching, volleyball (6-person, noncompetitive), golfing (pulling bag cart), archery, sailing (handling small boat), fly fishing (standing in waders), horseback riding (trotting), badminton (social doubles)
4–5 METs 14–18 ml/kg/min	Recreational activities promote endurance. Occupational activities must be continuous, lasting longer than 2 min	Painting, masonry, paperhanging, light carpentry, scrubbing floors, raking leaves, hoeing	Walking (3⅓ mph), bicycling (8 mph), table tennis, golfing (carrying clubs), dancing (foxtrot), badminton (singles), tennis (doubles), many calisthenics, ballet
5–6 METs 18–21 ml/kg/min	Yes	Digging garden, shoveling light earth	Walking (4 mph), bicycling (10 mph), canoeing (4 mph), horseback riding (posting to trotting), stream fishing (walking in *(continued)*

TABLE 8–1. *continued*

Intensity (70-kg Person)	Endurance Promoting	Occupational	Recreational
			light current in waders), ice or roller skating (9 mph)
6–7 METs 21–25 ml/kg/min 7–8 kcal/min	Yes	Shoveling 10 times/min (4½ kg or 10 lb), splitting wood, snow shoveling, hand lawn mowing	Walking (5 mph), bicycling (11 mph), competitive badminton, tennis (singles), folk and square dancing, light downhill skiing, ski touring (2½ mph), water skiing, swimming (20 yards/min)
7–8 METs 25–28 ml/kg/min 8–10 kcal/min	Yes	Digging ditches, carrying 36 kg or 80 lb, sawing hardwood	Jogging (5 mph), bicycling (12 mph), horseback riding (gallop), vigorous downhill skiing, basketball, mountain climbing, ice hockey, canoeing (5 mph), touch football, paddleball
8–9 METs 28–32 ml/kg/min 10–11 kcal/min	Yes	Shoveling 10 times/min (5½ kg or 14 lb)	Running (5½ mph), bicycling (13 mph), ski touring (4 mph), squash (social), handball (social), fencing, basketball (vigorous), swimming (30 yards/min), rope skipping
10+ METs 32+ ml/kg/min 11+ kcal/min	Yes	Shoveling 10 times/min (7½ kg or 16 lb)	Running (6 mph = 10 METs, 7 mph = 11½ METs, 8 mph = 13½ METs, 9 mph = 15 METs, 10 mph = 17 METs), ski touring (5+ mph), handball (competitive), squash (competitive), swimming (greater than 40 yards/min)

(From Fox, Naughton and Gorman,[5] pp. 26–27, with permission.)

facilitating compliance with a maintenance program once the patient leaves a formal program. Factors to consider include the patient's socioeconomic background, the availability of community facilities, the environmental conditions and terrain of the area in which the patient lives, orthopedic limitations, and the support of family members and friends. For example, a patient with limited funds is not likely to purchase a bicycle ergometer for later use and is less likely to join an athletic club or YMCA for the purpose of exercising. A geographic area with severe cold weather for a third of the year is not conducive to outdoor activities, and patients must be instructed in aerobic activities that can be performed indoors. Areas without designated bicycle paths and hilly, mountainous areas do not lend themselves well to cycling activities. A patient with severe arthritis of the knees and hips is likely to have more success in activities that take pressure off the weight-bearing joints.

Once the most suitable activities have been chosen for implementation, the appropriate intensity of the exercise must be determined for each individual.

Intensity of Exercise

There is an intensity or level of aerobic exercise that is necessary to improve cardiovascular fitness. This level of exercise, which is related to both exercise duration per session and the frequency of exercise sessions, is represented by the target zone or a target heart rate.

Generally, the target zone represents 50 to 85 percent of the estimated $\dot{V}O_2$max or the maximum METs achieved on the GXTT. A target heart rate (THR), on the other hand, generally represents 65 to 90 percent of the estimated or actual maximum heart rate achieved on the GXTT.[3]

To calculate the target zone for a specific patient, it is important to use the most accurate estimate of $\dot{V}O_2$max available. For GXTTs performed using the Bruce protocol, regression equations are available for use in estimating $\dot{V}O_2$max in specific populations (see Table 8-2).[7,8]

As yet, too few women with cardiovascular disease have been directly measured for $\dot{V}O_2$max to derive a reliable regression equation.[7]

As an example of the use of such equations, consider the case of a 48-year-old male cardiac patient who completes 6 min of a GXTT (Bruce protocol) and achieves a heart rate of 175 bpm (172 = AAMHR). In order to estimate the $\dot{V}O_2$max requirements of this patient in ml/kg/min, refer to Table 8-2. According to the formula for men with cardiac disease, his $\dot{V}O_2$max in METs may be derived as illustrated in Figure 8-1.

TABLE 8-2. Estimation of $\dot{V}O_2$max Requirement From Submaximal Treadmill Endurance Time Using the Bruce Protocol

Group	Equation
Sedentary men	$\dot{V}O_2$ (ml/kg/min) = (2.94 × time in min) + 8.33*
Cardiac men	$\dot{V}O_2$ (ml/kg/min) = (2.36 × time in min) + 10.16*
Trained men	$\dot{V}O_2$ (ml/kg/min) = (4.326 × time in min) − 4.66†
Normal women	VO_2 (ml/kg/min) = (2.74 × time in min) + 8.05*

*Bruce[7]
†Pollock, et al[8]

$$\dot{V}O_2 \text{ (ml/kg·min)} = (2.36 \times \text{treadmill time in min}) + (10.16)$$
For Male Cardiacs
$$\dot{V}O_2 \text{ (ml/kg·min)} = (2.36 \times 6) + 10.16$$
$$\dot{V}O_2 = 24.32 \text{ ml/kg·min}$$
$$\text{Max METs} = \frac{\dot{V}O_2}{3.5 \text{ ml/kg}} \cdot \text{min (1 MET)}$$
$$\text{Max METs} = \frac{24.32 \text{ ml/kg·min}}{3.5 \text{ ml/kg·min}}$$

$$\text{Max METs} = 6.95 \text{ or } {\sim}7$$

FIGURE 8-1. Determination of maximal aerobic capacity in METs from estimation of maximal aerobic capacity in ml/kg·min for a 48-year-old male cardiac patient.

The target zone or exercise intensity (50 to 85 percent of Max METs) should initially consider the Max MET level in order to give the patient a CR prescription which includes the speed of walking or cycling at which to begin. The prescription may specify 60 percent of the Max METs or less if the patient is very deconditioned. It has been suggested[9] that in order to maintain the cardiorespiratory system of older individuals, the training intensity should be between 40 and 70 percent of their maximum MET levels. Average maximum MET levels have been calculated for young-old (55 to 75 years of age) and old-old (over 75 years of age) individuals.[9,10] For men in the young-old group with a mean age of 72, the average MET level equals 5.75; for women in the same group with a mean age of 70, the average MET level equals 5.4. For the old-old men and women with a mean age of 85 years, the average Max MET level is 2.7.

The use of the chair-step test (see Chapter 7) for older adults (over 55 years of age) requires the use of a specific equation to predict maximum METS from the METS achieved on the test. To compute the estimated maximum MET level, one must first determine the percent of maximum heart rate (%MHR) from the formula in Figure 8-2.

$$\%MHR = \frac{(\text{Chair-step Max HR} - \text{Resting HR})}{(\text{AAMHR} - \text{Resting HR})} \times 100$$

FIGURE 8-2. Calculation of percent of maximum heart rate (%MHR).

The formula for estimating maximum MET level from the chair-step test MET level is given in Figure 8-3.

$$\text{Max METs} = (\text{Chair-step Max METs}) \times \frac{100}{\%MHR}$$

FIGURE 8-3. Estimation of Max METs from chair-step test MET level.

For example, consider the case of a 60-year-old male cardiac patient with a resting heart rate of 60 bpm. Because his actual maximum heart rate is not known, it must be estimated ($220 - 60 = 160$ bpm). Assume that he completes stage 4 of the chair-step test (3.9 METs from Table 7-9) with a heart rate of 138 bpm. His percent of MHR is computed in Figure 8-4.

$$\%MHR = \frac{(138 - 60)}{(160 - 60)} \times 100$$

$$\%MHR = \frac{78}{100} \times 100$$

$$\%MHR = 78$$

FIGURE 8–4. Computing %MHR for a 60-year-old male cardiac patient.

His estimated Max MET value is then determined by following the formula given in Figure 8–3 (Max METs = 3.9 METs × (100/78) = 5 METs).

Once the most accurate value for estimated maximum METs has been obtained for a specific patient, the target zone may be calculated by multiplying the maximum METs by 50 to 85 percent or, as in the case of older and/or cardiovascularly diseased patients, as low as 40 percent.[3] In addition, the target zone for an older patient should be formulated with the average maximum MET values in mind. Figure 8–5 gives an example of target zone calculation.

The initial target zone of approximately 50 to 60 percent of maximum METs may be increased gradually over several months to 65 to 70 percent of the patient's maximum aerobic capacity as training effects are exhibited.

Target heart rate (THR) is expressed as a value equal to 65 to 90 percent of maximum heart rate. THR provides the patient and the exercise supervisor with an easily measured indicator of the intensity required to promote training adaptation and a maximal safe exercise level. A heart rate which is 65 to 70 percent of the maximal heart rate attained on the GXTT is usually prescribed as the target heart rate for a beginning exercise program. As the patient's exercise capacity improves, usually after 12 weeks of CR training, heart rates in the range of 80 to 85 percent of maximum may be tolerated. As an example of how to determine the intensity of a cardiorespiratory prescription in terms of both target zone and target heart rate, consider a 48-year-old male cardiac patient who completes 6 min of the Bruce protocol, achieving a maximum heart rate of 175 bpm. He was taking no beta-blocking drugs and demonstrated no hypertensive response to exercise (Fig. 8–5).

$$Max\ METs\ from\ GXTT = 7\ (refer\ to\ Figure\ 8-1)$$
$$Target\ Zone = Max\ METs \times 50\%-70\%$$
$$= (7) \times (0.50-0.70)$$
$$= 3.5-4.9\ METs$$

$$Max\ Heart\ Rate\ on\ GXTT = 175\ bpm$$
$$Target\ Heart\ Rate\ (THR) = Max\ HR \times 70\%-80\%$$
$$= (175) \times (0.70-0.80)$$
$$= 122-140\ bpm$$

FIGURE 8–5. Calculating target zone and target heart rate for a 48-year-old male cardiac patient.

Generally, target heart rate is calculated using 70 to 80 percent of maximum heart rate, and target zone is calculated using 60 to 70 percent of maximum METs.

Other methods may also be used to calculate the level of intensity of prescribed exercise. According to Balke,[11] the formula in Figure 8–6 can be used to determine the Target Zone:

$$\text{Target Zone (METS)} = \frac{60 + \text{Max METs}}{100} \times \text{Max METs}$$

To calculate target zone using figures from Figure 8–4:

$$\text{Target Zone (METs)} = \frac{60 + 7 \text{ Max METs}}{100} \times 7 \text{ Max METs} = 4.69 \text{ METs}$$

Target Zone = 4.69 METs

FIGURE 8–6. Balke[11] formula for determining target zone.

Balke[11] also suggests that the minimum intensity level required to promote adaptation is 40 percent of Max METs and that the maximum training intensity for any adult should be limited to 85 percent of Max METs.

Another method of determining the target heart rate (THR) is to multiply the difference between the resting and maximal heart rates *by the same percentage used to determine the target zone in METS* and add this to the resting heart rate[12] (see Fig. 8–7).

Given: Maximum HR = 140 bpm
            Resting HR   = 70 bpm

Formula: Target HR   = (Max HR − Rest HR) × (60%) + (Rest HR)
            Target HR   = (140 − 70) × (0.60) + (70)
            Target HR   = 112 bpm

FIGURE 8–7. The Karvonen[12] formula for determining target heart rate.

The prescription of exercise intensity in METs should be adjusted often as CR endurance increases, but the target heart rate should remain relatively the same until the next GXTT. In other words, as training adaptation occurs, increases in workload will be necessary in order to maintain the workload at the prescribed target zone, even though the target heart rate will not change appreciably.

The methods for predicting exercise intensity just discussed are effective for producing CR training effects with exercise sessions 20 to 40 minutes in length, three times per week. However, as indicated by Balke,[11] the same metabolic effects can be obtained by exercising at lower intensities for longer durations. This is very important because a cardiac patient or a person with low functional capacity should begin with low-intensity exercise. Maximum aerobic capacity can then be increased by either increasing the target zone intensity or by extending the duration of the exercise session at the low-intensity level over a period of weeks. For the safety of the patient, the latter of the two methods is recommended.[3]

As patients become familiar with the feeling associated with exercising at the appropriate target zone, the need for an objective measurement of intensity declines. At this point, the phenomenon of "perceived exertion" provides a subjective monitor of exercise intensity.[13] Borg's[14,15] Perceived Exertion Scale may be used to monitor exercise intensity when objective pulse monitoring is inconvenient. The scale is used by the subject to rate, subjectively, the intensity of an activity during exercise. The Borg scale ranges from 3 to 19 at two-point intervals that relate to a perceived work intensity: 3, extremely light; 5, very light; 7, light; 9, rather light; 11, neither light nor hard; 13, rather hard; 15, hard; 17, very hard; 19, extremely hard (Table 8–3). The pulse rate and the rate of perceived exertion (RPE) increase linearly with increasing workloads. According to Borg's investigations, an RPE of 12 to 17 corresponds to a target zone intensity adequate for an exercise session of 20 to 40 min for most age groups.[14] Borg's RPE scale may be useful when evaluating patients on beta-blocking or calcium channel blocking medications and when supervising patients in atrial fibrillation. However, many clinicians report that patients with aggressive, competitive personality traits frequently deny that they perceive the exertion to be "hard," even though their exercise heart rates are at levels exceeding 85 percent of their maximum measured values. Denial of perceived exertion may limit the practical application of Borg's scale in some cases.

Other factors to consider in determining the intensity of the exercise include age, as previously mentioned, the sex of the patient, the blood pressure response during the GXTT, and orthopedic limitations. These factors are discussed in chapters 3 and 9.

Duration of Exercise

The duration of exercise is the amount of time allocated for activity per exercise session. Each CR exercise session should consist of a 5- to 10-min warm-up period,[4,5,16,17] a CR endurance training period of 20 to 60 min, during which time the heart rate is maintained continuously in the target zone,[11,12,18] and a 5- to 10-min cool-down period.[4,5,16,17]

WARM-UP

The warm-up period is divided into flexibility activities and low-intensity CR activities. The former may help to prevent muscle injury and soreness, and the latter prepares the cardiorespiratory system for additional work. Barnard and associates[19] reported that the CR warm-up period reduced the incidence of ST-segment depression during exercise.

TABLE 8–3. Borg's Original Rate of Perceived Exertion Scale and the Revised Scale

RPE		New Rating Scale	
6		0	Nothing at all
7	Very, very light	0.5	Very, very weak
8		1	Very weak
9	Very light	2	Weak
10		3	Moderate
11	Fairly light	4	Somewhat strong
12		5	Strong
13	Somewhat hard	6	
14		7	Very strong
15	Hard	8	
16		9	
17	Very hard	10	Very, very strong
18			Maximal
19	Very, very hard		

(From Borg,[15] p. 380, with permission.)

Stretching routines vary in length and may be performed prior to physical activity or after exercise because local warming of the joint increases extensibility[20] (see section on flexibility). In either case, the flexibility exercises must be individualized. Patients benefit from written as well as verbal instructions in the proper technique for performing the exercises. The CR warm-up should be performed at an intensity lower than the target zone, and the heart rate should be checked just prior to beginning the CR endurance training to ensure that adequate warm-up has occurred. Activities should include the same as those used for the CR endurance training but simply performed at a lower intensity, for example, slow walking or stationary cycling. A longer CR warm-up phase may be required for older and deconditioned patients, and a longer stretching and CR warm-up may be helpful for patients exercising at higher intensities during the CR endurance training. Wide variations exist among patients in regard to the length of CR warm-up time required. The 5 minutes indicated should be considered a guideline for the minimum amount of CR warm-up.

CR ENDURANCE TRAINING

The period of higher intensity exercise should immediately follow the CR warm-up. During warm-up, the body has been permitted to adjust slowly to increases in the amount of work performed. To produce CR adaptations leading to greater fitness (increased maximum aerobic capacity and decreased heart rate), the CR endurance training period should include 20 to 60 min of continuous exercise.[4,17] To achieve metabolic benefits from CR endurance training, such as improved carbohydrate tolerance and blood lipid profile, the exercise duration should be 40 min or longer.[17] Approximately 10 miles per week of jogging on a regular basis appears to be the minimum required to raise the high-density lipoprotein cholesterol level.[21] However, as previously stated, low-intensity exercise should be used initially for conditioning the cardiac patient. The intensity of the exercise should be increased by extending the duration of the exercise period and not the speed of the activity. To avoid injury, the initial CR endurance training periods should not exceed 15 to 20 min per exercise session unless the exercise is at an intensity below the target zone.[22] Pollock and associates,[22] in a study of novice joggers, reported the greatest frequency of injury (54 percent) in those initiating their training programs with exercise sessions of 45 min in duration. In comparison, the injury rate was approximately 23 percent in those beginning with training periods of 15 to 30 min.

COOL-DOWN

The CR endurance training period should be followed by a 5- to 10-minute cool-down period. Abrupt cessation of exercise causes pooling of blood in the exercising extremities. As a result of peripheral pooling, the brain, heart, or intestines may have insufficient blood supply. Thus, symptoms such as vertigo, syncope, palpitations, or nausea may result.[17] Exercises similar to those recommended for the CR warm-up are appropriate, as are continuous rocking from one foot to the other. The heart rate should be checked at least once during this period; it should be well below the target heart rate before the patient is considered to be cooled-down. If recovery is slow, the CR exercise intensity and/or cool-down activity must be modified to achieve a cool-down heart rate well below the target heart rate.

Frequency of Exercise

The frequency of exercise refers to the number of exercise sessions scheduled per week during the training program. To achieve CR training adaptations, exercise sessions must be scheduled at least three times per week with no more than 2 days between training sessions.[4,17] When beginning an exercise program, patients should be discouraged from exercising more than three times per week unless the exercise is of low intensity. This recommendation seems sensible in view of the increased injury rate reported for beginning joggers.[22]

After 2 to 3 weeks of exercising three times weekly, some improvement in CR functional capacity may occur. Generally, 6 to 8 weeks pass before significant physiologic changes take place (see Chapter 3). The patient then becomes aware of less fatigue, a lower resting heart rate and blood pressure, and perhaps a decrease in percent body fat. Maintenance of these physiologic changes requires a lifelong commitment to an exercise program. CR fitness rapidly declines when exercise is decreased or ceases.[4,17] By decreasing the frequency of exercise to one session weekly, half the fitness level gained will be lost in 10 weeks. If the program is discontinued completely, all gains will be lost in 5 weeks.[17]

In the following sections, the remaining fitness factors are discussed: percent body fat, muscular strength and endurance, and flexibility. The complete exercise prescription should make recommendations addressing all of these factors.

PERCENT BODY FAT

A large part of the total fat of the body is contained in many cells filled with fat molecules. After the age of 16, increases in the amount of body fat usually occur because of increases in the size of the cells[1,2,3,24] rather than in the number of fat cells. With weight loss, fat cell numbers do not decrease; rather, the size of the cells is reduced. The percentage of body fat in women aged 16 to 25 averages about 25 percent. For men of the same age, the average is about 13 to 15 percent. In women aged 30 to 68, the average body fat increases to about 29 to 34 percent, and in men aged 27 to 59, the average range is 22 to 27 percent.[23]

The average percentage body fat reported for older men and women does not mean that these values are ideal or compatible with health. It would appear that the percentage of body fat in young adults, that is, 15 percent for men and 25 percent for women, more nearly represent the values that should be maintained in middle and later adulthood. It is generally recognized that a percentage body fat value of greater than 20 for males and greater than 30 for females constitutes the degree of overfatness known as "obesity."[23,24]

Normalization of body weight and percentage body fat should be goals of any rehabilitation program. For most persons, regular exercise can be successfully used to help reduce body fat. It is also common for persons who have been sedentary for many months or years to increase their lean tissue weight after participation in an exercise program. Nearly all of this increase in lean tissue is due to an increase in muscle mass. Thus, exercise can alter body composition by increasing lean body mass as well as by reducing body fat. However, the most effective means of reducing body fat is through a combination of good nutritional habits and regular exercise.

MUSCULAR STRENGTH AND ENDURANCE

Any discussion of muscular strength and endurance training must consider the contribution that these factors make to an individual's total health or physical fitness and, therefore, the appropriate role they play in the rehabilitation of individuals with cardiovascular disease. Generally, the public has a tendency to confuse athletic performance with physical fitness and, in many cases, it tends to view the strong, heavily muscled, athletic individual as a prime example of physical fitness or health. The concept of a strong body not necessarily being a healthy body is one that most people have difficulty accepting. While muscular strength and endurance are important in athletic performance, their contribution to total health seems less significant than that of cardiorespiratory endurance. However, the development of muscular strength and endurance is desirable in the rehabilitation of patients with cardiovascular disease when patients' muscles have atrophied owing to prolonged hospitalization or their lives have been relatively free from physical work.

It is not uncommon for healthy adults as well as cardiovascularly diseased individuals to be so muscularly deconditioned that they require strength development to perform even low-level aerobic work. Also, many individuals require muscular strength and endurance training programs to enhance body contours and self-esteem following a considerable weight loss.

Therefore, since the development of muscular strength and endurance may be desirable in the rehabilitation of the cardiac patient, inclusion of these parameters in the exercise prescription must be carefully considered. One must be aware of the different training principles and various methods as well as the factors affecting strength and endurance gains in order to write the appropriate exercise prescription.

Muscular Strength Versus Muscular Endurance

In simple terms, muscular strength is defined as maximal one-effort force. Muscular strength can easily be measured and expressed as the maximum amount of weight that can be lifted correctly one time. Muscular endurance can be defined as the ability of the muscle group to perform localized muscular effort repeatedly.[25] Although many texts do not differentiate between the two parameters, and it is difficult to train for the development of one without also developing the other, it is important that one appreciate the difference in the physiologic demands made of the body in training for muscular strength versus muscular endurance.

Lifting a maximal or near maximal weight or straining to hold a maximal static contraction evokes the Valsalva maneuver (see Chapter 3) and causes rapid and significant increases in systolic and diastolic blood pressure and heart rate. Such physiologic changes may be undesirable in patients with coronary artery disease or with poor hemodynamic function.[26-28] Therefore, the discussion of training principles and methods will be limited to those that can be utilized for the development of muscular strength and endurance with less risk to the patient.

General Principles

In general, muscles produce force in four ways: isometric contraction (a static contraction), concentric isotonic contraction (shortening), eccentric isotonic contraction (lengthening), and isokinetic contraction in which the angular velocity of the limb segment is constant through the full range of motion. Exercises that produce isometric contractions should be eliminated from strength training programs for cardiac patients, as this type of contraction can evoke the Valsalva maneuver causing undesirable hemodynamic changes (see Chapter 3). Regardless of the type of training method (isotonic or isokinetic), there are general principles that should be followed in order to ensure that training adaptations and strength gains will occur with minimum risk to the patient.

PRINCIPLE 1

The training program should provide a progressive overload of the specific muscle groups that are to be strengthened.[29] The muscles will adapt only to the load placed upon them, and the loads must be progressively increased to keep pace with the acquisition of muscle strength. The amount of the overload should be decreased, relatively speaking, for cardiac patients, and the acquisition of strength should take place gradually over a longer period of time.

PRINCIPLE 2

Exercise large muscle groups before smaller ones. As muscles become fatigued, further training becomes less and less effective and eventually impossible. Most movements become fatiguing when the smaller muscles involved in the movement are fatigued. Hence, it is important to exercise the larger muscles first so that the capacities of those muscles can be overloaded before the smaller muscles become fatigued.

PRINCIPLE 3

Allow adequate recovery of the muscles between individual exercises and between exercise training sessions. Arrange a strength and endurance training routine so that successive exercises performed do not involve the same muscle groups. For example, knee extension-flexion exercise could be followed by arm curls, and vice versa. Studies indicate that the greatest training adaptation should occur when the muscle is best prepared to tolerate the greatest overload, that is, when it has almost fully recovered from a previous training session.[1-3,23,30] When working with severely deconditioned individuals, strength training exercises may initially be performed only twice a week, and then a third session may be added as the patient increases in strength.

Isotonic Training

It is important to remember that any overload of the muscles beyond their normal daily activities will improve muscular strength, but systematic application of the training principles previously described will enhance the strength and endurance gains achieved. Also, in rehabilitation the training methods are designed to improve strength and endurance, not maximal strength. Isotonic exercise involves the movement of a body limb through its full range of motion against gravity (concentric) or resisting the pull of gravity (eccentric); in either case, real work is performed (work = force × distance). In rehabilitation, the weight of the limb itself is often used to increase strength prior to adding weights (Fig. 8–8).

Isotonic training in the rehabilitation of cardiovascularly diseased patients is generally approached in a manner quite different from that of training for maximal strength. The goal is to assist the patient in attaining enough strength and muscular endurance to perform daily tasks easily, including his or her cardiovascular conditioning program, and to achieve a pleasing body symmetry.

Instead of straining while lifting a maximal or near maximal amount of weight, patients may utilize the overload principle by performing exercises with the major muscle groups in the body using the weight of the limbs themselves as the workload. Three sets of

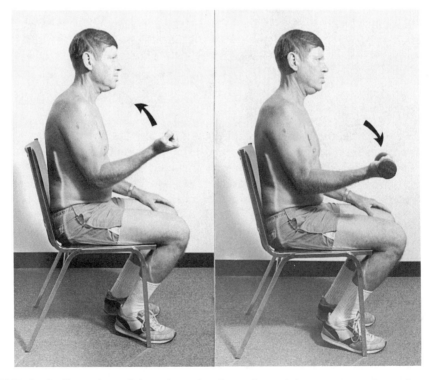

FIGURE 8–8. Examples of low intensity isotonic training—concentric and eccentric contractions.

each exercise are generally performed, and the number of repetitions is increased weekly from 5 to a maximum of 20 repetitions per set. After 20 repetition sets can be accomplished, a workload, such as a small dumbbell, is added and the repetitions are reduced again. This process is repeated until a maintenance load is achieved. Less recovery time is required between sets when minimal weight loads are used. Blood pressures and heart rates should be noted prior to the progressive resistive exercise (PRE) and *immediately* following the completion of the exercise. A significant increase in heart rate or blood pressure indicates that the training program must be changed to reduce the overload, increase the recovery time between sets, modify the exercise itself, or change the position in which the exercise is performed. If adaptation fails to diminish the heart rate or blood pressure response, then the exercise must be discontinued.

Once an individual's strength goals have been achieved, maintenance of that strength gain is possible with two training sessions per week.[29] If the frequency of training drops to less than two per week, the strength gains are lost after a few months. There appears to be no advantage to training with eccentric rather than concentric contractions.[1,29] Finally, most of the strength gained in isotonic training occurs at the weakest points in the range of motion and, as a result, the muscle is not maximally trained through the entire range.[1,2,3]

Isokinetic Training

Isokinetic training is a relatively new system that combines the features of both isometric and isotonic training. It can be used effectively with cardiac patients if the training is conducted using low-intensity workloads. Isokinetic exercise differs from isotonic training in that it provides overload of the working muscle or group of muscles at all points in the range of motion. This type of training can be implemented using the same methods as those previously described for isotonic training.

FLEXIBILITY

Flexibility can be most simply defined as the range of possible movement in a joint (as in the knee or hip) or series of joints (as in the wrist or spine). Although the importance of flexibility is apparent in various athletic endeavors (gymnastics, diving, hurdling, etc.), its importance is also evident in the performance of daily activities (putting on shoes, turning the head from side to side, etc.). The development of flexibility increases ease and efficiency of movement in walking and running and decreases the incidence of muscular injury. There is also considerable evidence that maintenance of good joint mobility can prevent or lessen the joint stiffness and soreness that often accompanies the aging process.[2]

The role that flexibility plays in the prevention of muscular injury and in the enhancement of efficiency and ease of movement makes it a valuable part of any cardiac exercise therapy program. Loss of range of joint motion is a major problem for most middle-aged and older persons (the majority of cardiac patients fall within this age group) and can contribute to injuries that will impede attempts to perform cardiorespiratory training. This problem should be resolved by including flexibility training as an integral part of cardiac exercise therapy.

In designing a flexibility or stretching program, it is important to recognize that the range of joint motion is specific to a given joint or combination of joints and that an individual is a composite of many joints of varying degrees of flexibility. There are mechanical factors that limit the range of possible movement in a joint. For example, the bony structures may prohibit the extension of the knee or elbow joint. Moreover, joint flexion may be limited by the intervening bulk of muscle in a heavily muscled individual. Although these mechanical factors exist in specific situations, in all joints the range of motion is affected by the soft tissues, including muscle and its fascial sheaths, connective tissue including tendons, ligaments, and joint capsules, and the skin. These structures are modifiable and therefore are the main concern in understanding the most effective way to develop or improve range of motion.[31]

In attempting to increase flexibility, a jerky stretching motion precipitates a muscle contraction, the amount and rate of which vary directly with the amount and rate of the stretching movement.[32] This is the result of the *myotatic or "stretch" reflex* that originates in the muscle spindle. Therefore, bouncing, bobbing, or ballistic types of stretching actually inhibit the desired effects of the stretching. On the other hand, a slow, steady, sustained, firm stretch evokes the inverse myotatic reflex which inhibits contraction of the muscle in which the tendon was stretched as well as the contraction of the entire functional group of muscles involved in the stretching movement. Through sustained, firm stretching, the soft tissue changes necessary for increased joint mobility can be made with less danger of exceeding the extensibility limits of the tissues involved, little or no muscular soreness (in fact, sustained stretching may even relieve soreness),[2] and less energy expenditure than ballistic stretching. Therefore, sustained, firm stretching appears to be the method of choice for improving flexibility.[1,2,32]

How to Stretch

As previously stated, slow, sustained, firm stretching is recommended to improve the range of joint motion. Because the development of flexibility is desirable, many exercise routines have been developed for use prior to and following exercise or sports participation.[4-6]

The type of stretching exercise performed should be specific to the functional groups of muscles involved in the performance of the physical activity. For example, as cardiorespiratory exercise involves rhythmic contraction and relaxation of the large muscles of the legs, thighs, and hips, the stretching program should be designed to increase flexibility in the prime movers of the ankle, knee, and hip joints. Stretching exercises must be performed within an individual's extensibility limits without straining or causing pain, yet they must be of appropriate intensity or no increase in flexibility will occur. A good stretching exercise involves two phases: (1) a slow, easy stretch held for a period of 10 to 30 sec while the individual relaxes and concentrates on relaxing the muscle or muscle group being stretched, and (2) an extension of the easy stretch into a moderate stretch in which the feeling of the stretch becomes more intense but does not actually cause pain.[33] The intense phase of the stretch is usually held for 30 sec or longer. Stretching to the point of actual pain or straining should not occur during a good stretching exercise. While stretching, breathing should be slow and rhythmic and an individual should never hold his or her breath. The position of the body is also to be considered in developing the flexibility program. During the stretching exercises, the individual should feel stable and comfortable, and exercises that may contribute to excessive stress on a joint or changes in blood pressure should be avoided. Any stretching exercise producing swelling or pain should be discontinued immediately; after careful evaluation, it may be either adapted or abandoned (see Appendix E for examples of basic flexibility exercise programs).

Stretching exercise routines vary in length and may be performed prior to physical activity as a part of the warm-up period and/or after exercise following a cool-down period. In general, basic stretching routines are completed in 5 to 10 min but may be extended if necessary. Ideally, stretching exercises should be performed as part of a patient's daily exercise program. Flexibility is affected by temperature (local warming of a joint increases flexibility).[20] This fact should be considered in selecting the time of day to schedule training sessions for older adults and for those patients with arthritic conditions. These patients may experience greater difficulty performing flexibility exercises early in the morning (owing to lower muscle temperature) or in a cooler environment. These patients may prefer to stretch after the muscle temperature has been raised, for example, following CR exercise. In general, changes that occur as a result of a flexibility training program persist for a considerable period of time (8 weeks or more) after stretching is discontinued,[20] in contrast to the length of time cardiorespiratory endurance is maintained after cessation of training.

WRITING THE EXERCISE PRESCRIPTION

The information presented in this chapter should serve as a guideline for writing a complete exercise prescription for the cardiovascularly diseased patient. The following examples (Tables 8 – 4 to 8 – 8) will illustrate a method of presenting standard information that should be contained in an exercise prescription, that is, the type, intensity, duration, and frequency of exercise. How these parameters are determined will vary among rehabilitation centers, as generally each rehabilitation center prefers to use its own methods for formulating CR intensity, percentage body fat, and other factors. The examples ought to clarify the procedures that should be followed in writing the prescription as well as the key elements for inclusion. The examples integrate the information presented in Chapters 7 and 8 and include case studies 1, 5, 6, and 7. The examples represent the initial exercise prescription written for these patients prior to beginning exercise therapy. Examples illustrating the adjustment of the exercise prescription during this period of time between evaluations is presented in chapter 9.

In writing an exercise prescription, using a standard form with adequate space for calculations and comments is helpful. This form becomes a part of each patient's permanent medical file and may be used to document changes made in the exercise prescription between evaluations (see Table 8 – 4).

TABLE 8–4. Sample Exercise Prescription Form

Exercise Rx

Name _____ F   M   Age _____ Date _____
                                            Ht. (in) _____ Wt. (lb) _____

Dx: _____

Meds: _____

Comments: _____
_____

GXT Data: Date Performed ____/____/____   Where: _____

          Rest HR _____   Protocol: _____

          Max HR _____   Max METs: _____

          Re-evaluation scheduled ____/____/____

C-R Rx:
    Target Zone (METs) = 50 to 85% of Max METs
                       = 0.50 to 0.85 × _____
                       = _____ METs
    Target HR (bpm) = (Max HR − Rest HR) (65% to 90%) + (Rest HR)
                    = (_____ − _____) (0.65 to 0.90) + (_____)
                    = _____ bpm
    Type of Exercise: _____ bike   _____ row   _____ walk   _____ walk/jog

    Length of session: _____ Frequency: _____
    Comments: _____
    _____
    _____

Flexibility Rx: _____
_____
_____

Muscular S & End Rx: _____
_____
_____

% Body Fat Rx:
    _____ %   Desirable M 15%
                                                     F   25%

Body Wt. _____ lb
         _____ kg   Desired Range _____ to _____ lb

TABLE 8–5. Exercise Prescription for Case Study #1 (see text)

Exercise Rx

Name ___Case Study 1___   Ⓕ M   Age _57_   Date _____
                           Ht. (in) _59_   Wt. (lb) _149.5_

Dx: ___CAD, CABG, Angina_____

Meds: ___Persantine, Synthroid_____

Comments: ST-T sagging — 2mm at Max HR GXT & Dyspnea, Fatigue _____

GXT Data: Date Performed _3/19/87_   Where: __X Hospital_____

　　　　　Rest HR   65   Protocol: _Adapted Bruce_____

　　　　　Max HR   118   Max METs: ___7_____

　　　　　Re-evaluation scheduled _6/20/87_

C-R Rx:

　　　Target Zone (METs) = 50 to 85% of Max METs
　　　　　　　　　　 = 0.50 to 0.85 × _7_
　　　　　　　　　　 = _3.5 to 6.0_ METs
　　　Target HR (bpm) = (Max HR − Rest HR) (65% to 90%) + (Rest HR)
　　　　　　　　　　 = (_118_ − _65_) (0.65) + (_65_)
　　　　　　　　　　 = _~99_ bpm
　　　Type of Exercise: _X_ bike ____ row _X_ walk ____ walk/jog

　　　Length of session: __20–30 min.__   Frequency: _2–3/wk_
　　　Comments: __Initial HR determined from Target Zone & THR = 99 bpm__
　　　RPP = 198
Flexibility Rx: __Begin with flex for calf, hamstring, quads, hip flexors.__
Hold 10 sec, progress to 30 sec. Add shoulder, trunk, neck and back exercises
as needed. 3Xs/week prior to Ex. 1X/day at home.
Muscular S & End Rx: __N/A Begin if needed p̄ re-evaluation 6/20/87__

% Body Fat Rx:
　___32___ %   Desirable M _15%_
                                           F _25%_

Body Wt. _149.5_ lb
　　　　 _68_ kg   Desired Range _115_ to _125_ lb
Referred also for nutrition education and weight reduction.

Page 204

TABLE 8–6. Exercise Prescription for Case Study #5 (see text)

Exercise Rx

Name __Case Study 5__   Ⓕ M   Age _70_   Date _____
                              Ht. (in) _59_   Wt. (lb) _180_

Dx: __Hypertension, Obesity, Arthritis (knees, wrists, spine)__

Meds: __HydroDIURIL, Aldomet__

Comments: __Severe hypertensive response to exercise Max BP 220/186,__
__severely deconditioned, orthopedic limitations.__

GXT Data: Date Performed _2/7/87_   Where: __Clinic X__
          Rest HR ___62___   Protocol: __Adapted Astrand-Rhyming__
          Max HR ___113___   Max METs: ___2___
          Re-evaluation scheduled __5/15/87__

C-R Rx:
    Target Zone (METs) = 50 to 85% of Max METs
                       = .50 to .85 × __2__
                       = ~1 to 2 __ METs ($\downarrow$40% due to age & BP = ~1 MET)
    Target HR (bpm) = (Max HR − Rest HR) (65% to 90%) + (Rest HR)
                    = (_113_ − _62_) (.65) + (_62_)
                    = _~95_ bpm
    Type of Exercise: _X_ bike ____ row ____ walk ____ walk/jog
                      (no arms on Schwinn Airdyne until adapt. occurs)
    Length of session: __20–30 min.__ Frequency: __3Xs/week__
    Comments: __Initial HR based on Target Zone and THR = 95 bpm.__
    __Limited by BP response. Intermittent CR exercise initially 2–3 min of__
    __exercise with 1–2 min rest. Progress to continuous. RPP = 248__

Flexibility Rx: __General program with emphasis on affected joints performed__
__3Xs/day.__

Muscular S & End Rx: __Mild strengthening program for quadriceps & hamstrings —__
__10 reps, 3Xs/day — no weights.__

% Body Fat Rx:
    ___44___ %   Desirable M _15%_
                                                  F _25%_

Body Wt. _180_ lb
         _82_ kg   Desired Range __115__ to __125__ lb

Referred also for nutrition education and weight reduction.

TABLE 8–7. Exercise Prescription for Case Study #6 (see text)

Exercise Rx

Name __Case Study 6__   F Ⓜ Age _73_   Date _____

Ht. (in) _67¾_   Wt. (lb) _190_

Dx: __Hypertension, COPD, Arthritis (hands, wrists, elbows, knees, spine)__

Meds: __Procainamide, Antivert, Ativan, Ecotrin, Tylenol__

Comments: Orthopedic limitations, Acute rectal sensitivity, PACs during
recovery on GXT, Mildly positive GXT II, III, AVF, Hypertensive response to exercise.

GXT Data: Date Performed _4/3/87_   Where: __Clinic X__
    Rest HR _76_   Protocol: _Adapted Bruce_
    Max HR _122_   Max METs: _5_
    Re-evaluation scheduled _7/7/87_

C-R Rx:
    Target Zone (METs) = 50 to 85% of Max METs
        = .50 to .85 × _5_
        = ~2.5 to 4 METs
    Target HR (bpm) = (Max HR − Rest HR) (65% to 90%) + (Rest HR)
        = (_122_ − _76_) (.65 to .90) + (_76_)
        = _~106_ bpm
    Type of Exercise: ____ bike ____ row _X_ walk ____ walk/jog

    Length of session: __20 minutes__   Frequency: 2–3×s/week
    Comments: __Initially limited by BP response, Target Zone & THR = 106 bpm__
    Intermittent CR ex. 2–3 min, 1–2 min rest. Progress to continuous. RPP = 268

Flexibility Rx: __General Flex. program emphasizing affected joints − performed__
2–3 ×s/day.

Muscular S & End Rx: __N/A Begin as needed after p̄ re-evaluation 7/7/87__

% Body Fat Rx:
    _30_ %   Desirable M _15%_
        F _25%_

Body Wt. _190_ lb
    _86_ kg   Desired Range _165_ to _175_ lb

Referred also for nutrition education and weight reduction.

TABLE 8–8. Exercise Prescription for Case Study #7 (see text)

Exercise Rx

Name ___Case Study 7___   F Ⓜ Age _51_   Date _____
                                 Ht. (in) _74_   Wt. (lb) _238_____

Dx: ___CAD, s/pMI, Hypertension, Rhythm Disturbance_____

Meds: ___Corgard, Procainamide_____

Comments: Mild hypertensive response GXT, PVCs, Coupling (1), Bigeminy
at Max HR on GXT._____

GXT Data: Date Performed _1/24/87_   Where: ___Hospital X_____

      Rest HR ___56_____   Protocol: _Bruce_____

      Max HR ___110_____   Max METs: ___7_____

      Re-evaluation scheduled _4/25/87_

C-R Rx:
    Target Zone (METs) = 50 to 85% of Max METs
                = .50 to .85 × _7_
                = 3.5 to 6 METs
    Target HR (bpm) = (Max HR − Rest HR) (65% to 90%) + (Rest HR)
                = (_110_ − _56_) (.65) + (_56_)
                = _~91_ bpm
    Type of Exercise: X bike ____ row X walk ____ walk/jog

    Length of session: ___20 – 30 min.___ Frequency: 3Xs/week
    Comments: ___Initial HR based on Target Zone, THR response = 91 bpm.___
    Patient referred to Physician for Med. change to stabilize Arrhythmia prior to
    beginning exercise therapy, RPP = 184

Flexibility Rx: ___Flex for calf, hamstrings, quads, hip flexors, 3Xs/week prior___
to therapy, 1X/day home, progress from 10 sec to 30 sec. Add shoulders, trunk,
neck as needed.

Muscular S & End Rx: ___N/A at this time._____

% Body Fat Rx:
    ___25___ %   Desirable M _15%_
                                             F _25%_

Body Wt. _238_ lb
        _108_ kg   Desired Range _200_ to _210_ lb
Referred also for nutrition education and weight reduction.

SUMMARY

Guidelines for writing a complete exercise prescription for the cardiovascularly diseased
patient have been presented. A discussion of the physiological factors essential to the
attainment and maintenance of physical fitness as well as the training principles associated with the development of each factor have been included. These fitness factors are:
cardiorespiratory endurance, body composition (percent body fat), muscular strength and

endurance, and flexibility. Each factor has been clearly defined, and training adaptations and methods have been described in detail. Emphasis has been placed on the importance of specificity of training and the need to standardize the exercise prescription in terms of the type, intensity, duration, and frequency of the exercise employed in rehabilitation. The rationale has been presented for adaptation of any training method that would prove unsafe for a cardiovascularly diseased patient. A discussion of the research regarding cardiorespiratory endurance training has been presented with recommendations for practical application. A sample exercise prescription form and four case histories have been included to assist the student in the application of the guidelines presented for writing a complete exercise prescription.

REFERENCES

1. Lamb, DR: Physiology of Exercise: Responses and Adaptations, ed 2. Macmillan, New York, 1984.
2. deVries, HA: Physiology of Exercise, ed 4. Wm C Brown, Dubuque, 1986.
3. American College of Sports Medicine: Guidelines for Exercise Testing and Prescription, ed 3. Lea & Febiger, Philadelphia, 1986.
4. American College of Sports Medicine: Position statement on the recommended quantity and quality of exercise for developing and maintaining fitness in healthy adults. Med Sci Sports 10:vii–x, 1978.
5. Fox, SM 3d, Naughton, JP and Gorman PA: Physical activity and cardiovascular health, 3., the exercise prescription: Frequency and type of activity. Mod Concepts Cardiovasc Dis 41:25–30, 1972.
6. Gibson, SB, Gerberich, SG and Leon, AS: Writing the exercise prescription: An individualized approach. Physician and Sports Med 11(No. 7):88–89, 1983.
7. Bruce, RA, Kusumi, F and Hosmer, D: Maximal oxygen intake and nomographic assessment of functional aerobic impairment in cardiovascular disease. Am Heart J 85:546–562, 1973.
8. Pollock, ML, et al: Am Heart J, 92:39–46, 1976.
9. Smith, EL and Gilligan, C: Physical activity prescription for the older adult. Physician and Sports Med 11:91–101, 1983.
10. Morse, CE and Smith, EL: Physical activity programming for the aged. In Smith, EL (ed): Exercising and Aging: The Scientific Basis. Enslow Publishing, Hillside, NJ, 1981, pp. 109–120.
11. Balke, B: Prescribing physical activity. In Ryan, AJ and Allman, FL: Sports Medicine. Academic Press, New York, 1974.
12. Karvonen, MJ, Kentala, E and Mustala, O: The effects of training on heart rate. Annales Medicinae Experimentalis et Biologiae Fenniae 35:307–315, 1957.
13. Borg, GA and Linderholm, H: Perceived exertion and pulse rate during graded exercise in various groups. Acta Med Scand [Suppl]472:194–206, 1967.
14. Borg, GA: Perceived exertion on a note on history and methods. Med Sci Sports 5:90–93, 1973.
15. Borg, GV: Psychophysical bases of perceived exertion. Med Sci Sports 14:377–87, 1982.
16. Wilson, PK, Fardy PS, and Froelicher, VF: Cardiac Rehabilitation, Adult Fitness, and Exercise Testing. Lea & Febiger, Philadelphia, 1981.
17. Zohman, LR: Beyond Diet: Exercise Your Way to Fitness and Heart Health. CPC (Corn Products Corp), Englewood Cliffs, NJ, 1974
18. Naughton, SP and Hellerstein, HK: Exercise Testing and Exercise Training. Academic Press, New York, 1973.
19. Barnard, RJ, et al: Ischemic responses to sudden strenuous exercise in healthy men. Circulation 48:936–942, 1973.
20. McCue, BF: Flexibility of college women. Res Q 24:316, 1953.
21. Williams, PT, et al: The effects of running mileage and duration on plasma protein levels. JAMA 247:2674–2679, 1982.
22. Pollock, ML et al: Effects of frequency and duration of training on attrition and incidence of injury. Med Sci Sports 9:31–36, 1979.
23. McArdle, WD, Katch, FI and Katch, VL: Exercise Physiology: Energy, Nutrition and Human Performance. Lea & Febiger, Philadelphia, 1981.
24. Oscai, LB: Obesity. In Stull GA (ed): Encyclopedia of Physical Education Fitness and Sports: Training, Environment, Nutrition, and Fitness. Brighton Publishing, Salt Lake City, pp. 356–361, 1980.

25. Brannon, FJ: Experiments and Instrumentation in Exercise Physiology, ed. 2. Kendall-Hunt, Dubuque, 1978.
26. Siegel, W, et al: Use of isometric handgrip for the indirect assessment of left ventricular function in patients with coronary atherosclerotic heart disease. Am J Cardiol 30:48–54, 1972.
27. Lind, AR: Cardiovascular response to static exercise. Circulation 41:173–76, 1970.
28. Wahren, J and Bygdemon, S: Onset of angina pectoris in relation to circulatory adaptation during arm and leg exercise. Circulation 44:432–441, 1971.
29. DeLorme, TL and Watkins, AL: Progressive Resistance Exercise. Appleton-Century-Crofts, New York, 1951.
30. Clarke, DH: Adaptations in strength and muscular endurance resulting from exercise. Exerc Sport Sci Rev 1:73–102, 1973.
31. Banus, MG and Zetlin, AM: The relation of isometric tension to length in skeletal muscle. J Cell Comp Physiol 12:403–20, 1938.
32. Astrand, PO. Textbook of Work Physiology, ed. 3. McGraw-Hill, New York, 1986.
33. Anderson, R: Stretching. Robert A. Anderson & Jean E. Anderson, Fullerton, CA, 1975.
34. Johns, RJ and Wright, V: Relative importance of various tissues in joint stiffness. J Appl Physiol 17:824–28, 1962.
35. Walker, SM: Delay of twitch relaxation induced by stress and stress relaxation. J Appl Physiol 16:801–6, 1961.
36. Kiphuth, RJH: Swimming. AG Barnes, New York, 1942.
37. deVries, HA: Evaluation of static stretching procedures for improvement of flexibility. Res Q 33:222–29, 1962.
38. Kirchner, G and Glines, D: Comparative analysis of Eugene, Oregon, elementary school children using the Kraus-Weber test of minimum muscular fitness. Res Q 28:16–25, 1957.
39. Wear, CL: Relationships of flexibility measurements to length of body segments. Res Q 34:234–38, 1963.
40. Wright, V and Johns, RJ: Physical factors concerned with the stiffness of normal and diseased joints. Bull Johns Hopkins Hosp 106:215–31, 1960.
41. Fletcher, GF and Cantwell, JD: Exercise and Coronary Heart Disease. Charles C Thomas, Springfield, IL, 1979.
42. Blocker, WP and Cardus, D: Rehabilitation in Ischemic Heart Disease. SP Medical and Scientific Books, New York, 1983.
43. Froelicher, VF: Exercise Testing and Training. LeJacq, New York, 1983.
44. Wenger, NK: Exercise and the Heart. FA Davis, Philadelphia, 1978.
45. Wiley, MJ: Significant variables associated with compliance in the Bio-Energetiks cardiac rehabilitation population. Master's Thesis, University of Pittsburgh, 1982. Unpublished material.
46. Haynes, RB: Strategies for improving compliance: A methodological analysis and review. In Sackett, DL and Haynes RB (eds): Compliance with Therapeutic Regimens. Johns Hopkins University Press, Baltimore, 1976, pp. 69–82.
47. Franklin, B: Motivating and Educating Adults to Exercise. JOHPER June 1978, 13–17.
48. Wenger, NK: Rehabilitation of the patient with symptomatic atherosclerotic coronary heart disease. In Hurst, JW, et al (eds): The Heart, ed 5. McGraw-Hill, New York, 1982.

CHAPTER 9

The Exercise Therapy Session

The preceding chapter gave specific recommendations for writing a complete exercise prescription and examples of written prescriptions based on case study information presented in Chapter 7. In this chapter, the principles and methods previously discussed are applied to the cardiac exercise therapy session.

During the normal course of a 12-week training period, a patient's exercise prescription is adjusted frequently to assure improvement in CR endurance and other physiological factors. The decision to change the prescription and the type of change made depends on several factors including heart rate, blood pressure, and respiration response, orthopedic problems, fatigue, medication changes, and other clinical symptoms, most of which are documented in the data obtained during each exercise session. The number of changes made cannot be predicted at the time the initial exercise prescription is written. Changes require feedback that can be obtained only from the patients' responses to the exercise therapy. Each patient presents a different set of problems to which there will be any number of solutions.

The process of writing an appropriate exercise prescription, implementing the training program, evaluating and re-evaluating patient progress, adjusting and readjusting the prescription, and finally evaluating the effects of the training program is a challenging aspect of cardiac rehabilitation.

This process tests clinicians' skill in applying their knowledge of principles and practices to each exercise therapy session and to the developmental progression of the training sessions that are implemented over a period of 12 to 24 weeks. For the inexperienced clinician, adjusting the exercise prescription as physiologic training adaptation occurs may be difficult, but this adjustment is imperative if the goals identified for each patient are to be attained.

To enhance the clinician's decision-making skills with regard to modification of the exercise prescription, this section includes case studies that describe a 12-week course of treatment for two cardiovascularly diseased patients. Each case study includes the initial exercise prescription and rationale as well as a summary of the data obtained during the exercise training sessions that justifies change in the exercise prescription. In this way, the developmental progression of the training sessions, as well as many of the factors that enter into the decision-making process for writing and adapting an exercise prescription, may be more easily understood. Additional guidelines for outpatient cardiac exercise are included in Appendix F.

In addition, this chapter will also present a discussion of patients requiring special consideration because of medical conditions not previously mentioned in the text. The conditions discussed are those that commonly occur in patients with CHD.

CASE STUDIES
Case Study 8

The following is a description of the course of rehabilitative treatment for Case Study 8. The initial exercise prescription written for this patient appears in Table 9 – 1. This prescription is based on the results of his GXTT (Chapter 7, Table 7 – 22) and the information gathered from his completed preliminary forms and interview.

Aspects of this 50-year-old, male cardiac patient's medical history that have particular significance in relation to his exercise prescription include his hypertensive response to exercise, ST-T depression of 3 mm in V5 with the absence of angina, bilateral leg claudication (pain level 1) at 3 METs, and ventricular arrhythmias that occur during the cool-down and recovery periods.

In formulating his training target heart rate (THR), both the heart rate derived from the target zone and the formula for THR must be considered. His target zone is 3.25 METs (65 percent of Max METS; see chapter 8). During the GXTT, at this MET level his heart rate was approximately 84 bpm and his BP was at least 146/90 (see Table 7 – 22); utilizing the Karvonen formula (Table 9-1), his THR results in a calculated THR of 80 bpm. Thus, a range of 80 to 93 bpm (93 = 90 percent) may be established for a training THR. However, considering his BP of 146/90 and his pain level at a heart rate of 94 bpm, as well as the significance of these responses in patients with peripheral vascular disease,[1] the initial prescription should be written for the lowest possible THR in the range given, 80 bpm or slightly lower. This prescription should be adjusted if the patient demonstrates signs that he is not tolerating the exercise well.

This patient should be monitored (see p. 226) continuously to ensure that his heart rate does not exceed the THR established for him. This is crucial to his safety, as the patient exhibited no angina or dyspnea when in an acute ischemic state (−3 mm in V5), and he exhibited PVCs and bigeminy during the cool-down and recovery phases of the GXTT. These responses also reinforce the need to begin his CR training at the lowest possible intensity. This patient's BP response to exercise should be monitored at regular intervals. The BP response to exercise is another indicator of the intensity of the exercise for any patient (see RPP, Chapter 7). A higher than normal BP response for this patient may require that the THR be lowered.

The bicycle ergometer and walking should be selected as the primary type or mode of exercise to be used in CR training because alternate bouts of walking and cycling will minimize his leg claudication (maintain a pain level of less than 2) and should not exacerbate his hypertensive response to exercise. The Schwinn Airdyne[2] or other bicycle

TABLE 9–1. Initial Exercise Prescription for Case Study 8

Exercise Rx

Name __Case Study 8__ F Ⓜ Age _50_ Date _____

Ht. (in) _69_ Wt. (lb) _160_

Dx: __CAD, Post-MI, Post CABG, Hyperlipidemia, PVD__

Meds: __Cardizem, Isordil, Transderm 5__

Comments: __Mild Hypertensive response on GXTT, ST-T depression of 3 mm in__
__V5 at Max HR on GXT, Leg claudication-bilateral at 3 METs on GXTT, PVCs,__
__bigeminy during cool-down and recovery.__

GXT Data: Date performed __2/4/87__ Where: __Clinic X__

Rest HR __48__ Protocol: __Adapted Bruce__

Max HR __98__ Max METs: __5__

Re-evaluation scheduled __5/7/87__

C-R Rx:

Target Zone (METs) = 50% to 85% of Max METs

= .50 to .85 × __5__

= __3.25__ METs

Target HR (bpm) = (Max HR − Rest HR) (65% to .90) + (Rest HR)

= (__98__ − __48__) (.65 to .90) + (__48__)

= __80__ bpm

Type of exercise: _X_ bike ____ row _X_ walk____ walk/jog

(Intermittent progressing to continuous as able.)

Length of session: __20–60 min__ Frequency __3 × s/week__

Comments: Initial HR: 80 bpm based on Target Heart Rate. Heart rate
corresponding to target zone is too high for this Pt. Longer cool-down.
Subjective gradation of pain = 2 at Max HR on GXT. RPP = 152

Flexibility Rx: __Stretching for calves, hamstrings, quads, hip flexors—__
__3 × s/week prior to exercise and daily on alternate days.__

Muscular S & End Rx: __N/A begin as needed p̄ re-eval. 5/7/87__

% Body Fat Rx:

__20%__ Desirable M __15%__

F __25%__

Body Wt. __160__ lb Desired Range __150__ to __160__ lb

__73__ kg

Referred for Lipid Lowering Diet Plan and Nutrition education.

---

ergometer may be used, and the patient should be instructed to refrain from using his arms to maintain his workload on the bike as this might increase his blood pressure response to exercise (see Chapter 3). The workload performed on the bicycle and the walking distance covered per exercise bout should be carefully recorded to give the patient and staff objective feedback about the intensity of the exercise. Accurate recording of the data makes it easier to identify the point at which training adaptations occur. Educating the patient regarding training adaptations and linking the adaptations to changes in daily exercise data help to motivate the patient to proceed with training.[3]

Initially, this patient may require longer than average warm-up and cool-down periods to prevent ventricular irritability. Also, his pain tolerance may not permit continuous exercise, and his walking and cycling bouts might have to be limited to 2 or 3 min of exercise followed by 1 or 2 min of rest. Intermittent exercise should be extended to continuous exercise as soon as possible. This is done by either gradually decreasing the rest period or increasing the exercise period, or both. The length of the total CR training period (excluding warm-up and cool-down) should be increased gradually from 20 to 45 min over a period of weeks. The patient should be encouraged to exercise at home in addition to the on-site therapy sessions, which should be scheduled a minimum of three times per week on alternate days.

The flexibility program for this patient should emphasize the muscles and joints of the legs and hips and exclude any exercises that may place excessive stress on a joint or change blood pressure. Stretching may be performed prior to or after CR training and the exercises should be clearly explained and demonstrated. This patient should be checked periodically to make sure that while stretching no straining or actual pain occurs and that he is breathing slowly and rhythmically and not holding his breath.

A muscular strength and endurance training program is not indicated for this patient at this time. The instability of his medical status would rule out, initially, any type of training other than CR and mild flexibility exercises.

This patient should be referred for nutrition education regarding cardiovascular disease and a lipid-lowering diet regimen (see Chapter 10). He is within his ideal weight range, and his percent body fat should decline as a result of the CR training.

A summary of this patient's course of treatment is recorded on a sample data sheet (see Table 9-2). Note that although the THR remained relatively the same (78 to 80 bpm), the workload was increased to compensate for the improvements made in CR endurance.

As the patient's BP response to exercise improved, the need for BP measurement during exercise bouts declined and BP during exercise was not measured again except for week 6, when he worked overtime and his resting values were unusually high. Note also that his unusually high BP at rest that week required an adjustment in both the THR and the workload.

By keeping the THR low and increasing the length of the cool-down period during the 12 weeks, the patient was able to tolerate the CR exercise well and exhibited no dysrhythmias. Gradual increases in the length of time he walked enabled him to exercise with manageable pain (<2 subjective gradation of pain).

Case Study 5

The following is a description of the course of rehabilitative treatment for Case Study 5. An initial exercise prescription written for this patient appears in Table 9-3. This prescription is based on the results of her GXTT (see Table 7-19) and the information obtained from her completed preliminary forms and interview.

Certain features of this 70-year-old cardiovascularly diseased female patient's medical history and response to the GXTT have special significance, namely, her age, arthritic condition (which limits her orthopedically), severe hypertensive response to exercise, and extremely deconditioned state (~2 Max METs on GXTT).

Her CR training heart rate should be determined after careful consideration of both the target zone and the result of calculations for THR as previously described.[4,5] Her target zone is approximately 1.5 METs. During the performance of her GXTT, the 1.5 MET level elicited a heart rate response of approximately 95 bpm and a BP response that was at least 146/92 (see Table 7–19). The THR calculations result in a THR of approximately 95 bpm. Thus, a range of 95 to 108 bpm (108 = 90 percent) may be established for a CR training THR. However, considering the rapid rise in both systolic and diastolic blood pressure (to 220/136 in 3 min), it is most likely that at a heart rate of 95 bpm her blood pressure response would make it unsafe for her to exercise (see Rate Pressure Product, Chapter 7). Therefore, her initial THR should be recalculated at a lower percentage (50 percent = ~88 bpm) or slightly lower. The intensity of the CR training should be adjusted by raising or lowering the THR as needed during the exercise session.

This patient's BP response to exercise should be monitored at regular intervals during the CR exercise session, as her BP response is another indicator of the intensity of her CR exercise and may be her limiting factor, not heart rate. Remember, a diastolic BP of 120 mmHg is considered to be a criterion for termination of exercise (see Chapter 7).

The bicycle ergometer is the mode of choice for CR training of this patient. Due to her arthritic condition and her obesity, it is important to reduce the pressure on her weight-bearing joints. Also, with the bicycle ergometer, lower initial workloads and smaller workload increments can be prescribed to avoid overtaxing her in this deconditioned state. The Schwinn Airdyne or other bicycle ergometer may be used, and the patient should be instructed not to use her arms to maintain her workload (see Chapter 3). The workload performed on the bicycle ergometer during each exercise bout should be carefully recorded. If weight loss and orthopedic conditions permit, walking may be added to her CR training program after initial improvements in strength and CR endurance are noted.

Initially this patient may require a shorter than average warm-up and cool-down period because of her deconditioned state. Her muscular weakness probably will not permit continuous exercise, and her cycling should be limited to bouts of 2 or 3 min of exercise followed by 1 or 2 min of rest. Intermittent exercise should be extended to continuous exercise as soon as possible (see p. 212). This patient should not be encouraged to perform CR exercise at home until her blood pressure response is under control.

The flexibility program for this patient should emphasize range-of-motion exercises for her affected joints. All stretching exercises should be performed in comfortable positions, most of which should be supported positions. A seated position should minimize the amount of strength required for stretching and permit the patient to concentrate on stretching technique. As muscular strength improves, the position in which the flexibility exercises are performed may be modified. The patient should be encouraged to perform the flexibility exercises daily.

Mild strengthening exercises should be prescribed for this patient because her quadriceps muscle weakness will limit her ability to perform CR training exercises. However, her BP response to even mild strengthening exercises must be evaluated when she performs the exercises for the first time (see Chapter 8). If her BP response is too high, these exercises should be added only after her BP response to exercise improves or her medication is adjusted.

This patient's medical problems are compounded by her obesity, and she should be

TABLE 9–2. Summary of 12-Week Cardiac Exercise Program for Case Study 8

Date	Rest HR	Rest BP	HR TARGET	HR W-UP	C-R Work Type-Min.*	C-R HR	Laps Wkload.	Cool-Down HR	Cool-Down BP	Wt. lb.	Comments (BPs, Arrhythmias, Med. Changes, Symptoms, etc.)
WEEK 1	50	140/84	78	72	B-3, R-2	76–72	0.8 KP	48	128/80	160	BP 1stB—144/82; BP 2ndW—138/82; 20' Inter. CRE$_x$. Pt. tolerance good. No pain on bike, pain level 1 walking. 7 min. cool-down. No arrhythmias
					W-3, R-2	78–74	3 Laps				
					B-3, R-2	76–72	0.8 KP				
					W-3, R-2	78–74	3 Laps				
WEEK 2	48	138/82	78	70	B-4, R-1	78	0.9 KP	68	118/78	159	BP 1stW—138/80; BP 3rdB—126/80; 25' Continuous CRE$_x$. Pt. tolerance good. Pain level 1 walking. 7 min. cool-down
					W-4, R-1	78	5 Laps				
					B-4, R-1	76	0.9 KP				
					W-4, R-1	80	6 Laps				
					B-4, R-1	78	0.8 KP				
WEEK 3	60	138/74	78–80	72	B-5	76	0.8 KP	70	126/70	158	BP 2ndB—132/72; 25' Continuous CRE$_x$. Pt. tolerance good. Pain level 1 to 2 walking. 6 min. cool-down. No arrhythmias
					W-5	80	6 Laps				
					B-5	78	0.8 KP				
					W-5	80	5 Laps				
					B-5	78	0.8 KP				
WEEK 4	60	126/74	78–80	72	B-5	78	0.9 KP	60	126/70	158	BP only prn; 25' Continuous CRE$_x$. Pt. tolerance good. 6 min. cool-down. No arrhythmias
					W-5	80	6 Laps				
					B-5	80	1.0 KP				
					W-5	80	6 Laps				
					B-5	80	0.9 KP				

Week												
WEEK 5	54	128/72	80	72	B-5 W-5 B-5 W-5 B-5 W-5	80 78 80 80 80 80	1.0 KP 6 Laps 1.0 KP 6 Laps 0.9 KP 6 Laps	60	124/70	158.5	BP only prn 30' Continuous CRE$_x$	Pt. tolerance good 6 min. cool-down No arrhythmias
WEEK 6	72	160/90	76	72	B-5 W-5 B-5 W-5	74 76 74 76 74 74	0.7 KP 4 Laps 0.7 KP 5 Laps 0.7 KP 4 Laps	70	128/80	158	BP p̄ 2nd Bike— 132/84 BP p̄ 2nd Walk— 130/80 30' Continuous CRE$_x$	↓Target Hr. Pt. tired, worked overtime all week 7 min. cool-down
WEEK 7	54	120/70	80	72	B-5 W-5 B-5 W-5	78 80 78 80 78 80	1.0 KP 6 Laps 1.0 KP 6 Laps 1.0 KP 6 Laps	62	118/70	157	BP only prn 35' Continuous CRE$_x$	Pt. tolerance good 6 min. cool-down No arrhythmias
WEEK 8	54	118/70	80	68	B-5 W-5 B-5 W-5	78 80 80 80 80 80 80 80	1.0 KP 6 Laps 1.1 KP 6 Laps 1.1 KP 6 Laps 1.1 KP 6 Laps	70	114/68	157	BP prn 40' Continuous CRE$_x$	Pt. tolerance good 6 min. cool-down No arrhythmias

TABLE 9-2. continued

Date	Rest HR	Rest BP	HR TARGET	W-UP	C-R Work Type-Min.*	C-R HR	Laps Wkload.	Cool-Down HR	Cool-Down BP	Wt. lb.	Comments — BPs, Arrhythmias, Med. Changes, Symptoms, etc.
	50	118/70	80	72	B-10	80	1.1 KP	68	112/68	156	BP prn — Pt. tolerance good 6 min. cool-down
					W-5	80	6-7 Laps				
					B-10	80	1.1 KP				40' Continuous CRE$_x$ — No arrhythmias
					W-5	80	7 Laps				
WEEK 9					B-10	80	1.1 KP				
	48	120/70	80	74	B-10	80	1.2 KP	64	114/68	156	BP prn — Pain Level 1 s/t cramping 5 min. cool-down
					W-7	80	10 Laps				
					B-10	80	1.2 KP				44' Continuous CRE$_x$ — No arrhythmias
					W-7	80	10 Laps				
WEEK 10					B-10	80	1.2 KP				
	48	118/68	80	68	B-10	78	1.2-1.3 KP	62	112/64	156	BP prn — Pt. tolerance good Pain level 1 5 min. cool-down
					W-10	80	13 Laps				
					B-10	80	1.3 KP				45' Continuous CRE$_x$ — No arrhythmias
WEEK 11					W-10	80	14 Laps				
	46	118/70	80	72	B-10	80	1.3 KP	64	110/60	156	BP prn — Pt. tolerance good Pain level 1 5 min. cool-down
					W-10	80	14-15 Laps				
					B-10	80	1.3 KP				45' Continuous CRE$_x$ — No arrhythmias
					W-10	80	14-15 Laps				
WEEK 12					B-5						

*B = Bike; W = Walk; R = Rest
Re-evaluation:

TABLE 9–3. Initial Exercise Prescription for Case Study 5

Exercise Rx

Name ___Case Study 5___ Ⓕ M Age _70_ Date _____
Ht. (in) _59_ Wt.(lb) _180_

Dx: __Hypertension, Obesity, Arthritis (knees, wrists, spine)__

Meds: __HydroDIURIL, Aldomet *Medication change 2nd week of therapy__

Comments: __Severe hypertensive response to exercise; Max BP 220/136;__
__severely deconditioned; orthopedic limitations.__

GXT Data: Date performed __2/7/87__ Where: __Clinic X__
Rest HR __62__ Protocol: __Adapted Astrand-Rhyming__
Max HR __113__ Max METs: __~2__
Re-evaluation scheduled __5/15/87__

C-R Rx:

Target Zone (METs) = 50% to 85% × Max METs
= .50 to .85 × __2__
= __1.3 or ~1–2__ METs
Target HR (bpm) = (Max HR − Rest HR) (65% to 90%) + (Rest HR)
= (__113__ − __62__) (.65 to .90) + (__62__)
= __95__ bpm
Type of exercise: _X_ bike ____ row ____ walk ____ walk/jog
(No arms on Schwinn Airdyne until adapt. occurs.)
Length of session: _20–30 min._ Frequency _3 × s/week_
Comments: Initial HR Range 95 bpm based on THR & Target Zone. ↓50% = 88 bpm
Limited by BP response. Intermittent CR exercise initially 2–3 min.
of exercise with 1–2 min. rest. Progress to continuous. RPP = 248

Flexibility Rx: __General program with emphasis on affected joints performed__
__3 × s/day—supported body positions__
Muscular S & End Rx: __Mild strengthening programs for quadriceps—10 reps,__
__3 × s/day—no weights.__
% Body Fat Rx:
__44%__ Desirable M _15%_
F _25%_

Body Wt. __180__ lb Desired Range __115__ to __125__ lb
__82__ kg

Pt. referred for nutrition education and weight reducing diet regimen.

referred for nutritional counseling (see Chapter 10). Fortunately, she is neither diabetic nor hyperlipidemic and should be able to tolerate a low-calorie general meal plan.

The following is a summary of this patient's course of treatment recorded on a sample data sheet (see Table 9–4). Note that the patient was unable to tolerate CR exercise bouts of 3 min and had to be referred to her physician regarding her continuation in the program (see example re-referral form in Appendix B). Her physician added Tenormin to her HydroDIURIL and eliminated Aldomet. Tenormin, a beta blocking drug, reduced her resting heart rate from 66 bpm to approximately 50 bpm. This medication change necessitated a change in her THR prescription. Although general guidelines exist regarding the effect of a beta blocking agent on maximum heart rate,[6] the true effect is difficult to predict, as it is influenced by both dosage and individual patient response. A practical

TABLE 9–4. Summary of a 12-Week Cardiovascular Exercise Program for Case Study 5

Date	Rest HR	Rest BP	HR TARGET	W-UP	C-R Work Type-Min.*	C-R HR	Laps Wkload.	Cool-Down HR	Cool-Down BP	Wt. Lb.	Comments: BPs, Arrhythmias, Med. Changes, Symptoms, etc.
WEEK 1	66	162/92	88	76	B-3, R-2	80	0.5 KP	78	160/90	180	B1st BP—170/103 Exercise terminated p 3rd bike due to hypertensive response to ex.
					B-3, R-3	82	0.5 KP				B2nd BP—172/106
					B-3, R-3	86	0.5 KP				B3rd BP—180/112 Pt. re-referred for BP control
					B-3, Terminate						9' CRE$_x$ Intermittent 10 minute cool-down
WEEK 2	52	152/84	78	68	B-2, R-2	72	0.5 KP	60	148/82	178	B2nd BP—160/86 Medication change: Tenormin Lower Target HR
					B-2, R-2	76	0.5 KP				B4th BP—168/90 Good tolerance
					B-2, R-2	78	0.5 KP				10' CRE$_x$ Intermittent
					B-2, R-2	75	0.5 KP				10' cool-down
					B-2, R-2	78	0.5 KP				
WEEK 3	52	140/78	78	66	B-3, R-1	70	0.5 KP	58	138/76	176	B2nd BP—156/82 Good tolerance, below THR
					B-3, R-1	70	0.5 KP				B4th BP—154/80 8' cool-down
					B-3, R-1	70	0.5 KP				12' CRE$_x$ Intermittent
					B-3, R-1	70	0.5 KP				
WEEK 4	50	152/74	78	68	B-5, R-1	78	0.6 KP	56	142/74	173	B2nd BP—148/76 Good tolerance, on target
					B-5, R-1	72	0.6 KP				B4th BP—144/74 8' cool-down
					B-5, R-1	78	0.6 KP				20' CRE$_x$ Intermittent
					B-5, R-1	78	0.6 KP				

WEEK 5	48	130/82	78	60	B-5	78	0.6–.7 KP	60	132/78	172	B3rd BP-132/80 20'CR Continuous	Good tolerance 6' cool-down
					B-5	73	0.6–.7 KP					
					B-5	78	0.6–.7 KP					
					B-5	78	0.6–.7 KP					
WEEK 6	50	136/74	78	66	B-5	72	0.7 KP	54	132/72	170	3rdB BP— 130/76 25'CR Continuous	Good tolerance 6' cool-down
					B-5	72	0.7 KP					
					B-5	73	0.7 KP					
					B-5	72	0.7 KP					
					B-5	78	0.7 KP					
WEEK 7	50	130/74	78	66	B-5	78	0.8 KP	58	128/72	168	BP's prn 30'CR Continuous	Good tolerance 6' cool-down
					B-5	76	0.8 KP					
					B-5	78	0.8 KP					
					B-5	76	0.8 KP					
					B-5	78	0.8 KP					
					B-5	78	0.8 KP					
WEEK 8	48	130/68	78	66	B-5	78	0.8–.9 KP	54	128/74	165	BP's prn 30'CR Continuous	Good tolerance 5' cool-down
					B-5	78	0.8–.9 KP					
					B-5	78	0.8–.9 KP					
					B-5	76	0.8–.9 KP					
					B-5	78	0.8–.9 KP					
					B-5	78	0.8–.9 KP					
WEEK 9	48	128/70	78	66	B-5	76	1.0 KP	50	110/70	163	BP's prn 30'CR Continuous	Good tolerance 5' cool-down
					B-5	76	1.0 KP					
					B-5	78	1.0 KP					
					B-5	76	1.0 KP					
					B-5	76	1.0 KP					
					B-5	76	1.0 KP					

TABLE 9–4. *continued*

Date	Rest		HR TARGET		C-R Training			Cool-Down		Wt.		Comments
	HR	BP	W-UP	C-R Work Type-Min.*	C-R HR	Laps Wkload.	HR	BP	Lb.	BPs prn / 30' CR Continuous	BPs, Arrhythmias, Med. Changes, Symptoms, etc.
WEEK 10	48	128/72	78 / 64	B-5	76	1.0 KP	50	114/70	160	BPs prn	Add walk to CR Ex.
				W-5	78	5 Laps				30' CR	Good tolerance
				B-5	76	1.0 KP				Continuous	
				B-5	78	5 Laps					5' cool-down
				W-5	78	1.0 KP					
				B-5	76	5 Laps					
WEEK 11	50	118/74	78 / 66	B-5	76	1.1 KP	48	110/70	158	BPs prn	Increase Walking to ½ of Cr Ex
				W-5	76	6 Laps				30' CR	Good tolerance
				B-5	76	1.1 KP				Continuous	
				W-5	78	6 Laps					5' cool-down
				B-5	76	1.1 KP					
				W-5	78	6 Laps					
WEEK 12	50	114/72	78 / 68	W-5	76	7 Laps	48	110/68	156	BPs prn	↑Length of CR bouts
				B-10	76	1.2 KP				30' CR	Good tolerance
				W-5	76	7 Laps				Continuous	
				B-10	76	1.2 KP					5' cool-down

*B = Bike; W = Walk; R = Rest.
Re-evaluation:

220

approach to changing the THR in this case is to exercise the patient at the same workload as prior to the medication change and establish a THR range based on the response. The patient's heart rate response to the same workload was approximately 8 to 10 bpm lower as a result of the beta blocking medication. Thus, her new THR range became 78 to 88 bpm.

As the patient's BP response to exercise improved, the need for frequent BP measurement during exercise bouts declined. BP was not measured during exercise after the sixth week of CR training. Her flexibility and muscular strength training was also adjusted at this time. Her improved recovery from CR exercise also resulted in a decrease in the time of her cool-down period.

The patient's compliance to her weight-reducing regimen was demonstrated by her weight loss of 24 pounds over the 12-week period. Her weight loss enhanced her CR training response and enabled her to tolerate more walking exercise and longer bouts of continuous cycling.

PATIENTS REQUIRING SPECIAL CONSIDERATION

Although some mention has been made of the problems arthritic or elderly cardiac patients may have in attempting an exercise program, a large number of patients seen in rehabilitation programs have multiple problems worthy of special consideration. This population includes the cardiovascularly diseased patient with one or more of the following conditions: angina pectoris, diabetes méllitus, peripheral vascular disease, pulmonary disease, arthritis or other orthopedic limitations, and obesity. In such cases, the exercise prescription must be modified to enable the patient to adjust physiologically and psychologically to exercise therapy.

Angina Pectoris

Patients with stable angina are excellent candidates for exercise therapy. The object of the exercise therapy is to increase the functional capacity of the patient so that more physical exercise can be performed before the onset of limiting angina. In this case, special consideration must be given to the ongoing evaluation of the angina, the extent of warm-up and cool-down periods, and the intensity of the cardiovascular endurance training period. Evaluation of the angina involves carefully documenting each episode as the patient describes it according to the type of pain, the location of the pain, factors which may have precipitated the episode, the duration and frequency of the episode and what methods were used to relieve the pain. Also, the therapist can usually observe and should record unique mannerisms or other subtle changes in coloring or demeanor exhibited by the patient during an episode. Ongoing evaluation of patients with stable angina is critical, as any change in either the frequency or the intensity of the episodes warrants immediate medical investigation. In addition, careful observation is required of patients for whom prophylactic use of nitroglycerin or long-acting nitrates has been prescribed as adverse hypotensive responses may occur.[8] Modification of the length of the cardiovascular exercise therapy session has been discussed. The patient's THR should remain below the anginal or ischemic threshold (see Chapter 3).

Diabetes Mellitus

There are two types of diabetes that must be identified in order to prescribe exercise properly. Type I or insulin-dependent diabetes (IDDM) is the result of a pancreatic deficiency in insulin production. The Type I diabetic is dependent upon the regular administration of exogenous insulin and 10 to 20 percent of the known diabetics in the United States are of this type.[24] In Type II or noninsulin-dependent diabetes (NIDDM), insulin levels may be normal, slightly depressed, or elevated. Usually, decreased cellular sensitivity or responsiveness to exogenous and endogenous insulin is present. Eighty to ninety percent of all known diabetics in this country are Type II. Although this form of diabetes can occur at any age, it is usually diagnosed after age 40 and is associated with obesity.[24] Type II diabetes is typically treated with dietary modification, exercise, oral hypoglycemic medication, and, in some cases, exogenous insulin.

Although more research is needed to determine the specific effects of exercise on Type I and Type II diabetics, existing research indicates that, provided certain guidelines are followed, increased physical activity has several actual and potential benefits to offer the diabetic patient: (1) improvement in insulin sensitivity and potential improvement in glucose tolerance in some individuals, (2) as an adjunct to diet therapy in the promotion of weight loss and the maintenance of body weight,[27] (3) improvement in peripheral hemodynamic function[25] and cardiovascular risk, including the enhancement of work capacity and reduction of body fat, (4) potential reduction in the dosage or need for insulin or oral hypoglycemic agents,[24,26] (5) enhancement of the quality of life and sense of well-being.

Again, it should be emphasized that more research is needed in regard to the actual benefits and actual risks and the establishment of specific guidelines for prescribing exercise for both the Type I and the Type II diabetic patient. At the present time, the following factors must be considered in writing an exercise prescription for a diabetic patient with known cardiovascular disease.

An exercise program is contraindicated for poorly controlled or uncontrolled diabetic patients (blood glucose greater than 300 mg/dl). Exercise may cause deterioration of metabolic control in such patients.[24]

One of the problems that exercising diabetics may encounter is the hypoglycemic effect of exercise. This effect occurs as a result of the increased mobilization of depot insulin during exercise. This condition may be exacerbated in the Type I diabetic if the insulin injection site is in the exercising muscle.[9] Because exercise creates an insulin-like effect, exercising diabetics may have to alter their insulin and carbohydrate intake in order to avoid hypoglycemic events.

All diabetics (Type I and Type II) should comply with the following recommendations to assure safe participation in an exercise program:

1. Carry a card or wear a bracelet at all times that identifies them as having diabetes mellitus; exercise with a partner when possible.
2. Be knowledgeable of and alert to the signs and symptoms of hypoglycemia (tachycardia, palpitations, increased sweating, hunger) during and up to several hours following exercise (hypoglycemic episodes may occur from 24 to 48 hours after an exercise session).
3. Have a source of readily absorbable carbohydrate (fruit juice, sugar cubes, glu-

cose tablets, or a solution equivalent to 5 to 20 grams of carbohydrate) available during and following exercise to prevent or treat hypoglycemia. (Intramuscular glucagon may be used to treat severe hypoglycemic reactions. The unconscious patient should be given an intravenous injection of glucose.)

4. Avoid the risk of dehydration (which may be a problem when metabolic control is less than satisfactory) by taking extra fluids or by skipping exercise on particularly warm days.

5. Have a careful evaluation of the feet performed by a qualified health professional prior to the initiation of an exercise program. Get instruction regarding the selection of proper footwear and foot protection.

Additional recommendations for the Type I (IDDM) patient are necessary.[9,24]

1. As individuals taking insulin vary considerably in their response to exercise, monitor blood glucose more frequently when beginning an exercise program to determine the response to the type, intensity, and duration of the exercise.

2. Choose an injection site, such as the abdomen, other than the actively exercising muscle.

3. Choose a time to exercise when the blood sugar level is above fasting value, perhaps 1 to 3 hours after a meal, not during peak insulin activity time.

4. It may be necessary to consume extra carbohydrate prior to, during, or following exercise to avoid hypoglycemic episodes.

5. Decreasing the insulin dose prior to an exercise bout may be necessary (*only as recommended by a physician*). For example,[24] if a patient is well controlled with a single dose of intermediate-acting insulin, the dose may be decreased on days when exercise is planned. Some patients may require a decrease in insulin dosage of 30 to 35 percent. If a patient is using a combination of intermediate- and short-acting insulin, the short-acting dose may be reduced or omitted and the intermediate-acting dose may need to be reduced by up to one third. Under these conditions, a patient may experience hyperglycemia later in the day and require a second injection of short-acting insulin.

Generally speaking, diabetic cardiac patients can participate in the same modes of activity as nondiabetic cardiacs. However, special precautions must be taken when the patient is taking drugs that potentiate exercise-induced hypoglycemia. For example, very high doses of salicylates may alone produce hypoglycemia and beta-adrenergic blocking agents may prevent the rapid response of the liver, which normally corrects the hypoglycemia.[24]

Type I (IDDM) diabetics should exercise daily, if possible, to assist in the maintenance of a regular pattern of diet and insulin dosage. Because the frequency of exercise is high, the duration may be decreased to 20 to 30 min. It is recommended that the intensity of exercise for the Type I diabetic be prescribed within the normal range (40 to 85 percent of functional capacity) and on the basis of heart rate in most cases. The diabetic with autonomic neuropathy, however, may demonstrate chronotropic insufficiency (altered heart rate response) during exercise. Such patients may also be unable to perceive angina or other symptoms of ischemia. Therefore, such patients must be carefully monitored, and the perceived exertion or MET (target zone; see Chapter 8) methods may prove to be helpful in prescribing their exercise intensity.

Type II (NIDDM) diabetic patients should exercise 5 days per week if possible to enhance caloric expenditure. The duration of exercise may be from 40 to 60 min in order, again, to assist in weight control. As the frequency and duration of exercise for Type II patients are high, the intensity of the exercise should be maintained in the lower end of the normal range.

Please note that the duration of the exercise sessions given for Type I and II diabetic patients represents the maintenance goal for such patients. Diabetic patients, just as all cardiac patients, must be carefully and developmentally progressed toward such goals.

The cardiac rehabilitation clinician must be knowledgeable concerning all of the aforementioned recommendations for Type I and Type II diabetic patients. Specific problems of diabetic patients in various stages of the disease must also be considered. The following examples serve to illustrate the importance of the clinician's need to individualize the exercise prescription for diabetic patients.

Patients with neuropathy have insensitive feet and should avoid exercises that involve running, a potentially traumatizing activity. Cycling and swimming are good alternatives. Recent research[28] indicates that patients with diabetic neuropathic skeletal disease (DNSD) may suffer from fractures of the ankle due to jogging. It has been recommended that jogging not be undertaken in diabetic patients with DNSD or advanced kidney, retinal, or peripheral nerve disease.[28]

Diabetic patients with active proliferative retinopathy, just as all cardiacs, should avoid strenuous activities associated with Valsalva-like maneuvers. Such activities cause an undesirable increase in blood pressure. In addition, such patients should avoid participation in activities associated with excessive jarring or jolting of the head.

Exercise for diabetic cardiac patients with hypertension should emphasize rhythmic exercise involving the lower extremities such as walking, jogging (except for patients with DNSD or advanced kidney, retinal, or peripheral nerve disease), or cycling, as intense exercise involving the arms and upper body causes greater increases in blood pressure than exercise involving the major muscle groups of the lower extremities.[24] This recommendation applies to all cardiac patients (Chapters 3 and 8).

The diabetic patient is a special challenge to the cardiac rehabilitation team and must always be observed for symptoms of hypoglycemia and further progression of the disease.

Peripheral Vascular Disease

In patients with claudication, the subjective gradation of pain is a useful technique for evaluating the pain over a period of time and, therefore, measuring slight improvements in exercise tolerance (see Table 9–5). This technique also aids in writing the exercise prescription when progressing the patient to higher work levels.

TABLE 9–5. Subjective Gradation of Pain in Patients with
Peripheral Vascular Disease

Grade 4 — Excrutiating and unbearable pain.
Grade 3 — Intense pain from which the patient's attention cannot be diverted except by cata-
strophic events (e.g., fire, explosion).
Grade 2 — Moderate discomfort or pain from which the patient's attention can be diverted by a
number of common stimuli (e.g., conversation).
Grade 1 — Definite discomfort or pain but only of initial or modest level (established but
minimal).

(From Unger, KM, Moser, K and Hansen, P: Selection of an exercise program for patients with
chronic obstructive pulmonary disease. Heart Lung 9:68–76, 1980, with permission.)

Patients with significant peripheral vascular disease are at a much higher risk of
having associated coronary and cerebral vascular disease than those without peripheral
impairment.[7] Therefore, an increase in systolic resting blood pressure warrants significant
reduction in the target heart rate for the exercise session. Failure of blood pressure to
normalize would justify termination of an exercise therapy session. The patient with
claudication may initially benefit from intermittent exercise but should be progressed to
continuous low-level exercise as soon as it can be tolerated. Exercise therapy sessions
should be increased in duration (to a maximum of 60 min) at a low level before the
intensity is increased. Two exercise periods per day may be beneficial if each session is
greater than 20 min in length.

Pulmonary Disease

Exercise for the patient with pulmonary disease is limited by reduced ventilatory capacity.
It has been suggested that the prescribed cardiorespiratory exercise therapy should not
lead to a ventilatory response greater than approximately 80 percent of the maximum
ventilation attained during the GXTT.[11] Although cardiorespiratory exercise may not
improve pulmonary function indices, chronic adaptations to aerobic exercise (see Chapter
3) will reduce the demands on limited pulmonary reserve during exercise. Upper body
aerobic exercise should not be used for patients with pulmonary disease because of the
high ventilation required at a given workload in this type of exercise.[11,12]

Osteoarthritis and Orthopedic Limitations

Any exercise that produces excessive stress on osteoarthritic or injured joints should be
avoided. The exercise prescription must emphasize exercises to increase both range of
joint motion and strength. Activities that place stress on the weight-bearing joints are
contraindicated during inflammatory periods. Intermittent cardiovascular exercise comprised of short bouts of exercise and rest intervals appears to be tolerated better than
continuous exercise by orthopedically limited patients.

Obesity

Exercise therapy for the obese patient should be of long duration (maximum of 60 min) and low intensity to avoid exercise that stresses the weight-bearing joints. The patient thus expends more calories while avoiding the orthopedic problems that may accompany higher intensity work.

MONITORING THE EXERCISE SESSION

There are a number of reasons for the wide variability in monitoring procedures that exist in the various rehabilitation programs in this country. Budget, staff composition, medical supervision, and size of the exercise area are important factors in the decision-making process for administrators of exercise therapy programs. Obviously, the more sophisticated the monitoring equipment, the higher the operating expense of the rehabilitation program.

Outpatient cardiac rehabilitation programs should have the equipment for continuous and/or intermittent ECGs and continuous and intermittent heart rate monitoring. This requires purchasing a cardiograph capable of obtaining 12-lead ECGs and an oscilloscope that permits monitoring by telemetry or through a hardwire connection. Patients can then be monitored continuously or intermittently, as indicated by their medical status. The usual procedure is to monitor a new patient continuously for approximately the first 6 or 12 weeks. If the patient proves to be stable, monitoring may continue on an intermittent basis using the equipment just described or through the paddles of a defibrillator (if the defibrillator unit has this capability). To detect subtle changes that occur over time, it is a good policy to obtain a rhythm strip on each patient every time he or she comes for exercise therapy, regardless of how long the patient has been in the rehabilitation program. This monitoring can be accomplished fairly economically and simply through the paddles of a defibrillator unit that also contains a chart recorder.

Again, the financial and supervisory circumstances in which a rehabilitation program operates will dictate the kind of equipment utilized in the therapy session. In making decisions of this nature, do so with the highest priority being that of patient safety.

ENVIRONMENTAL CONSIDERATIONS

Selected patients should be encouraged to exercise at home in addition to exercise therapy sessions. For these patients, it is important to teach them how to palpate their own pulses and to educate them about the effects various environmental factors may have on their ability to exercise. The major concerns are extremes of temperature and humidity. (Altitude and air pollution are not major factors for the majority of patients and should be discussed only with patients who travel extensively or expect to exercise regularly in areas where the air quality is poor.)

Heat

When ambient temperatures range between 40° and 75°F and the humidity is 65 percent or below, conditions are generally recognized as ideal for exercise.[12] In hot weather, however, the body temperature rises faster during exercise and extra precautions need to be observed. The harmful effect of higher temperatures is exacerbated by increases in relative humidity. In high heat and humidity the body struggles to dissipate heat and cool itself. The natural cooling of the body through the evaporation of sweat is ineffective due to the increased humidity. As the core temperature of the body rises, the heart rate increases (see Chapter 3). The volume of blood returning to the heart is reduced by the dilation of the peripheral veins. Therefore, stroke volume, cardiac output, and working capacity are reduced. In this situation, the extra effort demanded by exercise will precipitate ischemic changes and in some cases anginal pain. Patients should be instructed as to the best time of day to exercise, how to avoid excessive heat and humidity, the appropriate clothing, and the signs and symptoms of heat intolerance.

Cold

Obviously, patients should be informed of the appropriate clothing for cold weather exercise. Cold temperatures cause an increase in peripheral resistance at rest and during exercise. The peripheral vasoconstriction associated with cold produces an increase in arterial blood pressure that, when coupled with increased myocardial oxygen demand, causes the patient to reach ischemic threshold more rapidly and consequently may provoke anginal pain.[12]

Although ischemic responses are related to extremes in temperature and humidity, the same responses have been observed in cardiac patients with only moderate changes in temperature.[13] Therefore, all patients should be educated about the dangers associated with exposure to extremes in temperature. It should also be demonstrated to them that in addition to awareness of ambient temperature extremes during exercise, they should try to buffer the effects of temperature extremes in all aspects of daily living, including such situations as bathing and showering, going from air-conditioned buildings or cars out into extreme heat and vice versa, and drinking very cold or extremely hot beverages.

MOTIVATION/COMPLIANCE

The goals of an outpatient cardiac rehabilitation program are to develop the best possible prescribed therapeutic regimen (including modification of risk factors associated with life-style) for each patient and to enhance compliance with that regimen once it has been established. For the rehabilitation program to be successful, patients must adhere to their programs for months and years following the termination of the formal program. Therefore, all efforts must be made to understand the factors involved with compliant behavior, and plans must be made to incorporate successful strategies whenever and wherever possible.

Studies indicate that the various techniques utilized by health-care professionals to improve patient compliance can be grouped into three broad categories: educational methods, behavior modification methods, and a combination of the two methods.[14] Research also indicates that in terms of therapeutic success, the percent of compliance varies with each category. The lowest compliance rate has been associated with the educational method (50 percent), the highest by the behavioral method (82 percent), and an intermediate compliance rate of 75 percent has been demonstrated by combined methods.[15] There are many reasons for the variance. However, to improve patient compliance with exercise therapy, the rehabilitation staff apparently must not only teach patients about their disease, need for life-style change, and exercise requirements, but also *motivate* them to continue with their prescribed regimens with behavioral techniques.

The Rehabilitation Staff Instructors

The key to the success of any program is the competence of the instructional staff.[15] Individuals who work directly with patients must have a thorough and accurate knowledge of exercise physiology, the principles of assessment, exercise prescription, the principles of physical conditioning, and motivational techniques. Many of the techniques used to motivate patients are simple and almost instinctive to individuals who are sincere in their desire to help others to achieve goals to which they themselves are dedicated. The instructional staff must provide positive role models for the patients and must always maintain an enthusiastic attitude toward exercise and other life-style changes. This type of behavior reinforces patients' attitudes toward the rehabilitative process. They perceive that the changes they are making in their exercise and other habits can and must be a lifetime commitment.

Improving patient compliance involves breaking down barriers to compliance and motivating patient compliance by reinforcing, extrinsically and intrinsically, positive health behaviors. Methods employed to achieve these goals, again, fall into broad categories.

EDUCATIONAL TECHNIQUES

Education may be provided in a number of formal and informal situations. The type of educational experiences provided by a rehabilitation center will be limited by the staff, facilities, and location of the center. The types of experiences that might be provided include patient education manuals written at the appropriate reading level, informal patient education (discussions before, during, and after exercise therapy sessions; bulletin boards), and formal patient education (lectures; individual counseling sessions, with or without spouse).

BEHAVIORAL TECHNIQUES

To employ behavioral techniques effectively, an understanding of basic psychological principles is important. These basic principles may be expressed as follows: positive behavioral changes must be reinforced, reinforcement must be delivered immediately following the positive behavioral change, and negative responses should not be emphasized.[16] Some examples of how these principles might be applied are:

1. Measured improvement in percentage body fat, weight loss, vital signs, and functional capacity may be rewarded.
2. Chart or record miles completed, pounds lost, and attendance to break down the patient's goals into smaller goals that guarantee success and then reinforce or reward the patient for achieving each goal. Success breeds success!
3. Awards, T-shirts, pins, and certificates can be given for attainment of specific goals, such as completion of 50, 100, or 1000 miles.
4. Awards ceremonies and family nights are helpful in reinforcing positive attitudes.
5. Reinforcement of intrinsic motivation through education and role modeling.

Many different skills and factors must be properly combined to make a program successful. However, the most powerful motivating force lies in the knowledge, sincerity, enthusiasm, creativity, and dedication of the staff who are charged with direct patient care.

SUMMARY

Detailed case studies on two patients have been presented to help the clinician better understand the principles relative to target zone and THR and the application of these principles to the daily cardiac exercise therapy sessions. Examples of readjustments in the exercise prescription based on feedback obtained from the exercise session (such as blood pressure and medication changes) have been included. These examples will alert the clinician to the necessity for periodic adjustments to the THR when individual physiologic measurements seem to be atypical. Additional modifications of the exercise prescription may be necessary for the cardiovascularly diseased patient who also has angina pectoris, diabetes mellitus, peripheral vascular disease, orthopedic limitations and/or obesity.

Initially, patients should be monitored continuously. Rhythm strips should be obtained during each exercise session. Continuous monitoring may be tapered to intermittent monitoring as the patient progresses. Patients should be instructed as to the effects of environmental extremes on heart rate and blood pressure responses. They should be taught to palpate their own pulses so they can progress to a home exercise program and do so safely. Suggestions for maintaining patient compliance with the established exercise regimen include educational and behavioral techniques. Of prime importance to the long-term success of any CR program are the competency and sincerity of the instructional staff.

REFERENCES

1. American College of Sports Medicine: Guidelines for Graded Exercise Testing and Exercise Prescription, ed 2. Lea & Febiger, Philadelphia, 1980.
2. Schwinn Air-Dyne Owner's Manual. Schwinn Bicycle Co, Chicago 1984.
3. Blumenthal, JA, et al: Cardiac rehabilitation: A new frontier for behavioral medicine. Cardiac Rehab 3:637–656, 1983.

4. Balke, B: Prescribing physical activity. In Ryan, AJ and Allman FL: Sports Medicine. Academic Press, New York, 1974, pp. 505–523.

5. Karvonen, MJ, Kentala, E and Mustala, O: The effect of training on heart rate. Annales Medicinae Experimentalis et Biologiae Fenniae 35:307–315, 1957.

6. Lowenthal, DT, et al: The clinical pharmacology of cardiovascular drugs during exercise. J Cardiac Rehabil 3(No. 12):829–837, 1983.

7. Peterson, LH (ed): Cardiovascular Rehabilitation: A Comprehensive Approach. Macmillan, New York, 1983.

8. Cohn, JN: Drugs used to control vascular resistance and capacitance. In Hurst, JW (ed): The Heart, ed 6. McGraw-Hill, 1986, pp.1583–1586.

9. American College of Sports Mediciine: Guidelines for Exercise Testing and Prescription, ed 3. Lea & Febiger, Philadelphia, 1986.

10. Frishman, WH and Sonnenblick, EH: Beta-adrenergic blocking drugs. In Hurst JW (ed): The Heart, ed 6. McGraw-Hill, 1986, p. 1619.

11. Unger, KM, Moser, K and Hansen, P: Selection of an exercise program for patients with chronic obstructive pulmonary disease. Heart Lung 9:68–76, 1980.

12. deVries, HA: Physiology of Exercise, ed 4. Wm C Brown, Dubuque, 1986.

13. Astrand, P-O: Textbook of Work Physiology, ed 3. McGraw-Hill, New York, 1986.

14. Wiley, MJ: Significant variables associated with compliance in the Bio-Energetics cardiac rehabilitation population. Master's Thesis, University of Pittsburgh, 1982. Unpublished.

15. Haynes, RB: Strategies for improving compliance: A methodological analysis and review. In Sackett, DL and Haynes, RB (eds): Compliance with Therapeutic Regimens. Johns Hopkins University Press, Baltimore, 69–82, 1976.

16. Leventhal, H: Changing attitudes and habits to reduce risk factors in chronic disease. Am J Cardiol 31:571–580, 1973.

17. Lind, AR: Cardiovascular response to static exercise. Circulation 41:173–76, 1970.

18. Dennison, D: The Dine System. CV Mosby, St. Louis, 1982.

19. Connor, WE and Connor, SL: Dietary treatment of hyperlipidemia. In Rifkind, BM and Levy RI (eds): Hyperlipidemia: Diagnosis and Therapy. Grune & Stratton, New York, 1977.

20. Franklin, B. Motivating and educating adults to exercise. JOHPER June, 13–17, 1978.

21. Massie, JF and Shepard, RJ: Physiological and psychological effects of training. Med Sci Sports 3:110–117, 1971.

22. Wenger, NK: Rehabilitation of the patient with symptomatic atherosclerotic coronary heart disease. In Hurst, JW (ed): The Heart, ed 6. McGraw-Hill, New York, pp. 1032–1033, 1986.

23. Baile, WF and Engel, BT: A behavioral strategy for promoting treatment compliance following myocardial infarction. In Franck, CM and Wilson, GT (eds): Annual Review of Behavior Therapy. Brunner/Mazel, New York, pp. 399–428, 1979.

24. American Diabetes Association: The Physician's Guide to Type II Diabetes (NIDMM): Diagnosis and Treatment. American Diabetes Association, New York, 1984.

25. Cunningham, LN, et al: Peripheral hemodynamics and levels of endurance fitness in insulin-dependent diabetic patients. J Cardiopulm Rehabil 6(No. 10):421–429, 1986.

26. La Porte, RE, et al: Pittsburgh insulin-dependent diabetes mellitus morbidity and mortality study: Physical activity and diabetic complications. Pediatrics 78:1027–1033, 1986.

27. National Institutes of Health (NIH) Consensus Development Conference on Diet and Exercise in Non-Insulin-Dependent Diabetes Mellitus, draft statement. National Institute of Diabetes, Digestive and Kidney Diseases and the NIH Office of Medical Applications of Research, Bethesda, MD, 1986.

28. Duda, M: Some diabetics should cycle rather than jog. Physician and Sportsmedicine 14(No. 6):48–50, 1986.

CHAPTER 10

Risk Factor Modification

Scientific study has identified a number of risk factors, that is, circumstances or conditions, that contribute to the development or acceleration of atherosclerosis in humans.[1-4] Risk factors may be classified as primary or secondary, according to their effects, or as non-modifiable or modifiable.

The factors over which the patient has no control include age, gender, familial tendency toward developing coronary heart disease (CHD), and previous medical history. The risk of developing CHD increases with advancing age, is greater for males than females, and is greater for persons with a family history of CHD. Risk is also increased for persons with previous cardiovascular problems, congenital or otherwise. These factors are nonmodifiable.

The factors that are modifiable include blood lipid levels, hypertension, blood glucose, obesity, improper diet and exercise habits, stress, and smoking. These are the factors of greatest interest to the cardiac rehabilitation staff as these are the factors that must be modified if CHD patients are to function as optimally as possible once they leave the formal rehabilitation program and if they are to reduce their risk of the recurrence of myocardial infarction.[5-7]

STAFF INTERVENTION IN RISK FACTOR MODIFICATION

The first step in identifying the patients who are at greater risk is the assessment procedure (Chapter 7). Various questionnaires, surveys, and tests have been devised for this purpose.[1,8-11] Tables 10-1 through 10-5 are examples of health risk appraisals and stress appraisals. The analysis of the tests selected for use by the rehabilitation staff, along with information gathered from review of the patient's medical and personal history, should identify those risk factors that the patient has successfully modified and those that the patient must attempt to change in order to further reduce the risk of recurring coronary events (see Table 10-6).

TABLE 10–1. Example of a Cardiovascular Risk Appraisal*

AGE	1.	If you are over 55 years old	score	1
		If you are age 55 or younger	score	0
GENDER	2.	If you are a male	score	1
		If you are a female	score	0
FAMILY HISTORY	3.	For one or more close blood relatives who have had a heart attack or stroke before the age of 60	score	12
		For one or more who have had a heart attack or stroke after the age of 60	score	6
		Otherwise.	score	0
PERSONAL HISTORY	4.	If you have had one or more before the age of 50: A heart attack, heart or blood vessel surgery or a stroke	score	20
		If you have had one or more after the age of 50 ...	score	10
		If you have had none	score	0
DIABETES	5.	If you had diabetes before the age of 40 and are now on insulin	score	10
		If you had diabetes after the age of 40 and are now on insulin or pills	score	5
		If you have had no diabetes, or controlled diabetes with diet, or mild diabetes over the age of 55	score	0
SMOKING	6.	If you are a two-pack a day smoker or more	score	10
		If you smoke between one and two packs of cigarettes per day, or quit less than a year ago	score	6
		If you smoke less than one pack a day or quit from 1 to 10 years ago	score	3
		If you have never smoked, or quit more than 10 years ago	score	0
CHOLESTEROL	7.	If your cholesterol level is over 275	score	10
		If your cholesterol level is between 225 and 275 ..	score	5
		If your cholesterol level is below 225	score	0
DIET (If cholesterol count is not known answer 7a.)	7a.	In your regular eating pattern do you have at least one serving of red meat daily, more than seven eggs a week, use butter, whole milk and cheese daily? ...	score	8
		In your regular eating pattern do you eat red meat 5 to 6 times a week, eat 4 to 7 eggs a week, use margarine, low fat dairy products and some cheese?	score	4
		Do you eat poultry, fish and little or no red meat, 3 or fewer eggs a week, some margarine, skim milk, and skim milk products?	score	0
HIGH BLOOD PRESSURE	8.	If your blood pressure is above 160 over 105.....	score	8
		If your blood pressure is between 140 to 160 over 90 to 105	score	4
		If your blood pressure is lower than 140 over 90 ..	score	0

TABLE 10–1. *continued*

WEIGHT	9.	The ideal weight for men should be 110 pounds plus 5 pounds per inch over 5 feet. For women the ideal weight is 100 pounds, plus 5 pounds per inch over 5 feet. Calculate your weight on this formula and if you are 25 pounds overweight	score	4
		If you are 10 to 25 pounds overweight	score	2
		If you are less than 10 pounds overweight	score	0
EXERCISE	10.	If you engage in any aerobic exercise (brisk walking, jogging, bicycling, racketball, swimming) for more than 15 minutes less than once a week	score	4
		If you exercise that hard for 1 to 2 times a week . . .	score	2
		If you engage in that exercise for 3 or more times a week	score	0
STRESS	11.	If you are frustrated when waiting in line, often in a hurry to complete work or keep appointments, easily angered, irritable	score	4
		If you are simply impatient when waiting, occasionally hurried, or occasionally moody	score	2
		If you are relatively comfortable when waiting, seldom rushed, and easygoing	score	0

TOTAL YOUR POINTS

SCORE RESULTS

Tabulate your points. Compare them with the chart below.

Please note! A high score does not mean you will develop heart disease. It is a guide to make you aware of a potential risk. Since no two people are alike, an accurate prediction is impossible without further individual study.

High risk . . . . 40 and above
Medium risk . . . . 20 to 39
Low risk . . . . 19 and below

*Adapted from Dietrich.[1]

After the risk factors that need to be modified have been identified for the patient, intervention by the rehabilitation staff can proceed.

Patient Education

The patient must be made aware of the results of the risk factor analysis (preferably in writing) and must be instructed as to the negative effects associated with his or her modifiable risk factor(s). Attempts must be made to motivate the patient to change.

Planning a Strategy

The staff should prepare guidelines that include educational and behavioral objectives for risk factor modification for the patient. The staff psychologist and nutritionist should play

TABLE 10–2. Example of a Cardiovascular Risk Appraisal

Heart Attack Risk Score*
Developed by Stephen B. Guss, M.D., FACC

Is it possible to know whether you are likely to have a heart attack? *Cardiac Alert* has developed a "Heart Attack Risk Score" to better estimate whether a person is likely to sustain a heart attack within the next 10 years. Of course, the "Risk Score" is only an estimate, and a low score doesn't guarantee protection. Nor does a high score inevitably doom you. But taking the "Heart Attack Risk Score" test will tell you whether you have been taking care of your cardiac health and provide a guide for preventive measures you can take to lessen your chances of having a heart attack as you lower your risk score. The "Risk Score" test is not a substitute for good medical care, however.

Should your score be over 100, phone your physician and make an appointment to be examined thoroughly and instructed on ways of reducing your risk factors for developing a heart attack.

The first 16 questions provide a relative risk of having a heart attack during the coming 10 years for people without any known heart disease. If the answers to either questions 17 and 18 are yes, or if the answer to question 19 is anything but "negative," the likelihood of having coronary artery disease is quite high, and the risk for a subsequent heart attack is significantly greater.

QUESTIONS 1–16, NO KNOWN HEART DISEASE

1. How old are you?
    Greater than 60 years. Score 5 points.   _____
    50 to 59 years. Score 3 points.   _____
    40 to 49 years. Score 2 points.   _____
    Less than 40 years old. Score 0.   _____
    • Younger people are less likely to suffer a heart attack.

2. What sex are you?
    Male. Score 4 points.   _____
    Female (I have been through menopause). Score 2 points.   _____
    Female (I have not been through menopause). Score 0.   _____
    • Women still have fewer heart attacks than do men, but after menopause the risk
      becomes nearly even.

3. Do you smoke now?
    More than 2 packs a day. Score 20 points.   _____
    1 to 2 packs a day. Score 15 points.   _____
    ¼ to 1 pack a day. Score 10 points.   _____
    Less than ¼ pack a day. Score 5 points.   _____
    I do not smoke. Score 0.   _____
    • Cigarette smoking is one of the greatest causes of heart attacks. Even light
      smoking is bad for your health.

4. Have you ever smoked?
    I still smoke. Score 5 points.   _____
    I haven't smoked in 1 to 5 years. Score 3 points.   _____
    I haven't smoked in over 10 years. Score 1 point.   _____
    I have never smoked. Score 0.   _____
    • Discontinuing smoking is a must because some damage or cholesterol buildup in
      the coronary arteries will occur in heavy smokers. Years must pass before the ill
      effects of past smoking can be observed.

TABLE 10–2. *continued*

5. For how many years did you smoke? (Even if you have stopped)
   I have smoked for over 30 years. Score 6 points.   _____
   I have smoked between 10 and 20 years. Score 4 points.   _____
   I have smoked between 5 and 10 years. Score 3 points.   _____
   I have smoked less than 5 years. Score 2 points.   _____
   I have never smoked. Score 0.   _____
   • The cumulative effects of smoking, even at low quantities, can take their toll on
   the heart.

6. Does heart disease run in your family? (Including blood uncles, aunts, cousins)
   My mother or father had a heart attack before age 50. Score 25 points.   _____
   My brother or sister had a heart attack before age 55. Score 20 points.   _____
   Aunts, uncles, or cousins had heart attacks before age 60. Score 10 points. _____
   Heart attacks occur in the family but only after age 60. Score 6 points. _____
   Heart attacks occur only in aunts, uncles, cousins after age 60. Score 4 points. _____
   There is no heart disease in my family until after age 70. Score 0.   _____
   If several of the above apply, score only the one with the highest score.
   • Heart disease runs in families. Although you can do nothing about your ancestry,
   high scores on this question should motivate you to concentrate on changing
   other risk factors.

7. Do you have high blood pressure?
   Yes, and it is difficult to control even with medication. Score 25 points. _____
   Yes, but the doctor says it is under control with medication. Score 15 points. _____
   Yes, but it is under control with weight control, low salt diet, and exercise. Score
      10 points.   _____
   Yes, but only occasionally when the doctor takes my blood pressure. Score 8 points. _____
   No, but high blood pressure runs in my immediate family so I am limiting my salt
      intake and trying to keep an ideal weight to avoid developing hypertension.
      Score 3 points.   _____
   No, nor does it run in my immediate family. Score 0.   _____
   • Hypertension runs in families and predisposes to developing heart attacks. Blood
   pressure control (less than 140/90) can help prevent heart attacks. Salt avoidance
   and maintaining ideal weight may prevent the development of hypertension in
   susceptible individuals.

8. Is your blood cholesterol high?
   More than 350. Score 25 points.   _____
   300 to 350. Score 20 points.   _____
   260 to 300. Score 12 points.   _____
   240 to 260. Score 8 points.   _____
   220 to 260. Score 4 points.   _____
   Less than 200. Score 0   _____
   • If you don't know your blood cholesterol level, you really should have it checked.
   Perhaps your doctor has the results in your chart. Phone him or her. If you are
   unsure, score 12 (average American score). The higher your cholesterol, the
   greater the chance of having a heart attack.

9. Do you eat too much cholesterol?
   I eat red meat, dairy products, or egg yolks most days of the week. Score 8 points. _____
   I eat red meat, dairy products, or egg yolks 2–3 days a week. Score 3 points. _____
   I am a strict vegetarian. Score 0.   _____

(continued)

TABLE 10–2. *continued*

10. Do you have diabetes?
    Yes, and my blood sugar is usually out of control. Score 25 points.   _____
    Yes, but my blood sugar is well controlled on medications. Score 20 points.   _____
    Yes, but my blood sugar is controlled with diet alone. Score 15 points.   _____
    No, but it runs in my family. Score 10 points.   _____
    No, and it does not run in my family. Score 0.   _____

11. How long have you had diabetes?
    More than 20 years. Score 15 points.   _____
    10 to 20 years. Score 10 points.   _____
    0 to 10 years. Score 5 points.   _____
    I do not have diabetes. Score 0.   _____

12. How old were you when you first developed diabetes?
    Under age 20. Score 15 points.   _____
    20 to 40. Score 10 points.   _____
    40 to 60. Score 7 points.   _____
    Over 60. Score 3 points.   _____
    I do not have diabetes. Score 0.   _____
    • The earlier diabetes is developed, the longer it has been present, and the poorer is
      the diabetic control, the greater is the chance of having a heart attack.

13. Are you overweight?
    I am more than 50 pounds overweight. Score 10 points.   _____
    I am 25 to 50 pounds overweight. Score 7 points.   _____
    I am 15 to 25 pounds overweight. Score 2 points.   _____
    I am less than 15 pounds overweight. Score 0.   _____
    • It has been found that mild degrees of obesity are not by themselves contributory
      to developing a heart attack unless diabetes or hypertension are also present.

14. Are you a Type-A personality (aggressive, competitive, a slave to the clock)?
    Yes. Score 10 points.   _____
    No. Score 0.   _____
    • Type A people not only are driven but appear to drive their hearts so hard they
      have a higher incidence of heart attacks.

15. Do you exercise?
    No, I am totally sedentary. Score 15 points.   _____
    Only on weekends. Score 12 points.   _____
    I exercise 15 to 30 minutes 3–4 days a week. Score 5 points.   _____
    I exercise 30 to 45 minutes 4–5 days a week. Score 0.   _____
    • Exercisers have fewer heart attacks and live longer than nonexercisers.

16. What does your resting ECG (electrocardiogram) show?
    It is abnormal. Score 15 points.   _____
    It is normal. Score 0.   _____
    I don't know. Score 0.   _____
    • An abnormal resting ECG is a minor but definite risk factor in developing a heart
      attack.

(continued)

TABLE 10-2. *continued*

HEART DISEASE MOST LIKELY PRESENT

17. Have you had a heart attack?
    Yes. Score 30 points.   _____
    No. Score 0.   _____
    • People who have had a first heart attack have a high chance of having a second
      unless they take proper care of the heart.

18. Do you have chest pressure or heaviness when you exert yourself (angina)?
    Yes, but also at rest. Score 50 points.   _____
    Yes, but it has been occurring with greater frequency and with less exertion lately.
      Score 40 points.   _____
    Yes, but it seems to be stable. Score 30 points.   _____
    No. Score 0.   _____
    • Angina means the heart muscle is not receiving enough oxygen. The occurrence of
      angina at rest means the supplying coronary artery is almost totally blocked with
      cholesterol.

19. What does your stress test (treadmill stress test) show?
    ECG changes occurred quite early (very positive test). Score 50 points.   _____
    ECG changes occurred only after many minutes of exercise (mildly positive).
      Score 35 points.   _____
    My doctor told me the test was borderline. Score 25 points.   _____
    It was negative. Score 0.   _____
    Have not had a treadmill stress test. Score 0.   _____
    • A positive stress test at low levels of exercise is highly predictive of a heart attack
      in the near future.

    Tally your score and consult the guide below. Remember, high scores should encourage
you to work at lowering your score by changing lifestyle habits which are bad for the heart. A
very low score may make you feel good, but it should serve to reinforce the fact that you are
treating your heart properly and should continue to do so.

NO KNOWN HEART DISEASE

Score less than 20
    You are doing the right things and have an extremely unlikely chance of having a heart
    attack over the next 10 years.

Score 20 to 35
    Chances are unlikely that you will have a heart attack over the next 10 years.

Score 35 to 100
    There are life-style habits to work on, but a chance of a heart attack is small.

Score 100 to 150
    You need to modify your risk factors and consult a physician. Unless you change, you have
    a moderate chance of having a heart attack during the next 10 years.

Score more than 150
    You are at an extremely high risk for developing coronary artery disease and a heart attack.
    Consult your physician and work very hard to lower your score before it's too late.

                                                                    (continued)

TABLE 10–2. *continued*

If your answers to questions 17 and 18 were yes, or if your stress test answer to question 19 is abnormal, then you most likely have cholesterol narrowings in your coronary arteries and have at least triple the chance of having a heart attack compared to the group without known heart disease.

HIGH PROBABILITY OF HEART DISEASE

Score 30 or less on questions 17–19
    Although your chances of having a heart attack during the next 10 years are greater than the general population, the relative risk is still small, and you should work hard toward modifying your coronary risk factors. In addition, you should be under the care of a physician.

Score 31 to 50 on questions 17–19
    Chances of having a heart attack are moderately high. Stay under the care of a physician and reduce your other risk factors.

Score 50 or greater on questions 17–19
    Chances of having a heart attack are high. Consult your physician and work diligently to reduce your risk factors.

People in the "High Probability of Heart Disease" group also tally their score for the first 16 questions. It is even more important for the "High Probability" group to have as low a score as possible for the first 16 questions in order to reduce the chance of sustaining a heart attack.

*From Guss,[9] with permission.

TABLE 10–3. Example of a Coronary Risk Factor Questionnaire*

Risk Factor	Points
1. Cigarette Smoking	
a. 2 packs/day	7
b. 1–2 packs/day	6
c. ½–1 pack/day	5
2. Hypertension (systolic bp >150 or diastolic bp >90)	5
3. Elevated serum cholesterol	
a. 350	7
b. 300–350	6
c. 250–300	5
d. 225–250	3
4. Family history of coronary disease before age 55	4
5. Overweight >15%	3
6. Elevated serum triglyceride	
a. >300	5
b. 150–300	3
7. Diabetes mellitus	3
8. Type A personality	2
9. Abnormal ECG	2
10. Enlarged heart on chest x-ray	2
11. Low aerobic capacity (no regular [e.g., weekly] endurance as swimming, jogging, or bicycling)	3
12. Abnormal exercise stress test	17

Coronary Risk Categories	*Total Points*
I. Very low	(<6 points)
II. Low	(6–10 points)
III. Average	(11–15 points)
IV. Above average	(16–20 points)
V. Very high	(>20 points)

*From Fletcher and Cantwell,[11] with permission.

TABLE 10–4. Example of a Stress Inventory Commonly Used to Predict Health Change

Life Change Scale*
What events have happened to you in the past 12 months?

Event Rank	Event Value	Happened (✓)	Your Score	Life Event
1	100	_____	_____	Death of a spouse
2	73	_____	_____	Divorce
3	65	_____	_____	Marital separation
4	63	_____	_____	Jail term
5	63	_____	_____	Death of a close family member
6	53	_____	_____	Personal injury or illness
7	50	_____	_____	Marriage
8	47	_____	_____	Fired from a job
9	45	_____	_____	Marital reconciliation
10	45	_____	_____	Retirement
11	44	_____	_____	Change in health of a family member
12	40	_____	_____	Pregnancy
13	39	_____	_____	Sex difficulties
14	39	_____	_____	Gain of new family member
15	39	_____	_____	Business readjustment
16	38	_____	_____	Change in financial state
17	37	_____	_____	Death of a close friend
18	36	_____	_____	Change in different line of work
19	35	_____	_____	Change in number of arguments with spouse
20	31	_____	_____	Mortgage over $10,000
21	30	_____	_____	Foreclosure of mortgage or loan
22	29	_____	_____	Change in responsibilities at work
23	29	_____	_____	Son or daughter leaving home
24	29	_____	_____	Trouble with in-laws
25	28	_____	_____	Outstanding personal achievement
26	26	_____	_____	Wife begin or stop work
27	26	_____	_____	Begin or end school
28	25	_____	_____	Change in living conditions
29	25	_____	_____	Revision of personal habits
30	23	_____	_____	Trouble with boss
31	20	_____	_____	Change in work hours or conditions
32	20	_____	_____	Change in residence
33	20	_____	_____	Change in schools
34	19	_____	_____	Change in recreation
35	19	_____	_____	Change in church activities
36	18	_____	_____	Change in social activities
37	17	_____	_____	Mortgage or loan less than $10,000
38	16	_____	_____	Change in sleeping habits
39	15	_____	_____	Change in number of family get-togethers
40	15	_____	_____	Change in eating habits
41	13	_____	_____	Vacation
42	12	_____	_____	Christmas
43	11	_____	_____	Minor violations of the law

Your Total Score _____

Interpretation: 1466 points are possible.
150 points: "50–50" chance of a health change
300 points or more: 90 percent chance of a health change

The Scale is a version of the Social Readjustment Rating Scale, developed by Holmes and Rahe.

*From Gunderson, Rahe, and Rahe,[10] with permission.

TABLE 10–5. Example of a Stress Inventory and Profile*

Stress Cues List

Check items that occur frequently or often.

Emotional-Cognitive Cues:
   I become overexcited   _____
   I worry   _____
   I feel insecure   _____
   I have difficulty sleeping at night   _____
   I become easily confused or forgetful   _____
   I cry easily   _____
   I think about several things at once   _____
   I become easily irritable   _____
   I become very uncomfortable or ill at ease   _____
   I become nervous   _____
             Total Emotional-Cognitive Cues   _____

Physical Cues:
   I sweat profusely/hands get clammy   _____
   My face becomes "hot"   _____
   I shake or wiggle my feet when I sit   _____
   I have frequent headaches   _____
   My muscles become tense or stiff   _____
   I feel my heart pounding   _____
   I have difficulty saying what I want to say   _____
   My stomach becomes upset or cramped   _____
   I have diarrhea or have colitis   _____
   I have twitches   _____
             Total Physical Cues   _____

Behavioral Cues:
   I act impulsively   _____
   I walk rapidly   _____
   I eat when I'm nervous or bored   _____
   I smoke when I'm nervous   _____
   I drink to make me less nervous   _____
   I often do two things at once   _____
   I work later than others   _____
   I'm more responsible than others   _____
   I am more competitive than others   _____
   I am frequently late or rushing to be on time   _____
             Total Behavioral Cues   _____

SCORING:
             Sum of Three Scores   _____

Type A Behavior Inventory

The following statements are similar to those associated with Type A behavior. Circle the appropriate letter for each question.

(continued)

TABLE 10–5. *continued*

	Frequently	Sometimes	Never
1. Do you have problems getting along with your superiors at work?	F	S	N
2. Do you bring work home more than once a week?	F	S	N
3. Do you consider yourself keenly competitive or hard-driving at work?	F	S	N
4. Do you feel uncomfortable or upset when you have to wait in a long line?	F	S	N
5. Do you eat rapidly?	F	S	N
6. Do you generally prefer to do things yourself rather than have others do them for you?	F	S	N
7. Do you engage in two things at once, e.g., reading the newspaper while eating?	F	S	N
8. Are you easily irritated?	F	S	N
9. Do you become upset when others observe you while you are working on a task?	F	S	N
10. Do you go back to your work during your time off?	F	S	N
11. Do you try harder than most at what you do?	F	S	N
12. Do you feel like hurrying someone who takes too long to come to the point?	F	S	N
13. Do you generally walk faster during the day than you would if you were walking on a beach?	F	S	N
14. Do you believe yourself to be more responsible than others around you?	F	S	N
15. Do you think about other things when someone is talking to you?	F	S	N

SCORING:
Number of "F" answers _____ × 2 = _____
Number of "S" answers _____ × 1 = _____
Number of "N" answers _____ × 0 = _____
Add these three for a total of   _____

Relaxation Scale

Put a checkmark in the column that most accurately answers each question.

	Frequently	Sometimes	Never
1. Do you take regular naps or relaxation breaks at least once per day?	___	___	___
2. Do you plan "alone time" for yourself to engage in some pleasant activity at least once a day?	___	___	___
3. Do you regularly engage in some play activity?	___	___	___
4. Do you spend some time regularly in which you concentrate fully on only one task for an extended period of time?	___	___	___
5. Do you wear clothing that fits well and you feel good in?	___	___	___
6. Do you plan or organize your day's activities ahead of time?	___	___	___
7. Are you able to effectively "come down" at the end of the day in order to fall quickly asleep?	___	___	___

(continued)

TABLE 10-5. *continued*

	Frequently	Sometimes	Never
8. Do you actively attempt to create regular changes in your environment, for example, take different routes to and from work or do routine tasks in different rooms?	___	___	___
9. Do you regularly monitor your tension behavior and take steps to reduce it, i.e., sit back in your chair and take several deep breaths, slow down your walking pace?	___	___	___
10. Do you engage in some exercise activity at least 20 minutes daily?	___	___	___
11. Do you allow time for yourself to daydream about your goals and future plans?	___	___	___
12. When worried do you know how to put troublesome thoughts into perspective to reduce their potency?	___	___	___
13. Do you regularly spend time planning vacations and entertainment activity?	___	___	___
14. Do you actively seek out humor in your life and spend some time laughing every day?	___	___	___
15. Do you frequently act and respond in a spontaneous manner rather than in a controlled and calculated fashion?	___	___	___

SCORING:

Number of "F" answers _____ × 2 = _____
Number of "S" answers _____ × 1 = _____
Number of "N" answers _____ × 0 = _____
Add these three for a total of   _____

Stress Thinking Scale

Put a checkmark in the column that most accurately answers each question.

	Frequently	Sometimes	Never
1. Polyphasic Thinking: Do you think of several things at a time, or find it difficult to concentrate on or persist with a thought to its completion?	___	___	___
2. Low Self-Confidence: Do you think about yourself in depreciating terms or make negative self-statements?	___	___	___
3. Excessive Responsibility: Do you think of yourself as being the only one or best one capable of carrying the burden of completing tasks or projects?	___	___	___
4. Self-Reference: Do you think predominantly in "I" terms with you at the center of attention, that is, do the words "I" or "me" occur frequently in your language and thoughts?	___	___	___
5. Confusion: Do you become easily confused?	___	___	___
6. Catastrophizing: Do you think of the worst possible outcomes for unfortunate events or circumstances?	___	___	___

(continued)

TABLE 10–5. *continued*

	Frequently	Sometimes	Never
7. Dichotomous Thinking: Do you think of things as being either one extreme or another, good or bad, right or wrong, best or worst?	____	____	____
8. Negativistic Thinking: Do you think badly of events or circumstances or hold negative thoughts about people?	____	____	____
9. Angry Thinking: Do you think about things or people in your past, the present, or the future that generate anger or revenge in you?	____	____	____
10. Hypochondriacal Thinking: Do you concern yourself or worry about your body or your health?	____	____	____

SCORING:
Number of "F" answers _____ $\times 3$ = _____
Number of "S" answers _____ $\times 1.5$ = _____
Number of "N" answers _____ $\times 0$ = _____
Add these three for a total of _____

Time Use Scale

Circle the appropriate letter for each question.

	Frequently	Sometimes	Never
1. Do you put things off until the last minute?	F	S	N
2. Would others consider you, or do you feel, harried or rushed?	F	S	N
3. Do you feel that you have made the best use of your time after completing an activity?	F	S	N
4. Do you plan your activities ahead of time?	F	S	N
5. Are you successful at ending time-consuming events easily, such as telephone calls, meetings, conversations, or activities?	F	S	N
6. Do you tell others beforehand how much time you have allotted for what you are about to do?	F	S	N
7. Are you an accurate judge of the amount of time an activity will take?	F	S	N
8. Do you plan for yourself a certain amount of "alone time" every day?	F	S	N
9. Do you plan time to be with others who are helpful or are willing to give to you?	F	S	N
10. Do you delegate tasks to others easily?	F	S	N

SCORING:
Number of "F" answers _____ $\times 3$ = _____
Number of "S" answers _____ $\times 1.5$ = _____
Number of "N" answers _____ $\times 0$ = _____
Add these three for a total of _____

(*continued*)

TABLE 10–5. *continued*

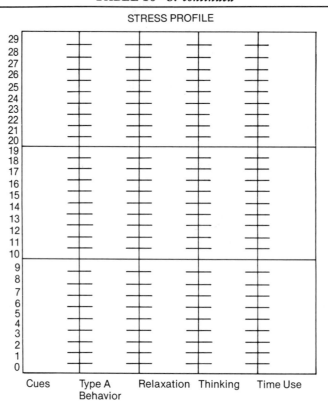

STRESS PROFILE

Cues Type A Behavior Relaxation Thinking Time Use

*From Dietrich,[1] pp. 80–88, with permission.

TABLE 10–6. Results of Evaluation and Risk Factor Analysis with Behavioral Objectives

Patient Name: ___John Smith___   Date: __8-15-87__
Address: ___123___
Referring Physician(s): ___Robert Jones, M.D.___
Diagnosis(es): __CAD, S/P MI (6-15-87), Hypertension__
Medications and dosages: ___Corgard, Procainamide___

Smoking Habits: __Cigarettes — 1 ppd, a decrease from 2 ppd__

	Current	Prior	Percent Change
Exercise Tolerance Test (Adapted Bruce Protocol)			
Max Heart Rate (bpm)	80	N/A	
Max O_2 Consumed (ml/kg/min)	17.5		
Max Systolic BP (mmHg)	158		
Max Diastolic BP (mmHg)	94		
Total Exercise Time (min)	9		

(continued)

TABLE 10-6. *continued*

Body Composition/Blood Profile: (Ht: 5'10")	Current	Prior	Percent Change
Body Weight (lbs)	182		
Percent Body Fat	24		
Total Cholesterol (mg/dl)	160		
HDLs (mg/dl)	35		
Triglycerides	250		
Blood Glucose	92		
Stress/Tension			
Cues (emotional, physical, behavioral)	15		
Type A Behavior	23		
Relaxation	22		
Thinking	9		
Time Use	10		

Cardiovascular Risk Factor Analysis

Scientific studies have identified risk factors that contribute to the development and progression of coronary artery disease. The risk factors over which you have no control include age, being male or female, having a family history of coronary disease, and your previous medical history. Risk factors that you can control include smoking, obesity, elevated blood fats and blood sugar, physical inactivity, and excessive stress.

Risk factors you must modify in order to reduce the risk of recurring coronary events include: cessation of smoking, lowering of triglycerides by adherence to dietary guidelines established for you, decrease body weight through proper nutrition, increase your cardiovascular endurance (exercise tolerance) through prescribed aerobic exercise, and learn how to decrease your stress and tension level through stress management group counseling.

Desirable Levels for Risk Factors

Smoking: Total abstinence, none.

Exercise Tolerance: Increase activity level to attain and maintain a maximum of 30 to 60 minutes of cardiorespiratory work, 3 to 5 times/week at your prescribed target heart rate.

Body Weight: Your present weight is __182__ lbs. A __Lowfat Modified__, 1800 cal, diet has been recommended in order that your lipid levels may be controlled and an ideal body weight of __160-168__ lbs. may be achieved/maintained. (If you need to lose weight, set a goal of losing 1 to 1½ lbs. per week until you achieve your ideal weight.)

Percentage Body Fat: Your present percentage of body fat, __24__, is a more accurate way of determining how close you are to your ideal weight for your own body type. Although age affects the desirable level of body fat, in general, men should try to maintain levels <20 percent and women <30 percent.

Blood Profile: Desirable lipid levels (these levels may be altered somewhat by age or recent occurrence of heart attack or myocardial infarction):

Cholesterol	200
Triglycerides	160
HDLs	45

Stress Profile: The stress profile has helped to identify those areas that are particular problems for you. These are the areas that will be addressed in your stress management sessions.

primary roles in establishing these guidelines. However, the entire rehabilitation staff must be aware of the goals established for each patient to effect appropriate reinforcement.

Implementing the Plan

The patient must be instructed in the proper technique, for example, relaxation techniques for controlling stress or specific dietary changes. This instruction may be given individually or in groups. Individual counseling may be very effective but is also time consuming. A combination of both types of instruction appears to be the most feasible in most situations. Staff time devoted to instructing the patient varies with the intent of the instruction.

Evaluation of Patient Risk Factor Modification

Regular evaluation of patient compliance with risk factor modification is a standard procedure while the patient is participating in the formal supervised program. However, once the patient leaves the program and is exercising independently at home, compliance to the prescribed plan for risk factor modification and exercise can be assessed through regularly scheduled evaluations. These evaluations are scheduled at intervals determined by the medical status of the patient. After "graduation" from the formal program, the patient should be evaluated at least annually.

Rehabilitation staff should note that in the initial stages of rehabilitation, too much change will defeat the purpose of behavior modification. Patients must not be overwhelmed by the considerable changes that must be made in their lifestyles. Care must be taken to apply developmental principles to the establishment of goals to ensure success in modifying behavior.

The following discussion of the major modifiable risk factors in addition to the lack of cardiorespiratory exercise (smoking, improper diet, and stress) will be limited to the primary physiologic effects and current trends in the management of these factors.

SMOKING

For the past 20 years, Americans have become increasingly aware of the health risks associated with smoking. Nevertheless, approximately 54 million Americans continue to smoke. The number of male smokers has declined by an average of 15 percent since the Surgeon General's first warning in 1964. However, the number of female smokers has increased.[3,12-14] This behavior is difficult to comprehend in light of the evidence demonstrated by numerous studies that smoking of any kind (cigarette, pipe, or cigar) is hazardous to one's health.

Physiologic Effects. The physiologic effects of smoking are complex and too numerous for the scope of this text. However, the major effects of smoking will be described in relation to the substances absorbed by the body (nicotine and carbon monoxide) and the actual physical effects of the smoke itself.

Nicotine may be absorbed through the skin and mucous membranes of the body and, through stimulation of various chemoreceptors and nerve cells, acts to increase blood pressure and heart rate and indirectly enhances platelet aggregation. The inhalation of tobacco smoke directly or indirectly (side-stream smoke) permits carbon monoxide (CO) to be absorbed into the blood stream via the lungs. The concentration of CO is greater in side-stream smoke than in directly inhaled smoke. As the red blood cell has greater affinity for CO than it has for oxygen, the oxygen-carrying capacity of the blood is decreased. The increased concentration of CO triggers production of red blood cells, which in turn increases the viscosity of the blood and, therefore, the peripheral resistance increases. Consequently, blood pressure rises and the heart is forced to work harder and is adversely affected. Recent research also indicates that CO may be directly related to the development of atherosclerotic lesions[12] and has been demonstrated to cause degenerative effects on the myofibrils and mitochondria of the myocardium.[12] In addition, tobacco smoke eventually destroys the cilia in the lungs and reduces the ability of the lungs to clear themselves of dust, germs, and other debris. Smoke in the lungs also impairs oxygen exchange.

Smoking Cessation. Assisting the cardiac patient in the process of smoking cessation should be a high priority for the rehabilitation staff. In lay terms, the patient should be informed about the adverse effects of smoking. The information may be contained in a patient education manual or provided as supplemental material for distribution during individual or group counseling. Various guidelines and suggestions are available to assist the patient in his or her efforts. A most helpful and complete publication is provided by the U.S. Department of Health and Human Services.[15] Videotapes are available from the National Audio Visual Center. Most formal guides to smoking cessation recommend the following procedures:

1. An analysis of why the patient smokes that includes identification of specific behavioral and psychological states that accompany the smoking habit.
2. Reinforcement of the reasons why the patient may want to stop smoking.
3. Assisting the patient with the selection of a method for cessation of smoking.
4. Enrolling the patient in a structured program that utilizes small-group counseling under the guidance of a qualified counselor or therapist.

Formal group therapy is not always required to help a patient stop smoking. In fact, many cardiac patients will have stopped smoking already on the advice of their physicians prior to beginning an exercise program. Therefore, the role of the rehabilitation staff becomes primarily one of reinforcing the patient's compliance with his or her self-motivated behavioral change. Compliance with positive behavioral change may be reinforced by reminding the patient of the reason(s) that motivated the patient to stop smoking. The most common reasons are as follows:

1. Concern over the effects of health (particularly fear of recurring coronary events).
2. Desire to set an example for others.
3. Recognition of the unpleasant aspects of smoking, e.g., nicotine stains, foul-smelling clothing, halitosis.
4. Desire to exercise self-control.

As smoking is one of the most serious of the risk factors associated with CHD, the rehabilitation staff needs to make a concentrated effort to motivate patients to stop smoking and to educate and encourage patients who have stopped so that the chances of their resuming the habit are significantly reduced.

DIETARY RECOMMENDATIONS

Few areas of scientific investigation have as great an impact on the population as a whole as nutritional research, the result of which is intense scrutiny by the mass media with apparently continuous controversy. Therefore, this discussion of nutritional considerations in cardiovascular disease needs to be prefaced by several comments regarding dietary advice and how it should be interpreted.

In light of the diversity of expert opinion, it is no wonder that patients are confused. However, patients should learn to expect that dietary advice will change as the results of new research are reported.

Patients should be made aware that scientists will continue to differ in both their interpretation of the scientific evidence relating to the effect of dietary changes and their recommendations for the application of new scientific information. Consumers need to make informed, common-sense decisions about their diets based on their own individual needs and priorities. Patients should be taught that dietary recommendations developed by experts are generally more scientifically based and associated with fewer health risks than those formulated by groups or individuals who may receive financial gain as a result of the advice that they are giving. Therefore, patients should be taught to interpret information in a critical and thoughtful manner (see Appendix G).

DIETARY INTERVENTION

In most cases, rehabilitation of the cardiac patient involves major dietary changes. Generally, the goals of dietary intervention are to decrease blood lipid levels in hyperlipidemic patients, to reduce hypertension or maintain normal blood pressure, and to reduce or normalize body weight. These goals are basically accomplished through reduction in dietary consumption of cholesterol-rich foods and saturated fats, restriction of sodium intake, and reduction in total caloric intake.

Justification for such intervention is based primarily on the associations among total serum cholesterol, diet, and mortality rates owing to CHD as demonstrated by numerous studies, including long-term epidemiological investigations such as the Framingham[2] and Chicago[16] studies that followed the progression of the disease in populations that were initially free of CHD.

A basic understanding of the current theory regarding dietary intervention is necessary for the cardiac rehabilitation staff to reinforce behavioral change effectively and provide informal patient education regarding dietary recommendations. For this reason, the following information concerning blood lipids and antihyperlipidemic dietary regimens is included.

Lipids. Basically, there are three types of lipids (or fats) that circulate in the blood. The most common type, triglycerides, make up 95 percent of the total plasma lipid content, and the remaining 5 percent is comprised of sterols (cholesterol) and phospholipids (lecithin).

Transportation and function of the lipids in the plasma is made possible by the attachment of the lipid molecule to protein molecules; consequently, triglycerides, cholesterol, and other fatty substances in the plasma are known collectively as lipoproteins. The lipoprotein molecules exist in various sizes and molecular weights and also differ in the amount of cholesterol and other lipid material that they contain.

High Density Lipoproteins (HDLs). HDLs are the heaviest of this class of substances and have the highest proportion of protein. HDLs are important in the removal of fat from the plasma and away from body cells by transporting fats to the liver, where they are metabolized (into bile) and excreted from the body via the intestines. Hence, the HDLs have been labeled "good" cholesterol, as they tend to inhibit the acceleration of atherosclerosis by preventing the deposition of cholesterol and other fats in arterial walls.

Research has demonstrated that high plasma levels of HDL are associated with lower risk of atherosclerosis, myocardial infarctions and cerebrovascular accidents.[17-20] HDL levels above 65 mg per dl suggest a decreased risk of coronary heart disease. Values less than 35 mg per dl suggest an increased risk.[21] Generally, women have higher HDL levels than men. Regular, continuous aerobic exercise performed for extended periods of time produces an increase in HDL levels in both men and women.[22,23] Scientific evidence suggests that HDL levels are adversely affected by smoking and positively affected by moderate consumption of alcohol.[24] However, recent investigation suggests that the increase in HDL levels due to alcoholic consumption may be the result of the inability of the liver to metabolize HDLs.[25-27]

Low Density Lipoproteins (LDLs). These molecules, as their name implies, are smaller and lighter in molecular weight than the HDLs. Among lipoproteins, the LDLs contain the highest percentage of cholesterol and have been identified as a major factor in the deposition of cholesterol in arterial atheromas.[18,28,29] A direct relationship has been demonstrated between LDL plasma levels and the incidence of CHD and strokes.[28] Hence, the LDLs have been labeled "bad" cholesterol. LDL levels are significantly affected by diet. Excessive consumption of dietary cholesterol has been shown to increase LDL levels.[30] In epidemiological studies, total serum cholesterol and LDL levels appear to be related to cultural differences in the incidence of CAD.[19] The results of a recent study suggest that dietary fiber may be effective in reducing LDL levels while HDL levels remain unchanged.[30]

Very Low Density Lipoproteins (VLDLs). These molecules are the lightest of the three lipoproteins discussed. VLDLs are the primary transporters of triglycerides and play a role in the production and transportation of other lipoproteins as well. VLDL is a precursor of LDL. High levels of VLDLs may tend to elevate LDL levels and lower HDL levels. The risk of future myocardial infarction, CAD, and stroke is directly related to levels of total serum cholesterol and LDLs.[28]

In Western societies, the average total serum cholesterol level is 220 to 280 mg per dl. Cultures associated with a lower incidence of CAD report average levels of 100 to 140 mg per dl. Generally, a total serum cholesterol level of 200 mg per dl or lower maintained throughout adult life is associated with a relatively low risk of developing CAD, while levels exceeding 300 mg per dl are associated with high risk.[31,32]

Reduction of Total Serum Cholesterol. Investigation of various experimental diets developed for the treatment of all types of hyperlipidemia has yielded specific information about dietary modification. A 10 percent reduction in total serum cholesterol has been reported as a result of therapeutic diet regimens that limit the total dietary cholesterol to

200 mg per day and also limit fat to 30 percent of the total caloric intake, with the ratio of polyunsaturated fat to saturated fat (P/S ratio) 2.0 or greater.[30] Therapeutic diets for hyperlipidemic patients must have a P/S ratio greater than 1.0 and diets with a P/S ratio of 2.0 have been demonstrated to be hypocholesterolemic in effect.[30] In contrast, the average American daily diet contains 500 mg of cholesterol and has a P/S ratio of 0.4.[24] Even greater declines in serum cholesterol (as much as 24 percent) have been reported with therapeutic regimens of 25 mg of cholesterol per day, 10 percent fat (P/S ratio of 1.24), and little protein intake from animal sources[30] (see Table 10–7).

Further reductions in total serum cholesterol may be achieved by increasing the fiber in the diet. This is particularly true of fiber in the form of pectin, which is derived from plant material. Cholesterol reductions in the range of 10 percent have been achieved by substituting vegetable protein for animal protein and changing the composition of the diet to include complex carbohydrates.[30]

Moderate weight reduction may also decrease total serum cholesterol (15 mg per dl) and triglyceride levels. There is some suggestion that an antihyperlipidemic diet regimen may lead to the regression of atheromatous lesions in laboratory animals and humans. However, these investigations are limited and require further study.

EXAMPLES OF ANTIHYPERLIPIDEMIC REGIMENS

Although a variety of diets are currently in use throughout the country, most cardiac rehabilitation centers use the "Alternative Diet"[30] or a modification of this plan. This diet has been recommended for initial use in the treatment of all types of hyperlipidemia. Basically, this diet restricts the daily intake of cholesterol to 100 mg, dietary fat to 20 percent of total calories (high P/S ratio), and meat consumption to 3 to 4 ounces per day and encourages the exclusive use of polyunsaturated fats, complex carbohydrates, and low-cholesterol cheeses.

In comparison, the experimental diet reported by Barnard and associates[33] (Pritikin Longevity Center Diet) restricts the daily intake of cholesterol to 25 mg, dietary fat to 10 percent of total calories (P/S ratio 1.24), and meat consumption; all protein requirements (13 percent of total calories) are derived from vegetable sources, with the exception of nonfat milk and small amounts of fish or fowl. All remaining calories (77 percent) are consumed in the form of complex carbohydrates. In addition, no caffeine or alcohol is permitted.[33]

In contrast to the Pritikin Diet are the recommendations of the American Heart Association (AHA).[31] The guidelines for dietary modification recommended by the AHA

TABLE 10–7. A Comparison of the Average American Diet
to the Lowfat Modified Diet

	Average American Diet	Lowfat Modified Diet
% Fat	42 (P/S ratio 0.4)	30 (P/S ratio 1.0–2.0)
% Protein	15 Animal	15 Vegetable and animal
% Carbohydrate	42 Simple	55 Complex
	100	100
Cholesterol Content	500 mg/day	300 mg/day or less

TABLE 10–8. A Comparison of Diet Plans for CHD Patients

Name of Plan	Cholesterol (mg)	% Fat	P/S Ratio	Meat (oz)	Alcohol	Caffeine	High in Complex Carbohydrates
Alternative	100	20	1.0–2.0	3–4	0–rarely	0	Yes
Pritikin	25	10	1.0–2.0	0–rarely	0	0	Yes
AHA	300 or less	30–35	1.0–2.0	4–6	0–rarely	0	Yes

have come to be known as the "prudent" diet. The AHA diet restricts the daily intake of cholesterol to less than 300 mgs, dietary fat to 30 to 35 percent of total calories (P/S ratio 1.0), and meat consumption to 4 to 6 ounces per day. Table 10–8 summarizes the differences among the three diet plans.

The staff dietitian or nutritionist and the referring physician play the major role in determining each patient's dietary regimen. However, everyone shares the responsibility of keeping abreast of current trends and research in dietary management of CHD patients. (See Tables 10–9, 10–10, 10–11, and 10–12 for examples of dietary regimens, a summary of lowfat dietary objectives, and a list of the cholesterol content of common foods.)

OTHER DIETARY CONCERNS

The attainment of the therapeutic goals of controlling or reducing hypertension and normalizing body weight in known CHD populations may be thwarted by dietary intake of excessive sodium, caffeine, or alcohol. Alcohol provides excess calories with little or no nutritive value. It should be restricted from weight reduction diet plans. In addition to the excess calories alcohol supplies, alcohol exerts many direct and indirect adverse effects on the cardiovascular system, as do sodium and caffeine.

Sodium. Sodium is an element found in the blood and other body fluids and is naturally occurring in many foods. Sodium concentration in the blood and body fluids is precisely controlled by hormones that are secreted in response to fluctuations in sodium levels at various body sites. These hormones signal the kidneys to eliminate or retain sodium in accordance with body needs.

The major source of sodium in the American diet is sodium chloride, table salt. The average adult consumption of salt is 6 to 18 grams per day. The nutritional requirement for sodium alone ranges from .5 to 1 gram per day, which is easily met by a daily intake of 2 to 4 grams of sodium chloride. Excessive consumption of salt contributes to high blood pressure and, therefore, increases the risk for recurring coronary events. (See Table 10–13 for food sources high in sodium.)

Caffeine. Caffeine is classified chemically as a methylxanthine. It is generally recognized as safe (GRAS) according to the U.S. Code of Federal Regulations.[34-36] Caffeine is found in coffee (40 to 150 mg per 5 oz., depending on the method of preparation), cola drinks (30 to 59 mg per 12 oz.), chocolate, and over-the-counter preparations such as pain relievers, diuretics, and weight-control aids.

Caffeine exerts a mild stimulating effect on the central nervous system. The degree of stimulation may be related to an individual's previous caffeine consumption, dietary

TABLE 10-9. Summary of Diets for Hyperlipoproteinemias, Types I to V*

	Type I	Type IIa	Type IIb and Type III	Type IV	Type V
Diet prescription	Low fat (25–35 g)	Low cholesterol PUF increased	Low cholesterol Approximate calorie breakdown: 20% protein 40% fat 40% CHO	Controlled CHO Approximately 45% of calories Moderately restricted cholesterol	Restricted fat (30% of calories) Controlled CHO (50% of calories) Moderately restricted cholesterol
Calories	Not restricted	Not restricted	Achieve and maintain "ideal" weight, i.e., reduction diet if necessary	Achieve and maintain "ideal" weight, i.e., reduction diet if necessary	Achieve and maintain "ideal" weight, i.e., reduction diet if necessary
Protein	Total protein intake is not limited	Total protein intake is not limited	High protein	Not limited other than control of patient's weight	High protein
Fat	Restricted to 25–35 g	Saturated fat intake limited; PUF intake increased	Controlled to 40% of calories (PUF recommended in preference to saturated fats)	Not limited other than control of patient's weight (PUF recommended in preference to saturated fats)	Restricted to 30% of calories (PUF recommended in preference to saturated fats)
Cholesterol	Not restricted	As low as possible; the only source of cholesterol is the meat in the diet	Less than 300 mg (the only source of cholesterol is the meat in the diet)	Moderately restricted to 300–500 mg	Moderately restricted to 300–500 mg
Carbohydrate	Not limited	Not limited	Controlled, concentrated sweets are restricted	Controlled, concentrated sweets are restricted	Controlled, concentrated sweets are restricted
Alcohol	Not recommended	May be used with discretion	Limited to 2 servings (substituted for CHO)	Limited to 2 servings (substituted for CHO)	Not recommended

*PUF-polyunsaturated fat; CHO-carbohydrate.

TABLE 10–10. Quantitative Guidelines for the AHA and Alternative Diet Plans

Food Group	AHA	Alternative
I. Meat Poultry Fish	No more than 2 servings/day One serving = 2–3 oz. meat, fish, poultry	No more than 2 servings/day One serving = 0–2 oz. meat, fish, poultry (If vegetarian, B_{12} supplement may be required)
Legumes Nuts Eggs	1 c. cooked legumes 4 T. peanut butter 3 eggs/week	1 c. cooked legumes No nuts except chestnuts No yolks, 7 whites/week
II. Fruits and Vegetables	4 or more servings/day One serving = ½ c. fruit juice or vegetable juice 1 medium fruit or vegetable ½ c. cooked fruit or vegetable	4 or more servings/day One serving = 1 medium fruit, fresh No fruit juice Avoid canned and processed fruits Use fruit juice and dried fruits as a substitute for sugar in recipes
III. Breads and Cereals	4 or more servings/day One serving = 1 slice bread, french, rye, pumpernickel, pita, containing 1.5 g. fat/slice 1 c. dry cereal ½ c. cooked cereal ½ c. pasta, rice, noodles (no yolk) 1 tortilla, corn 2 graham crackers 1 c. popcorn 1 bagel made without eggs	4 or more servings/day One serving = (same as Lowfat) Use whole grains and unprocessed whole grain products rather than defined products 2 or more different grains/day
IV. Milk Products	2 or more servings/day One serving = Nonfat milk or buttermilk (8 oz.) Lowfat cheese (1 oz.) Lowfat yogurt (8 oz.) ⅓ c. lowfat cottage cheese	2 servings/day One serving = Nonfat milk or buttermilk (8 oz.) Nonfat cheese (2 oz.) Nonfat yogurt (2 oz.) Nonfat milk powder (5 T.) Tofu (2 oz.) Soybeans (2 oz.)
V. Fats	2–4 T. polyunsaturated/day	No processed fats or oils Avoid avocados and olives

history, and medical status. Adding caffeine to the diet of caffeine-free individuals may produce modest increases in blood pressure, heart rate, stroke volume, and basal metabolic rate.[35] Apparently, the enzyme systems responsible for caffeine metabolism decrease in activity with advancing age. However, it remains to be seen if this decline in enzyme activity is directly related to caffeine tolerance. Caffeine has been reported to trigger cardiac arrhythmias in some individuals. For these reasons, caffeine consumption is generally not recommended for CHD patients.

TABLE 10–11. Summary of Lowfat Diet Objectives*

1. Reduce the consumption of beef, pork, and lamb.
2. Substitute poultry, fish, and meat substitutes for beef, lamb, and pork.
3. Prepare poultry and seafood without added fat.
4. Increase consumption of meatless meals.
5. Prepare rice, macaroni, and other grains without added fat.
6. Prepare vegetables without added fat.
7. Reduce the consumption of margarine and peanut butter as spreads for breads and rolls. Eliminate butter totally.
8. Use only fat-free salad dressings.
9. Use only skim and lowfat dairy products.
10. Use only lowfat breads and cereals.
11. Avoid commercial baked goods (cakes, pies, cookies).
12. Avoid egg yolks.
13. Avoid foods high in sodium, and do not add salt at the table.
14. Limit the use of sugar in coffee and tea and on cereal.
15. Substitute fruit toppings for jams, preserves, jellies, honey, syrup, and molasses.
16. Use only recommended dessert recipes.
17. Drink decaffeinated coffee and caffeine-free herb teas.
18. Limit alcoholic beverages.

*From Frye, et al: A Comprehensive Guide to Cardiac Rehabilitation. The Methodist Hospital, Houston, TX, 1982, with permission.

TABLE 10–12. Cholesterol Content of Foods*

Item	Portion	Cholesterol (mg)
Dairy Products		
Cheese, cheddar	1 oz.	30
Cottage cheese, 4% fat	1 cup	34
Cottage cheese, 2% fat	1 cup	19
Cottage cheese, <½% fat	1 cup	10
Cheese, mozzarella, part skim	1 oz.	15
Pasteurized process American	1 oz.	27
Half-and-half	1 tbsp.	6
Cream, sour	1 tbsp.	5
Milk, whole (3.3% fat)	1 cup	33
Milk, skim	1 cup	4
Buttermilk	1 cup	9
Ice cream, regular (11% fat)	1 cup	59
Ice cream, rich (16% fat)	1 cup	88
Ice cream, soft serve (3% fat)	1 cup	13
Sherbet (2% fat)	1 cup	14
Yogurt, plain	8 oz.	14
Eggs		
whole, without shell	1 egg	274
Scrambled (milk added) in butter	1 egg	282
Fats and Oils		
Butter	1 tbsp.	31
Vegetable oils	1 tbsp.	0

(continued)

TABLE 10–12. *continued*

Item	Portion	Cholesterol (mg)
Margarine	1 tbsp.	0
Salad dressings:		
Mayonnaise	1 tbsp.	8
Blue cheese	1 tbsp	15
Italian	1 tbsp.	0
Fish and Shellfish		
Clams (raw meat only)	3 oz.	43
Flounder or Sole, baked	3 oz.	59
Oysters (raw, 13–19 med.)	1 cup	120
Salmon (baked)	3 oz.	60
Shrimp (canned)	3 oz.	128
Tuna (water pack)	3 oz.	48
Desserts		
Cake (cake mix): 1/16 of cake	1 piece	74
Fruitcake: 1/32 of cake	1 piece	20
Pound cake: 1/17 of loaf	1 piece	32
Cheesecake: 1/12 of cake	1 piece	170
Brownies: 1¾ × ⅞ in.	1 brownie	18
Cookie, choc. chip	4 cookies	5
Meat and Meat Products		
Beef, lean and fat	3 oz.	87
Beef, ground, lean	3 oz.	74
Liver, fried	3 oz.	410
Bacon, regular slices	3 medium	16
Ham, lean only	2.4 oz.	37
Ham, cooked, regular	2 slices	27
Pork chop, broiled lean & fat	3.1 oz.	84
Bologna, slice	2 slices	31
Frankfurter, 10 per lb.	1 frankfurter	23
Salami, cooked-type	2 slices	37
Poultry and Poultry Products		
Chicken, breast, roasted	3.0 oz.	73
Turkey, light meat, 4 × 2 × ½ in.	2 pieces	59

*Adapted from: Nutritive Value of Foods, U.S. Department of Agriculture, Home and Garden Bulletin No. 72, 1985.

Alcohol. It is beyond the scope of this text to review comprehensively the effects of alcohol on the body. However, persons working with CHD patients should have a basic understanding of the major effects of alcohol on the cardiovascular system.

As the blood alcohol level rises, it has a diuretic effect. The loss of fluids during this period impairs the electrolyte balance (hypokalemia and hypomagnesemia are common), which results in secondary cardiac effects (increased irritability of the myocardium). Alcohol has both direct and indirect effects on the cardiovascular system. The heart's ability to pump is decreased with alcohol consumption. The effect of alcohol on heart rate

TABLE 10–13. Sodium Content of Popular Foods

Item	Amount	Mg of Sodium
Beverages		
Cola	12 fl. oz	30
Diet Pepsi	12 fl. oz.	62
Diet 7-Up	12 fl. oz.	48
Ginger ale	12 fl. oz.	45
Campbell's Tomato Juice	6 fl. oz.	292
Bread and Cereals		
Pepperidge Farm White Bread	1 sl.	117
Fresh Horizons Wheat	1 sl.	153
Pepperidge Farm Whole Wheat	1 sl.	107
Kellogg's Corn Flakes	1 oz.	260
Crackers and Chips		
Ritz Crackers	9	288
Lays Potato Chips	14 chips	191
Cheese and Dairy		
Breakstone Cottage Cheese	½ c.	435
Kraft Processed American	1 oz.	238
Kraft Cheddar	1 oz.	190
Milk, whole	8 fl. oz.	130
Breakstone Low Fat Cottage Cheese	4 oz.	435
Dannon Low Fat Fruit-flavored Yogurt	1 cup	147
Condiments		
Herb-Ox bouillon	1 packet	818
Heinz dill pickles	1 large	1,137
Heinz mustard	1 T.	212
Heinz ketchup	1 T.	154
Desserts		
Jello Instant Chocolate Pudding	½ c.	404
Jello Wild Cherry gelatin	½ c.	95
Cake donut, plain	1 donut	291
Pillsbury sugar cookies	3	210
Sara Lee frozen apple pie	1 piece	555
Hostess Twinkies	1	240
Fast Foods		
McDonald's Big Mac	1	1,510
McDonald's Egg McMuffin	1	914
McDonald's apple pie	1	414
McDonald's chocolate shake	1	328
Fish		
DelMonte Tuna	3 oz.	430
Flounder fillets, broiled	2 oz.	355
Bumble Bee Albacore Tuna	3¼ oz.	628

(continued)

TABLE 10–13. *continued*

Item	Amount	Mg of Sodium
Nuts		
Planter's Cocktail Peanuts	1 oz.	132
Jif Peanut Butter	2 T.	178
Skippy Creamy Peanut Butter	2 T.	167
Meats and Poultry		
Oscar Mayer Bologna	3 sl.	672
Oscar Mayer Bacon	3 sl.	302
Chicken, roasted	2 pcs.	57
Chuck steak, lean, cooked	8.4 oz.	381
Swanson's Fried Chicken Dinner	1	1,152
Pasta and Pizza		
Chef Boy-ar-dee Beefaroni	7.5 oz.	1,186
Celeste Frozen Pizza	2 oz.	328
Soups, Sauces, Salad Dressings		
Campbell's Tomato Soup	10 oz.	950
Herb-Ox broth, beef	1 packet	818
Wishbone Italian Dressing	1 T.	315
Vegetables		
DelMonte green beans, canned	1 cup	925
DelMonte sweet peas, canned	5¼ oz.	349

and cardiac output is influenced by the quantity of alcohol consumed. With increasing blood levels, the heart rate slows and cardiac output decreases as a result of stimulation of the vagus nerve. This decrease in cardiac output has the net effect of causing dilation of the peripheral vascular system owing to the accumulation of lactic acid and the ensuing tachycardia. Alcoholic cardiomyopathy is one long-term development of alcohol consumption. It occurs as a direct result of the toxic effects of alcohol on heart muscle. Cardiac conduction abnormalities and rhythm disturbances are common findings, but the major characteristic associated with alcohol-related myocardial disease is inappropriate tachycardia.[37]

Alcohol consumption has similar adverse effects on the respiratory, musculoskeletal, and hematologic systems that also increase in direct proportion to the quantity of alcohol consumed. The physiologic and biochemical toxicities of alcohol affect all aspects of blood cell development, length of life, and function. All these effects are potentially dangerous to the cardiac patient. Further complications imposed by medications and their side effects make abstinence from alcohol the prudent choice for most cardiac patients.

Patients should be informed about the dangers associated with alcohol consumption. The decision as to whether or not a patient is permitted to consume alcohol is one that must be made in conjunction with the primary physician. However, patients should be encouraged to abstain or to select alcoholic beverages containing lower percentages of alcohol per volume, such as light beer or wine.

Stress Management and Type A Behavior Modification

"Stress" is a term that is used rather indiscriminately today to describe a host of physiologic and psychological parameters. Simply stated, though, "stress" may be defined as a stressor (physical, social, psychological) reacting with an individual's unique personality to form a perception of stress. What is stressful to one is not necessarily stressful to another although certain stressors appear to be universally effective in producing perceived stress. Stress is believed to be a causative factor in the development of CHD. (See Tables 10–4 and 10–5 for examples of stress inventories.)

Type A behavior refers to a number of psychologic traits, behaviors, and response tendencies. Type A individuals are ambitious, competitive, aggressive, and impatient, whereas Type B individuals possess relatively few of these traits. Research has linked Type A behavior to the development of CHD[38] and to increased rates of reinfarction.[39]

The physiologic mechanisms occurring in response to chronic stress are central to understanding the role of stress in the development of degenerative disease.

PHYSIOLOGIC BASIS OF THE STRESS REACTION

Until recently it was not considered possible for an individual to exert conscious control over involuntary functions (gastrointestinal, vascular, hormonal). However, research has demonstrated that individuals can learn to control such functions to a certain extent, and stress management techniques are based on this principle. Through the use of methods such as biofeedback and progressive muscle relaxation, individuals can learn to avoid or reduce the effects of stress.

Any description of the body's response to stress must differentiate between acute and chronic stress. Although the physical reaction to acute stress is often extreme, it is not generally considered harmful to normal individuals because the body returns to prestress homeostasis within a relatively short period of time. In patients with CHD, however, a full-blown stress reaction could prove harmful. Attempts should be made through self-regulation to avoid triggering such states. The most insidious form of stress for the known CHD patient is chronic stress, as the effects are not necessarily physically evident.

ACUTE STRESS RESPONSE

Although the body responds voluntarily in stressful situations, the involuntary or autonomic nervous system response is largely responsible for the body's stress reaction. In response to conscious or subconscious perception of stress, the sympathetic branch of the autonomic nervous system initiates the following physiologic adaptations:

1. The hypothalamus through direct neural innervation stimulates the posterior lobe of the pituitary gland to secrete vasopressin.
2. Vasopressin acts directly, causing arterial constriction.
3. Simultaneously, secretions from the hypothalamus stimulate the anterior portion of the pituitary gland, which in turn activates the endocrine system.
4. Through a series of precise and complex feedback mechanisms, the hypothalamus, pituitary gland, and endocrine system work to inhibit or stimulate sympathetic nervous action.

5. The pituitary gland's anterior lobe secretes ACTH (adrenocorticotropic hormone), TTH (thyrotropic hormone), and GTH (gonadotropic hormone).
6. ACTH stimulates the cortex of the adrenal glands, which produces the glucocorticoid or anti-inflammatory hormones cortisone and cortisol, as well as the mineralocorticoid or pro-inflammatory hormones of deoxycorticosterone and aldosterone.
7. ACTH also stimulates the adrenal medulla, which secretes epinephrine and norepinephrine.
8. TTH stimulates the thyroid gland, which secretes primarily the hormone thyroxin.
9. GTH stimulates activity in the gonad or genital glands.

A summary of the physical changes created by stimulation of the sympathetic system during acute stress is as follows (Figure 10-1):

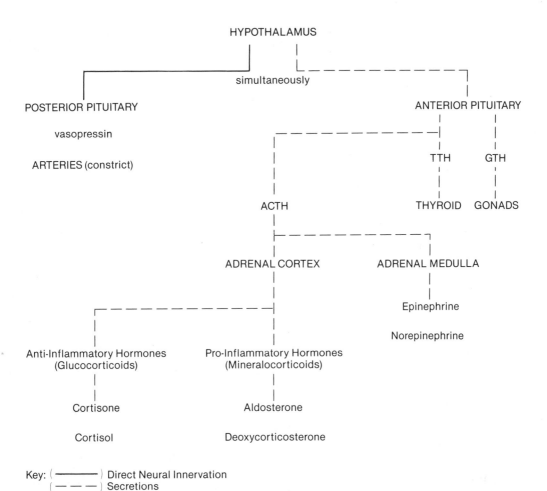

FIGURE 10-1. Diagram of the biochemical mechanisms associated with acute stress.

1. Heart rate, blood pressure, and cardiac output increase.
2. Respiration rate increases, and the bronchial muscles dilate.
3. Blood glucose levels rise.
4. Muscle tension increases.
5. All senses are sharpened.
6. Perspiration increases.
7. Basal metabolic rate increases, and free fatty acids are mobilized in the blood.
8. Blood coagulation time is decreased.

These physiologic changes are primarily the result of ACTH stimulation of the adrenal medulla and the subsequent secretion of epinephrine and norepinephrine (the other glands in the endocrine system as previously described are secondary in their effect). This adaptation is known as the "fight or flight" response.

CHRONIC STRESS RESPONSE

Sympathetic stimulation in chronic stress involves primarily the secretions of the adrenal cortex and the thyroid gland (Figure 10 – 2). The glucocorticoids raise blood sugar and the

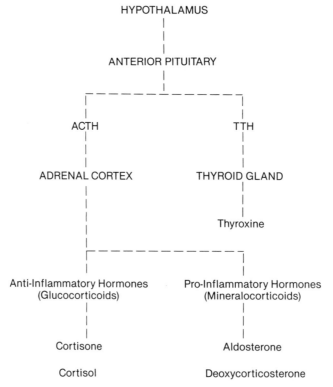

FIGURE 10–2. A diagram of the biochemical mechanisms associated with the chronic stress response.

mineralocorticoids stimulate the retention of sodium and chloride and increase the excretion of potassium. When the pro-inflammatory mineralocorticoids circulate in the blood for long periods of time, the water-mineral balance of the blood and tissues is upset, and blood pressure increases. High blood pressure increases the number of small tears in the arterial walls that then become sites for atheromaotus lesions and plaque formation. In some cases, hypertension results in permanent kidney damage, which leads to even higher blood pressure and an acceleration of the atherosclerotic process.

Presence of both pro-inflammatory and anti-inflammatory hormones in the blood for prolonged periods of time upsets the body's chemical balance and results in the following physiologic adaptations:

1. Increase in blood glucose
2. Increase in blood pressure
3. Increase in acceleration of atherosclerosis
4. Decrease in response of the immunologic system to disease or contamination
5. Increase in cardiac arrhythmias

The thyroid gland also plays a key role in chronic stress. Thyroxin is produced more during chronic stress than in stages of acute stress. Thyroxin creates many of the same effects that epinephrine and norepinephrine cause. These effects are summarized as follows:

1. Increased basal metabolic rate
2. Increased heart and respiration rate
3. Increased perspiration
4. Increased sensitivity to epinephrine
5. Increased fatigue (relative)

CONTROLLING STRESS

In light of the adverse affects of both the acute and chronic physiologic adaptations to stress, numerous investigators have initiated evaluations of comprehensive treatment programs designed to reduce stress and modify Type A behavior.

Suinn,[40] one of the first to attempt modification of Type A behavior, used a treatment program comprised of four techniques. Variations of the same techniques are currently in use in cardiac rehabilitation centers throughout the country. Suinn's program for post-MI patients consisted of the following:

1. Progressive muscle relaxation
2. Identification of various levels of muscle tension and accompanying stress
3. Practice of relaxation as a coping strategy in response to visual imagery that was perceived as stressful
4. Use of visual imagery to practice behavior patterns that are inconsistent with Type A behavior

In addition to such techniques, stress profiles should evaluate physical cues, time management, style of thinking (negative/positive), and coping mechanisms. Many different types of relaxation techniques are effective, and patients should be aware of alternatives in order to choose the technique most suitable for the individual. Alternative techniques include:

1. Meditation — phrases, breathing
2. Biofeedback
3. Progressive muscle relaxation
4. Cardiovascular endurance training combined with meditation
5. Guided mental or visual imagery

CONCLUSIONS

In the future, the present emphasis on surgical and pharmacologic treatment of CHD patients will shift to the behavioral treatment of this population. Currently, efforts to treat CHD patients have extended beyond the traditional approaches to include new efforts in risk factor modification as adjuncts to medical and surgical treatment. Justification for behavioral treatment is based on prevention of both initial cardiac events and recurring events. Future goals must be directed toward the identification of factors that positively affect motivation and compliance, as well as toward effective procedures and evaluation processes. Long-term investigations are required if the efficacy of behavioral medicine is to be determined.

SUMMARY

Risk factors associated with increased incidence of CHD have been identified. The modifiable risk factors, including blood lipid levels, hypertension, blood glucose, improper diet and exercise habits, and smoking, are significant to the cardiac rehabilitation clinician. Suggestions have been presented for cardiac rehabilitation staff intervention including the preparation of written guidelines for patient risk factor modification. The major modifiable risk factors (in addition to lack of cardiorespiratory exercise) of smoking, improper diet, and stress have been discussed in regard to their primary physiologic effects and current trends in the management of these factors. Examples of inventories for assessment of stress have been included, as well as examples of antihyperlipidemic diet regimens and a summary of low-fat dietary objectives. Emphasis has been placed on the current need for the identification of factors that influence patient motivation and compliance as well as identification of effective standard procedures and evaluation processes that can make behavioral medicine an efficacious adjunct to medical and surgical treatment of the CHD patient in the future.

REFERENCES

1. Diethrich, EB: The Arizona Heart Institute's Heart Test. Cornerstone Library, Simon and Schuster, New York, 1982.
2. Dawber, TR: The Framingham Study: The Epidemiology of Atherosclerotic Disease. Harvard University Press, Cambridge, 1980.

3. Multiple Risk Factor Intervention Trial. In Public Annual Report No. NIH 76-1000. Department of Health, Education and Welfare, Bethesda, MD, 1974–75.
4. Multiple Risk Factor Intervention Trial (MRFIT): A national study of primary prevention of coronary heart disease. JAMA 235:249–258, 1976.
5. Mulcahy, R, et al: Factors affecting the five-year survival rate of men following acute coronary heart disease. Am Heart J 93:556–559, 1977.
6. Coronary Drug Project Research Group: Implications of findings in the Coronary Drug Project for Secondary Prevention Trials in Coronary Heart Disease. Circulation 63:1342–1349, 1981.
7. Coronary Drug Project Research Group: Influence of adherence to treatment and response of cholesterol on mortality in the Coronary Drug Project. N Engl J Med 303:1038–1041, 1980.
8. Friedman, M and Ulmer, D: Treating Type A Behavior and Your Heart. Knopf, New York, 1984.
9. Guss, B: Heart Attack Risk Score. Cardiac Alert. November 1982.
10. Gunderson, EK, Rahe, E and Rahe, RH: Life Stress and Illness. Charles C Thomas, Springfield, IL, 1974.
11. Fletcher, GF and Cantwell, JD: Exercise and Coronary Heart Disease: Role in Prevention, Diagnosis, Treatment, ed 2. Charles C Thomas, Springfield, IL, 1979.
12. Kjeldsen, K: Smoking and carbon monoxide uptake as a risk factor in atherosclerotic cardiovascular disease. In Kritchevsky, D, et al (eds): Lipids, Lipoproteins and Drugs. Plenum Press, New York, 1975.
13. Astrup, P, et al: The effects of exposure to carbon monoxide hypoxia and hyperoxia on the development of experimental atheromatosis in rabbits. In Jones, RJ (ed): Atherosclerosis: Proceedings of the Second International Symposium. Springer-Verlag, New York, 1970.
14. Sparrow, D, et al: The influence of cigarette smoking on prognosis after a first myocardial infarction. J Chronic Dis 31:425–432, 1978.
15. Smoking and Health. U.S. Department of Health and Human Services, Publication No. PHS 79-50066, Bethesda, MD, 1979.
16. Truett, J, Cornfield, J and Kannel, W: A Multivariate analysis of the risk of coronary disease. J Chronic Dis 20:511–524, 1967.
17. Gordon, R, et al: High density lipoprotein as a protective factor against coronary heart disease — The Framingham Study. Am J Med 62:707, 1977.
18. Greten, H, et al (eds): Lipoproteins and Coronary Heart Disease: New Aspects in the Diagnosis and Therapy of Lipid Metabolism. International Symposium, Vienna, May 1979. Gerhard Witzstrock Publishing, New York, 1980.
19. Garrison, RJ, et al: Epidemiology of coronary heart disease. In Greten, H, et al: Lipoproteins and Coronary Heart Disease. International Symposium, Vienna 1979. Gerhard Witzstrock Publishing, New York, 1980.
20. Hietanen, E (ed): Regulation of Serum Lipids by Physical Exercise. CRC Press, Boca Raton, 1982.
21. HDL Normal Values. Clinical Pathology Facility. Associated Pathologists Laboratories, 1985.
22. Enger, S, et al: High density lipoproteins (HDL) and physical activity: The influence of physical exercise, age and smoking on HDL cholesterol and the HDL–total cholesterol ratio. Scand J Clini Lab Investig 37:251, 1977.
23. Hartung, GH, et al: Relation of diet to high-density lipoprotein cholesterol in middle-aged marathon runners, joggers, and inactive men. N Engl J Med 302:357, 1980.
24. Levy, RI, et al (eds): Nutrition, lipids, and coronary heart disease: A global view. In Nutrition in Health and Disease. Raven Press, New York, 1979.
25. Haskell, WL, et al: The effect of cessation and resumption of moderate alcohol intake on serum high-density lipoprotein subfractions. N Engl J Med 310(13):405, 1984.
26. Dyer, AR, Stamler, J and Paul, O: Alcohol consumption and 17-year mortality in the Chicago Western Electric Study. Prev Med 9:78–90, 1980.
27. Lieber, CS: To drink (moderately) or not to drink? N Engl J Med 310(13):846–7, 1984.
28. Shekelle, RB, et al: Diet, serum cholesterol, and death from coronary heart disease. N Engl J Med 304:65–70, 1981.
29. Wissler, RW: Nutrition, plasma, lipids, and atherosclerosis. In Laver, RM and Shekelle, RB (eds): Childhood Prevention of Atherosclerosis and Hypertension. Raven Press, New York, 1980.
30. Connor, WE and Connor, SL: Dietary treatment of hyperlipidemia. In Rifkind, BM and RI Levy (eds): Hyperlipidemia: Diagnosis and Therapy. Grune & Stratton, New York, 1977.
31. American Heart Association: Heartbook: A Guide to Prevention and Treatment of Cardiovascular Diseases. Dutton, New York, 1980.
32. Gasner, D, et al (advisors): The AMA's Book of Heart Care. Random House, New York, 1982, p. 220.
33. Barnard, JR, et al: Effects of an intensive exercise and nutrition program on patients with coronary artery disease: Five year follow-up. J Cardiac Rehabil 3:183–190, 1983.
34. Dews, PB: Caffeine. Am Rev Nutr 2:323–41, 1982.
35. Morgan, KJ, Stults, VJ and Zabik, ME: Amount and dietary sources of caffeine and saccharine intake by individuals ages 5–18 years. Regul Toxicol Pharmacol 2:296–307, 1982.

36. Oser, BL and Ford, RA: Caffeine: An update. Drug Chem Toxicol 4:311–329, 1981.
37. Marmot, MG: Alcohol and coronary heart disease. Int J Epidemiol 13(2):160–7, 1984.
38. Blumenthal, JA, et al: Type A behavior pattern and coronary atherosclerosis. Circulation 58:634–639, 1978.
39. Williams, RB, et al: Type A behavior, hostility, and coronary atherosclerosis. Psychosom Med 42:539, 1980.
40. Suinin, RM: The Cardiac Stress Management Program for Type A patients. Cardiovasc Rehabil 5:13–15, 1975.
41. Conti, RC, et al: Unstable angina: A national cooperative study comparing medical and surgical therapy. Cardiovasc Clin 8:167–178, 1977.
42. Watts, DT: The effects of nicotine and smoking on the secretion of epinephrine. Ann NY Acad Sci 90:1, 1960.
43. Burt, A, et al: Stopping smoking after myocardial infarction. Lancet 1:304–306, 1974.
44. Bruce, RA: The benefits of physical training for patients with coronary disease. In Ingelfinger, FJ et al (eds): Controversy in Internal Medicine. WB Saunders, Philadelphia, 1974.
45. Wood, PO, et al: The distribution of plasma lipoproteins in middle-aged male runners. Metabolism 25:1249, 1976.
46. Diamond, EL: The role of anger and hostility in essential hypertension and coronary heart disease. Psychol Bull 92(2):410–33, 1982.
47. Smith, TW: Type A behavior, anger, and neuroticism: The discriminant validity of self-reports in a patient sample. Br J Clin Psychol 23(2):147–8, 1984.
48. Dzvonik, ML: Alcohol intake, blood lipids, and mortality from coronary heart disease. Clin Nutr 3(4):139–42, 1984.
49. Baile, WF and Engel, BT: A behavioral strategy for promoting treatment compliance following myocardial infarction. In Franck, CM and Wilson, GT (eds): Annual Review of Behavior Therapy. Brunner/Mazel, New York, 1979.
50. Leventhal, H: Changing attitudes and habits to reduce risk factors in chronic disease. Am J Cardiol 31:571–580, 1973.
51. Frye, N, et al: A Comprehensive Guide to Cardiac Rehabilitation. The Methodist Hospital, Houston, 1982.
52. Nutritive Value of Foods. Home and Garden Bulletin No. 72, U.S. Department of Agriculture. 1985.
53. Dennison, D: The Dine System. CV Mosby, St. Louis, 1982.
54. Society of Actuaries and Association of Life Insurance Medical Directors of America: 1979 Build Study. 1980.
55. Peterson, LH (ed): Cardiovascular Rehabilitation: A Comprehensive Approach. Macmillan, New York, 1986.

Appendices

APPENDIX **A**

Patient Program Application Forms

Dear

Enclosed are the preliminary application forms that we discussed via telephone. Please complete the enclosed forms as indicated (x).

_____ Medical and Personal History Form
_____ Dietary Profile Form
_____ Insurance Information Form
_____ Medical Release Authorization Form

These forms must be completed by you and returned to _____ before your therapy can be initiated. Referral forms will be forwarded to your personal physician, cardiologist, and/or other medical specialist for specific medical information that we require.

Upon receiving your forms and the physician referral forms, we will contact you to schedule an orientation/observation session. Instructions for the session are enclosed in this mailing. When you are contacted to schedule your orientation/observation session, record the date and time of your appointment on this form.

_____ offers complete rehabilitative services. Whether you are a patient (cardiac, diabetic, arthritic, post-surgical, etc.) requiring a prescribed rehabilitation program, or a person seeking help in beginning an exercise and/or weight-control program, the staff works as a team to design and supervise an individualized program for you. Our staff of physicians, exercise and medical physiologists, registered nurses, physical therapists, nutritionists, and other health professionals work together to promote health through lifestyle modification and applied education.

The specific needs of each individual are considered; therefore, the appropriate treatment, as well as the cost of treatment will vary among patients. Your medical/health insurance will pay for the major portion of your treatment; however, the percentage of reimbursement is dependent upon individual insurance policies. Transportation costs incurred during treatment are also tax-deductible.

Please do not hesitate to contact me if you have any questions regarding our services or the completion of the enclosed forms.

Sincerely,

Director

PLEASE COMPLETE AND RETURN TO:

Medical and Personal History Forms: <u>PLEASE PRINT</u>

NAME: _____AGE ____SEX ____BIRTHDATE ____/____/____

I. Conditions which you have had/or currently have:

	Yes	No	Unknown	Date Occurred
Allergies	—	—	_____	_____
Specify			_____	
Congenital heart defect	—	—	_____	_____
Rheumatic fever	—	—	_____	_____
Heart murmur	—	—	_____	_____
Vascular diseases:	—	—	_____	_____
Coronary artery disease	—	—	_____	_____
Artery diseases, other	—	—	_____	_____
Varicose veins	—	—	_____	_____
Leg cramps (claudication)	—	—	_____	_____
Phlebitis	—	—	_____	_____
Heart attack(s)	—	—	_____	_____
High blood pressure	—	—	_____	_____
Hyperlipidemia (elevated cholesterol, triglycerides)	—	—	_____	_____
Obesity (MORE THAN 20 lb above ideal weight)	—	—	_____	_____
Diabetes	—	—	_____	_____
Gout	—	—	_____	_____
Hernia(s)	—	—	_____	_____
Epilepsy	—	—	_____	_____
Arthritis	—	—	_____	_____
Specify (knees, elbows, spine, etc.)			_____	
Injuries to:				
Back	—	—	_____	_____
Muscles	—	—	_____	_____
Bones	—	—	_____	_____
Joints	—	—	_____	_____
Lung disease	—	—	_____	_____
Kidney disease	—	—	_____	_____
Liver disease	—	—	_____	_____
Psychological/emotional problems	—	—	_____	_____

II. Operations: Date Occurred

  1. _____ _____

  2. _____ _____

  3. _____ _____

  4. _____ _____

  5. _____ _____

III. Other medical problems:

_____

_____

_____

IV. Current medications & dosages:

MEDICATIONS   DOSAGES

_____   _____

_____   _____

_____   _____

_____   _____

_____   _____

_____   _____

V. Risk Factors:

   A. <u>Family History</u>: Have any of your relatives had?

	Yes	No	Unknown

   Heart attacks   —   —   _____
      Specify relative   _____
   High blood pressure   —   —   _____
      Specify relative   _____
   Hyperlipidemia   —   —   _____
      Specify relative   _____
   Heart operations   —   —   _____
      Specify relative   _____
   Diabetes   —   —   _____
      Specify relative   _____
   Other diseases   _____

   B. <u>Smoking</u>: Did you smoke in the past? _____ Age when you started smoking _____ Do you smoke now? _____ If you have stopped smoking, when did you and why? _____

      Currently smoking: cigarettes   cigars   pipe   (please circle)
      Number per day? _____.

   C. <u>Diet</u>: Present weight _____ lb   Weight 1 year ago _____ lb
      Weight at age 21 _____ lb
      Are you dieting presently? _____ Why? _____
      What type of diet? _____

   D. <u>Employment/Occupation</u>:
      Current employment status:
      Full time _____   Retired _____   Unemployed _____
      Part time _____   Disabled _____
      Occupation _____ Number of years _____
      Employer _____
      Do you plan to return to this job or continue in the occupation? _____
      Physical activity required in occupation:

(continued)

	Almost All	(½)+	(½)	−(½)	Almost None
Time spent sitting					
Time spent walking					
Time spent standing					
Time spent standing/sitting with arm work					

Lifting or carrying heavy objects: Seldom   Sometimes   Often
(please circle one)

Approximate weight range _____ to _____ lb

Transportation to and from work: (please circle one of the following)
    car   bus   railroad   ferry   subway   walking
If walking to work: (please circle one)
    Less than 1 block   1–2 blocks   3–4 blocks   5–9 blocks
    10–19 blocks   1 mile   2 miles+
Working hours per week: (please circle one)
    Less than 25   25–35   36–40   41–50   51+

E. Physical Activity:

In addition to your occupation, do you exercise on a regular basis? _____
If so, list your activities:

ACTIVITY   NUMBER OF TIMES PER WEEK

_____   _____

_____   _____

_____   _____

Have you previously participated in an exercise class or program? _____
If so, describe the activities you performed: _____

_____

F. Stress:

Are you: Yes   No

   Frustrated when waiting in line, often in a hurry to complete
      work or keep appointments, easily angered, irritable?   ____   ____
   Impatient when waiting, occasionally hurried, or occasionally
      moody?   ____   ____
   Comfortable when waiting, seldom rushed, and easygoing?   ____   ____

PLEASE COMPLETE AND RETURN TO:

Name _____

Dietary Information Form

1. Are you on a specialized diet at this time? _____ yes _____ no
2. If so what type of diet? (e.g., low salt, low fat, number of calories, etc.)
   _____
3. Who recommended this diet? _____
4. Have you recently gained or lost weight? _____ yes _____ no
5. If yes, how much gained? _____ lost? _____
6. Describe your use of salt. _____
7. Check all of the following commercially prepared foods which you use:
   _____ Canned, dehydrated, or frozen soups or stews
   _____ Canned or frozen casseroles
   _____ Frozen dinners
   _____ Pretzels, chips, or snack crackers
   _____ Fast-food chain foods
8. Do you eat meals out frequently (3 times per week or more)? _____
9. Name any foods you *cannot* eat. _____
10. What foods would be particularly hard for you to give up? _____
    _____

Daily Dietary Habits

List foods and beverages commonly consumed. Include ALCOHOL, sugar, milk, or cream
used in beverages, butter or margarine used, and dressing used on salads.

Breakfast:

Lunch:

Dinner:

Snacks:

Food preference: <u>Check</u> the foods that you eat almost every day. <u>Circle</u> the foods that you
eat at least once a week.

Milk and Dairy Products:
— whole milk   — 2% milk   — skim milk   — buttermilk
— evap. milk   — cream   — cheese   — prc. cheese and spreads
— cottage cheese   — yogurt   — ice cream   — low-fat cottage cheese

Vegetables:
— green and yellow beans   — carrots   — lettuce and salad greens
— beets   — corn   — broccoli, brussel sprouts
— sweet potatoes   — peas   — lima beans
— squash   — potatoes   — cabbage
— tomatoes   — baked beans

Fruits and Juices:
— citrus fruits   — citrus juice   — pineapple   — pineapple juice
— apples   — peaches   — bananas   — apple juice
— grapes   — grape juice   — cherries
— berries   — prune juice   — plums

Breads/Cereals/Pasta:
— cereal, dry, unsweet.   — cereal, dry, sweet.   — cereal, cooked
— muffins   — bread   — rice
— biscuits   — crackers   — rolls
— macaroni   — spaghetti   — noodles

Meat/Fish/Poultry/Eggs:
— eggs   — beef   — poultry   — fish
— liver   — pork   — bacon   — shellfish
— cold cuts   — dried beans   — frankfurters   — peanut butter

Fats/Oils/Snacks:
— salad dressing   — pastries   — peanuts and other nuts
— margarine   — cookies   — potato chips and other chips
— butter   — candy   — popcorn
— oil   — pie   — cake

PLEASE COMPLETE AND RETURN TO:

Insurance Information Form

Patient's Name _____ Date _____ / ___ / _____
       (Last, First, MI)
Address _____ Phone: Home _____
_____ Work _____
       Zip Code
Patient's Date of Birth _____
Insurance Company _____
Address _____
Telephone Number _____
Insured's Name _____ Insured's Date of Birth _____
      Last, First, MI   SS# ____-____-____
Insured's Employer _____ Occupation _____
Insured's relationship to patient __ self __ spouse__ child __ other
Insurance ID Number _____
Group Name or Number _____
Are you covered by any other plans which provide medical benefits or
services? __ yes __ no
If "yes," list all other insurance companies or service plans providing coverage:
Company Name _____ Insured's Name _____
Company Address _____ ID Number _____
_____ Group Name or Number _____
      Zip Code
Referring Physician: _____
Most recent diagnosis/symptoms   Date illness/injury
1. _____   _____
2. _____   _____
3. _____   _____
4. _____   _____
Date of first treatment _____
I certify that the above information is correct to the best of my knowledge.

_____
         SIGNATURE

PLEASE COMPLETE AND RETURN TO:

Medical Records Release Authorization

TO: _____

_____
(Physician's Address)

I HEREBY AUTHORIZE AND REQUEST YOU TO RELEASE TO:

Records and/or pertinent information in your possession concerning my
illness/treatment.

Name _____ Date _____ / ___ / ___

Address _____

Signature: _____
(If relative, state relationship)

Witness: _____

Instructions for Orientation/Observation Sessions

Name _____

Appointment   _____   _____   _____
                   Month   Date   Time

Clothing
    Bring soft-soled shoes, e.g., tennis or walking shoes, socks, cotton shorts and a cotton shirt; and wear no unnecessary jewelry. (If you are more comfortable in slacks, feel free to wear them.)

    DO NOT WEAR A NYLON SHIRT.

Day of the Orientation/Observation Session:
1. Do not eat for at least two hours preceding the session.
2. Do not vary your medications (regular).
3. Do not ingest coffee, tea, coke, or other stimulants.
4. Do not engage in excessive physical activity.
5. Do not ingest alcohol or other depressants.
6. Do not smoke for at least two hours preceding the session.

    The procedures will take approximately one hour and are not particularly stressful or uncomfortable to most people. You should try to remain as relaxed as possible during all of the procedures.

APPENDIX **B**

Referring Physician Forms

To _____ M.D.

We have been contacted by _____
concerning participation in one of our rehabilitation programs.

The enclosed form must be completed and returned to us prior to the initiation of therapy. Your recommendations concerning your patient's participation in the program will be adhered to completely. Please do not hesitate to contact us should you have any questions regarding your patient's therapy.

Thank you for your time and consideration.

PLEASE COMPLETE AND RETURN TO:

Referring Physician Form

Patient's Name ——————————————————————— Age ————
Etiology: ——————————————————————————————
Diagnosis(es): ————————————————————————————
Medications: —————————————————————————————
Blood Analysis: Date ———— CBC: Hgb — HCT — WBC — Diff —
                            Lipids: Trig — Chol — HDL — LDL — HDL/Chol —
Urinalysis: Date ———   Alb ————   Glucose ————   Micro ————
Other Tests (please attach findings) ——————————————————————
Treadmill Report (if applicable):

    Date of test   ——— / ——— / ———   Protocol   ——————————

    Resting heart rate ———————————   Resting BP ——— / ———

    MAX heart rate   ——————— bpm   MAX BP   ——— / ———

    Maximum METs ——————————
12-Lead ECG Interpretation/Comments (Rhythm/abnormalities): ———————
——
——

STAT and PRN Orders
    1. Nitroglycerin 1/150 gr. SL PRN for chest pain.
    2. Lidocaine 50 mg. bolus IVP for PVCs 6–7/min. or V-bigeminy or V-tachycardia.
    3. Atropine 0.6 mg. IVP q 2–3 hrs. PRN for heart rate 40/min.
    4. Oxygen Intranasal 2–6 liters/min. PRN.
    5. Hang 250 D_5W and run at KVO rate.
    6. Defibrillate for ventricular fibrillation:
     Start at: 200–300 joules delivered energy; if no results 360 joules delivered energy;
    7. Additional (specify): ———————————————————————
——
——
——

                                  ————————————————————, M.D.
                                              Signature
                            Date ——— / ——— / ———

Physician Re-Referral Form

Patient's Name _____ Date _____ / /
Address _____ Telephone _____
Date of conducted laboratory evaluation or exercise session episode _____
_____
_____
_____

YOU RECOMMEND:
_____ 1. Discontinue participation in the cardiac rehabilitation program.
_____ 2. Temporarily discontinue participation in the cardiac rehabilitation program
while further investigation procedures are conducted. Probable date of renewed
participation _____.
_____ 3. Continue participation in the cardiac rehabilitation program while further in-
vestigative procedures are conducted. Probable date of completion of investiga-
tive procedures _____.
_____ 4. Continue participation in the cardiac rehabilitation program. No further inves-
tigative procedures to be conducted.

Physician's Name _____ Date _____ / /

Physician's Signature _____

APPENDIX C

Informed Consent Forms

Graded Exercise Tolerance Test Informed Consent

I, the undersigned, authorize the _____ Diagnostic Laboratory to administer and conduct the Exercise Tolerance Test. This test is designed to measure my fitness for work and/or sport; to determine the presence or absence of clinically significant heart disease; and/or to evaluate the effectiveness of my current therapy.

I understand that the test will require that I either walk on a motor-driven treadmill or pedal a bicycle ergometer. During the performance of physical activity, my electrocardiogram will be monitored and my blood pressure will be measured at periodic intervals and recorded. Exercise will be progressively increased until I attain a predetermined endpoint corresponding to a moderate work level, or become distressed in any way, or develop an abnormal response the administrator of the test considers significant, whichever of the above occurs first.

Every effort will be made to conduct the test in such a way as to minimize discomfort and risk. However, I understand that in performing diagnostic tests on individuals with pre-existing medical problems (diagnosed or undiagnosed) that there are potential risks associated with such tests. In particular, an exercise tolerance test may elicit episodes of transient light-headedness, fainting, chest discomfort, or leg cramps, and very rarely heart attack or death may occur. I further understand that emergency equipment, drugs, and trained personnel are available to provide usual and customary care in unusual situations that may arise including: basic and advanced life support and transportation of a patient by ambulance to the nearest hospital.

Questions: _____

_____

Reply: _____

_____

_____ ___/___/___   _____ ___/___/___
       Witness   Date   Signature of Patient   Date

Informed Consent/Release

1. Explanation of Program

You will be participating in a rehabilitation program that will include physical exercise, nutritional counseling, and patient education and may include stress management/relaxation therapy. The intensity and type of exercise you will perform will be based on your cardiovascular response to an initial graded exercise tolerance test that will be performed at the _____ clinic or by your personal physician within one month prior to beginning your exercise therapy. You may also be given other tests as needed to estimate body composition, desirable weight, lung function, various physiological parameters, personality traits, and stress levels. You will be given instructions regarding the amount and kind of regular exercise you should do. Exercise treatment visits will be available on a regularly scheduled basis. Your exercise prescription may be adjusted by the staff depending on your progress. You will be given the opportunity for re-evaluation at regularly scheduled intervals after beginning the rehabilitation program. Other re-evaluations may be recommended as needed. Progress reports will be sent to your personal physician on a regular basis.

2. Monitoring

Your blood pressure will be monitored regularly as part of your program. You will be taught to monitor your own pulse rate before, during, and after each exercise session. In addition, ECG monitoring will be performed as a routine part of your program and according to individual needs.

3. Risks and Discomforts

In rehabilitating individuals with pre-existing medical problems (diagnosed or undiagnosed), there exists the possibility of certain physiological changes occurring during the exercise treatment visits. These changes include abnormal blood pressures, fainting, and irregular heart beats, and in rare instances a heart attack or death may occur. We emphasize that every effort will be made to minimize the danger associated with the aforementioned changes by review of referring physician information, preliminary examination, and through observations of your exercise sessions. Emergency equipment, drugs, and trained personnel are available to provide basic life support at times when unusual situations arise. A registered nurse, physician, or emergency medical technician are available to provide advanced life support within a reasonable period of time. If required, patients may be transported by ambulance to the nearest hospital.

4. Benefits to be Expected

Participation in the rehabilitation program may not benefit you directly in any way. The results obtained may help in evaluating the types of activities in which you might engage safely in your daily life. No assurance can be given that the rehabilitation program will increase your functional capacity, although widespread research and experience indicates that improvement is usually achieved.

5. Responsibility of the Participant

To gain expected benefits you must give priority to <u>regular attendance and adherence to prescribed amounts of intensity, duration, frequency, and type of activity</u>.

To assure the safest exercise environment:

DO NOT: A. Withhold any information pertinent to symptoms from the professional staff.
          B. Exceed target heart rate.
          C. Exercise when you do not feel well.
          D. Exercise within 2 hours after eating.
          E. Exercise after drinking alcoholic beverages.
          F. Expose yourself to extremes in temperature; e.g., hot shower after exercising, saunas, steam baths, and similar extreme temperatures, as well as iced or hot drinks.
          G. Undertake isometric or straining exercise.

DO: A. Report any unusual symptom you experience before, during, or after exercise.
          B. Before leaving the site, check out with a member of the staff.

6. Use of Medical Records

The information obtained during evaluation performed at the clinic and/or while I am a participant in the rehabilitation program will be treated as privileged and confidential. It is not to be released or revealed to any person except my referring physician without my written consent. The information obtained, however, may be used for statistical analysis or scientific purpose with my right to privacy retained.

7. Inquiries

Any questions about the rehabilitation program are welcome. If you have doubts or questions, please ask us for further explanation.

8. Freedom of Consent

Your permission to engage in this rehabilitation program is voluntary. You are free to deny consent if you so desire, both now and at any point in the program.

I acknowledge that I have read this form in its entirety or it has been read to me and that I understand the rehabilitation program in which I will be engaged. I accept the rules and regulations set forth. I consent to participate in the _____ rehabilitation program.

Questions: _____

Response: _____

9. Release

I have read the foregoing and I understand it. Any questions that have occurred to me have been answered to my satisfaction. Therefore, for guidance and supervision in exercise therapy, life-style change counseling, and/or diet therapy, I hereby for myself, my heirs, Executors and Administrators, waive and release any and all rights and

claims for damages I may now and hereafter have against the staff of the
_____ Rehabilitation Program, its Agents, Representatives or
Assigns and Consultants.

_____   _____   _____
  Signature of Patient   Signature of Director   Signature of Witness
Date _____   Date _____   Date _____

APPENDIX D

Emergency Procedures, Medications, and Basic Emergency Equipment

Standing Emergency Orders

The following emergency procedures have been adapted to make the procedures more practical to the real environment of the prehospital setting and are presented as guidelines only. Keep in mind that the prehospital setting is very different from the hospital setting in terms of the advanced surgical procedures used in the care of cardiac and other trauma patients. Also, it should be noted that there is more than one acceptable way to manage most situations. Clinicians must get advice from the medical director as to how emergency situations might best be handled in specific areas of the country.

General Procedures

The following orders delegate authority to the nurse to initiate emergency and resuscitative treatment in the absence of a physician. All patients participating in rehabilitation programs provided by _____ shall be covered under these orders — with or without a written order by the physician.

The following is the basic outline of all procedures and medications covered by this policy:

A. Initial response to emergency
   1. Evacuation of the exercise area. When an emergency situation arises, the staff shall immediately order evacuation of the exercise area. Patients should exit to the hallway area and proceed to cool-down. Patients should remain outside the exercise area until the endangered patient has been safely transported out of the building.
   2. Notify the _____ ambulance authority. Use the emergency message posted by the phone.
   3. Notify the physician in charge.
B. CPR, PRN: All nursing personnel must be certified in basic life support (BLS) as

described by the AHA or Red Cross. Certification must be current and evidence of certification must be on file at each clinic.

C. Defibrillation: For ventricular fibrillation (VF) and
                                    ventricular tachycardia (VT)
     Start at 200 joules; if no change in cardiac rhythm, 200–300 joules; if no change, 200–300 joules; if no change, 360 joules, maximal output.

D. Initiating IV therapy: All patients in a life-threatening situation must have a route whereby IV therapy can be administered if necessary. The nurse may start an IV of 250 ml D5/W, KVO, using an angiocath.

E. ECG: In an emergency or a justifiably abnormal situation, e.g., patient experiencing persistent chest pain, obtain an ECG and monitor continuously PRN.

F. Oxygen: Give intranasal O_2, PRN 2 L/min rate. To increase flow rate, notify physician.

Procedures for Specific Situations Including the Administration of Medications

A. Hypotension: Systolic BP <90 mmHg
                                Symptomatic
                                HR >60 bpm
     1. Elevate feet
     2. Notify physician
     3. Obtain ECG

B. Fainting:
     1. Lay flat; elevate feet
     2. Use ammonia ampules
     3. Give O_2 PRN
     4. Notify physician
     5. Obtain ECG

C. Bradyarrhythmias: Ventricular rate <60 bpm
                                        Symptomatic
     1. Notify ambulance and physician
     2. Assure adequate airway and ventilation; O_2 PRN
     3. IV therapy
     4. If HR <50 bpm, give atropine: 0.5 or 0.6 mg IV bolus
     5. Obtain ECG
     If circulatory collapse and loss of consciousness occur, proceed to BLS measures appropriate to shock and/or other dysrhythmia.

D. Asystole: Carotid pulse = 0; Respiration rate <2/min
     1. Begin BLS, notify ambulance and physician
     2. Obtain ECG and give O_2
     3. Continue BLS until spontaneous respiration and circulation are established (presence of carotid pulse)
     4. If no response:
          a. IV therapy
          b. Give epinephrine: 5–10 ml of a 1:10,000 solution IV
          c. Give sodium bicarbonate: 1 mEq/kg IV Bolus

5. If a change in cardiac rhythm occurs, proceed to appropriate cardiac dysrhythmia protocol.
6. If asystole persists:
   give calcium chloride: 5 ml of a 10% solution IV
7. If asystole persists:
   give atropine: 0.5 mg IV bolus
8. Continue the following sequence if asystole persists:
   a. Epinephrine: 0.5 mg (5 ml) q 5 min IV bolus
   b. Sodium bicarbonate: ½ mEq/kg q 10 min IV
   c. Calcium chloride: 0.5 mg 10% (5 ml) IV bolus q 10 min. Do not mix calcium chloride with sodium bicarb.
   d. Atropine: 0.5 mg IV bolus q 5 min to maximum 2 mg
9. If a change in rhythm occurs, proceed to appropriate dysrhythmia protocol
10. Obtain ECG

E. Symptomatic PVCs: New onset of PVCs, PVCs >6/min, R on T phenomenon, change in mental status with symptomatic PVCs, salvos
   1. Notify physician
   2. Assure adequate airway and ventilation, O$_2$ PRN
   3. IV therapy
   4. Obtain ECG strips, 12-lead if possible
   5. Give lidocaine: 50–100 mg IV bolus, int. dose (1 mg/kg)
   6. Begin lidocaine drip, premixed 2g/500ml D5/W at 2–3 mg/min (30 ml/hr) (30 mcgtts/min)
   7. Additional 50 mg bolus (0.5 mg/kg) may be given q 5 min if necessary to total of 225 mg
   8. Increase infusion by 1 mg/min with additional bolus to a maximum of 4 mg/min (60 ml/hr) (60 mcgtts/min)
   9. Watch for signs of toxic RXN—slurred speech, altered consciousness, muscle twitches, seizures
   10. If change in rhythm occurs, follow appropriate cardiac rhythm sequence

F. Symptomatic PVCs: Ventricular rate <60 bpm
                       Patient symptomatic
                       Systolic BP <90 mmHg
   1. Notify physician and ambulance
   2. Assure adequate airway and ventilation
   3. Give atropine: 0.5 mg IV bolus, repeat q 5 min to total dosage of 2 mg
   4. If ineffective in increasing hr to >60 bpm and overriding PVCs, start isuprel drip. Mix 1 mg in 250 ml D5/W (4 mcg/ml): titrate between 2–20 mcg/min to maintain hr 60–100 BPM and override PVCs

G. Ventricular Tachycardia: Patient conscious and symptomatic
   1. Notify ambulance and physician
   2. Provide adequate airway and ventilation and give O$_2$ PRN
   3. IV therapy
   4. Obtain ECG strips and 12-lead if possible
   5. Give lidocaine: 50–100 mg IV bolus int. dose (1 mg/kg)
   6. Begin lidocaine drip premixed 2 g/500 ml D5/W (Start at 2 mg/min, 30 ml/hr)

    7. Additional 50 mg bolus (0.5 mg/kg) may be given q 5 min if necessary to a total of 225 mg
    8. Increase infusion by 1 mg/min with additional bolus to a maximum of 4 mg/min
    9. Watch for CNS signs of toxic RXN — slurred speech, altered consciousness, muscle twitching, seizures
  10. If change in rhythm occurs, follow appropriate cardiac rhythm sequence

H. Ventricular Tachycardia: Patient unconscious $\overline{p}$ max lidocaine infusion
    1. Witnessed and monitored: give precordial thump
    2. Begin BLS and continue until spontaneous respiration and circulation are established
    3. Give lidocaine 50–100 mg IV bolus (1 mg/kg)
    4. Defibrillate: 200–300 joules
    5. If change in rhythm occurs, follow appropriate cardiac rhythm sequence and:
    6. Begin lidocaine infusion: 2 g/500 ml D5/W (0.4%) at 2 mg/min (30 ml/hr) (30 mcgtts/min)
    7. Repeat step 5
    8. If ineffective:
      a. Give sodium bicarbonate 1 mEq/kg IV
      b. Give lidocaine 0.5 mg IV bolus
      c. Increase lidocaine infusion to max 4 mg/min (60 ml/hr) (60 mcgtts/min)
      d. Cardiovert with 200–300 joules

If no change in cardiac rhythm occurs $\overline{p}$ max of 10 min lidocaine infusion, follow sequence for recurrent ventricular tachycardia

I. Recurrent Ventricular Tachycardia: Patient unconscious p max lidocaine infusion
    1. Continue BLS until spontaneous respiration and circulation are established
    2. Discontinue lidocaine infusion

J. Ventricular Fibrillation:
    1. Notify ambulance and physician
    2. Obtain ECG strips, 12-lead if possible
    3. If onset of VF witnessed, give precordial thump
    4. If ineffective or if patient is found in VF, begin CPR and defibrillate immediately: 200–300 joules
    5. If change in cardiac rhythm occurs, follow appropriate cardiac sequence
    6. If first defibrillation is unsuccessful, deliver second countershock of 360 joules immediately
    7. Repeat step 5
    8. If ineffective:
      a. Give epinephrine: 0.5 mg (5 ml of 1 : 10,000) IV bolus
      b. Give sodium bicarbonate: 1 mEq/kg IV
      c. Continue CPR for 2 min
      d. Defibrillate with 360 joules
    9. Repeat step 5
  10. If ineffective, or if VF recurs after successful defibrillation,
      a. Give lidocaine 50–100 mg IV bolus and start infusion of 2–3 mg/min
      b. Continue CPR for 2 min
      c. Defibrillate with 360 joules

11. Repeat step 5
12. Repeat steps 10b and 10c
13. Repeat step 5
14. If no change in cardiac rhythm:
    a. Continue CPR for 2 min
    b. Defibrillate with 360 joules
15. Repeat step 5
16. If no change in cardiac rhythm:
    a. Continue CPR
    b. Give sodium bicarbonate ($\frac{1}{2}$ mEq/kg) if 10 min have elapsed
    c. Defibrillate with 360 joules
17. Repeat step 5
18. If no change in cardiac rhythm occurs:
    a. Continue CPR
    b. Give epinephrine: 0.5–1 mg (5–10 ml of 1:10,000) IV bolus q 5 min
    c. Give sodium bicarbonate: $\frac{1}{2}$ mEq/kg q 10 min
K. Supraventricular Tachycardia: Patient symptomatic; i.e., change in mental status, Systolic BP <90 mmHg

1. Notify physician
2. Assure adequate airway, ventilation and O_2 PRN
3. Obtain ECG
4. Instruct patient to perform Valsalva maneuver
5. Perform carotid massage (under direct physician supervision only)
6. IV therapy

Medications

1. Atropine Sulfate: 0.1 mg/ml in 10 ml syringe
   Dosage: 0.5 mg–1.0 mg = 5–10 ml
   Repeat at 5 min intervals to achieve desired HR generally, do not exceed 2 mg

2. Calcium Chloride: 10% solution, 100 mg/ml in 10 ml syringe
   Dosage: 500 mg = 5 ml
   May repeat dose q 10 min PRN

3. Dopamine: 200 mg in 5 ml ampule
   Dosage: 200 mg in 250 ml D5/W = 800 mcg/ml
   Infusion: 2–10 mcg/kg/min

4. Epinephrine: 1:10,000 solution, 0.1 mg/ml in 10 ml syringe
   Dosage: 0.5 mg–1.0 mg = 5–10 ml IV
           Repeat dose q 5 min PRN in cardiac arrest
   Infusion: 1 mg in D5/W (4 mcg/ml in 250 ml; 2 mcg/ml in 500 ml)
           Rate: 1 mcg/min for maintenance of BP

5. Isoproterenol (Isuprel): 0.2 mg/ml in 5 ml ampule
   Dosage: 1 mg in D5/W (4 mcg/ml in 250 ml; 2 mcg/ml in 500 ml)
   Infusion: 2–20 mcg/min; titrate; beware of PVCs

6. Lidocaine: 1% (10 mg/ml; 100 mg/10 ml) and 2% (20 mg/ml; 100 mg/5 ml) for IV bolus
   for infusion after bolus: 4% (40 mg/ml; 1 g/25 ml)
   Dosage: 1%: 75 mg = 7.50 ml
   2%: 75 mg = 3.75 ml
   2 g/500 ml D5/W or 1 g/250 ml D5/W premixed = 4 mg/ml
   Infusion: 1–4 mg/min
   For breakthrough ventricular ectopy, additional 50 mg bolus q 5 min to suppress ectopy—total 225 mg; increase drip: 4 mg/min

7. Procainamide: 100 mg/ml in 10 ml ampule for IV bolus
   500 mg/ml in 2 ml ampules for infusion p bolus
   Dosage: 20 mg/min until:
   a. Dysrhythmia suppressed
   b. Hypotension ensues
   c. QRS widens by 50%
   d. Total of 1 g given
   1 g/250 ml D5/W = mg/ml; infusion: 1–4 mg/min
   Monitor ECG and BP. Give cautiously in patients with acute MI.

8. Sodium Bicarbonate: 1 mEq/ml in 50 ml = 50 mEq
   Dosage: 1 mEq/kg or 75 ml initial dose for average-sized adult
   Repeat according to pH. If not available, use ½ initial dose q 10 min

9. Dextrose: 5% in water premixed 250 ml bag

All Orders and Medication Instructions Approved

_____ M.D. _____

Medical Director   Date
_____ Clinic

Basic Emergency Equipment
Portable Cart
Defibrillator
IV lines, needles, syringes
Ambu bags
Airways and O_2 tank
ECG equipment
Stethoscope
Sphygmomanometer

APPENDIX E

Flexibility Exercises

Stretching I

Discontinue any exercise that causes you pain or discomfort.
Don't hold your breath—breathe slowly and deeply.
Stretch slowly and gently––no bouncing.
Try not to strain. Relax while you stretch.

1. Wall Stretch

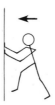

Stand facing wall with feet a shoulder-width apart. Take one step forward with right leg, bending knee. Keep back heel on floor. Place hands a shoulder-width apart on the wall for support. Hold. Repeat with other leg.

2. Stand and Reach

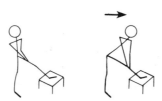

Using a bench or stool, place one foot up on bench, keeping leg straight. Slowly extend arms down leg. Hold. Repeat with other leg.

3. Standing Foot Hold

Stand with left hand on chair or wall for support. Bend right leg and grasp foot with right hand. Gently pull foot toward body. Repeat with other leg.

4. Groin Stretch

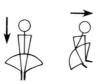

Sit on mat with feet together. Place hands on ankles. Gently pull them in close to hips. Slowly bend forward, keeping back straight. Relax. Repeat.

5. Straddle

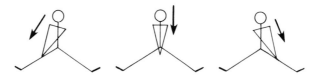

Sit on mat with legs apart extended straight out. Extend arms out, reaching toward right foot. Return to center. Reach toward left foot. Return to center and reach forward. Relax. Keep back straight.

6. Spinal Twist

Sitting on mat, extend right leg to front, and place left foot on mat on other side of right knee. Reach over left leg with right arm. Use left hand behind you for balance. Turn upper body to left, looking over left shoulder. Repeat to other side.

7. Curl Stretch

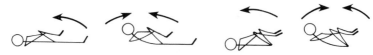

Lie on back on mat with legs extended. Bring right knee up to chest. Hold hands just below knee. As you stretch slowly, bring head up toward knee. Relax. Repeat with other knee. Relax. Bring both knees up and slowly curl head up. Relax.

8. Neck Limber

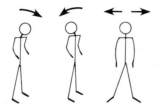

Seated or standing, pull head down toward chest and hold for 10 seconds. Return to starting position and then pull head back and hold for 10 seconds. Repeat for left and right side and as many angles in between as you wish.

9. Arm Circle

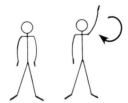

Seated or standing, begin with right arm, depressing shoulder down toward floor with arm extended. Continue to raise arm slowly up toward ceiling and around toward back. Keep arm extended and stretch throughout movement. Repeat with other arm.

Flexibility and Muscular Strength and Endurance Data Sheet

Name ——————

Kinetic Activities

| | Flexibility Exercises | | | | | | Muscular Strength and Endurance | | | | | | |
Date	Calf	Hamstring	Quads	Groin	Trunk	Shoulder	Neck	1	2	3	4	5	6	BP

APPENDIX F

Coronary Outpatient Exercise Guidelines

Coronary Outpatient Exercise Guidelines

Level	Approx. No. of Weeks after Event	Calisthenics No. of Repetitions	Medically Supervised			Unsupervised (85% of Supervised)	
			Bicycle Ergometer	Arm Ergometer	Treadmill or Walk-Jog	Bicycle Ergometer	Walk
Phase II (Therapeutic)							
1	3–4	6	8 min (×2) 35% MET-ET or 50 r/min at 150 KPM	8 min (×2) 30% MET-ET or 100 T at 150 KPM	12 min* 50% MET-ET† or 22-min time	8 min (×2) 50 r/min at 130 KPM	12 min* 25-min mile
2	3–4	7	8 min (×2) 40% MET-ET or 50 r/min at 225 KPM	8 min (×2) 35% MET-ET or 125 T at 225 KPM	12 min* 60% MET-ET† or 22-min mile	8 min (×2) 50 r/min at 190 KPM	12 min* 25-min mile
3	3–4	8	8 min (×2) 45% MET-ET or 50 r/min at 300 KPM	8 min (×2) 45% MET-ET or 125 T at 300 KPM	12 min* 70% MET-ET† or 20-min mile	8 min (×2) 60 r/min at 225 KPM	12 min* 22-min mile
4	5	10	12 min 45% MET-ET or 60 r/min at 300 KPM	8 min (×2) 45% MET-ET or 150 T at 300 KPM	12 min* 75% MET-ET† or 18-min mile	12 min 60 r/min at 225 KPM	12 min* 20-min mile
5	5	10	15 min 45% MET-ET or 70 r/min at 300 KPM	8 min (×2) 45% MET-ET or 150 T at 300 KPM	12 min* 75% MET-ET† or 18-min mile	15 min 70 r/min at 225 KPM	12 min* 20-min mile
6	5	10	15 min 45% MET-ET or 70 r/min at 300 KPM	8 min (×2) 45% MET-ET or 150 T at 300 KPM	12 min* 75% MET-ET† or 18-min mile	15 min 70 r/min at 255 KPM	12 min* 20-min mile
7‡	6	12	15 min 60 r/min at 300 KPM or 3.7 MET	175 T at 300 KPM or 4.5 MET	1.5 min§ 3.9 MET, 16-min mile walk; or 6.0 MET, 14-min mile walk; or 8.6 MET, 12-min mile jog; or 10.2 MET, 10-min mile jog	15 min 60 r/min at 255 KPM or 3.1 MET	1.5 min 3.9 MET or 16-min mile walk

8‡	7	18	15 min 60 r/min at 450 KPM or 4.9 MET	200 T at 375 KPM or 5.5 MET	2.0 min§ 3.9 MET, 16-min mile walk; or 6.0 MET, 14-min mile walk; or 8.6 MET, 12-min mile jog; or 10.2 MET, 10- min mile jog	15 min 60 r/min at 380 KPM or 4.2 MET	2.0 min 3.9 MET or 16-min mile walk
9‡	9	18	15 min 60 r/min at 450 KPM or 4.9 MET	200 T at 450 KPM or 6.4 MET	2.25 min§ 6.0 MET, 14-min mile walk; or 8.6 MET, 12-min mile jog; or 10.2 MET, 10-min mile jog; or 11.0 MET, 9- min mile jog	15 min 60 r/min at 380 KPM or 4.2 MET	2.25 min 3.9 MET or 16-min mile walk
10‡	11	18	15 min 60 r/min at 600 KPM or 6.1 MET	250 T at 450 KPM or 6.4 MET	2.5 min§ 6.0 MET, 14-min mile walk; or 8.6 MET, 12-min mile jog; or 10.2 MET, 10-min mile jog; or 11.0 MET, 9- min mile jog	15 min 60 r/min at 500 KPM or 5.2 MET	2.5 min 6.0 MET or 14-min mile walk
11‡	12	18	15 min 60 r/min at 600 KPM or 6.1 MET	250 T at 450 KPM or 6.4 MET	2.75 min§ 6.0 MET, 14-min mile walk; or 8.6 MET, 12-min mile jog; or 10.2 MET, 10-min mile jog; or 11.0 MET, 9- min mile jog	15 m 60 r/min at 500 KPM or 5.2 MET	2.75 min 6.0 MET or 14-min mile walk

Coronary Outpatient Exercise Guidelines—*continued*

Level	Calisthenics No. of Repetitions	Medically Supervised			Unsupervised	
Approx. No. of Weeks after Event		Bicycle Ergometer	Arm Ergometer	Treadmill or Walk-Jog	Bicycle Ergometer	Walk
					(85% of Supervised)	
Phase II (*Therapeutic*)						
12‡ 13	18	15 min 60 r/min at 600 KPM or 6.1 MET	250 T at 450 KPM or 6.4 MET	3.00 min§ 6.0 MET, 14-min mile walk; or 8.6 MET, 12-min mile jog; or 10.2 MET, 10-min mile jog; or 11.0 MET, 9-min mile jog	15 min 60 r/min at 500 KPM or 5.2 MET	3.00 min 6.0 MET or 14-min mile walk
Phase III (*Maintenance*)						
13‡ 14 on	18	15 min 60 r/min at 600 KPM or 6.1 MET	250 T at 450 KPM or 6.4 MET	3.00 min 9–12-min mile or 11.0–8.6 MET jog-walk	15 min 60 r/min at 500 KPM or 5.2 MET	3.00 min 6.0 MET or 14-min mile walk

Levels 1–6 typically accomplished in a 2-week period. Telemetry ECG monitoring may aid in heart rate and rhythm evaluation during this period. Supervised programs, 3 sessions weekly. Unsupervised programs 3–4 sessions weekly. MET-ET = MET level on treadmill test. KPM = bicycle resistance in kilo and meters. T = turns of 60–75 revolutions per minute (r/min). Event = myocardial infarction, coronary bypass surgery, or coronary angioplasty.

*Plus an additional 1-min warm-up and 1-min cool-down.

†As designated on exercise treadmill (calibrated).

‡Levels 7–13, rowing machine may be used for 3–5 min, progressing from slight to moderate resistance.

§Select pace on an individual basis considering activity level in previous weeks and patient's cardiovascular status.

(From Fletcher, GF and Cantwell, JD: Exercise and Coronary Heart Disease, ed 2. Charles C Thomas, Springfield, IL, 1979, p. 175, with permission.)

APPENDIX G

Dietary Goals for the United States

1. To avoid overweight, consume only as much energy (calories) as is expended; if overweight, decrease energy intake and increase energy expenditure.

2. Increase the consumption of complex carbohydrates and "naturally occurring" sugars from about 28 percent to about 48 percent of energy intake.

3. Reduce the consumption of refined and other processed sugars by about 45 percent to account for about 10 percent of total energy intake.

4. Reduce overall fat consumption from approximately 40 percent to about 30 percent of energy intake.

5. Reduce saturated-fat consumption to account for about 10 percent of total energy intake and balance that with polyunsaturated and monounsaturated fats, which should account for about 10 percent of energy intake each.

6. Reduce cholesterol consumption to about 300 mg per day.

7. Limit the intake of sodium by reducing the intake of salt (sodium chloride) to about 5 g per day (2 g sodium).

(From Select Committee on Nutrition and Human Needs, U.S. Senate: Dietary Goals for the United States, ed 2. December 1977.)

Index

An *italic* page number indicates a figure; a "T" following a page number indicates a table.